# THE ENDURING ASYLUM
## Cycles of Institutional Reform at
## Worcester State Hospital

**Joseph P. Morrissey, Ph.D.**
Senior Research Scientist (Sociology)
Bureau of Special Projects Research
New York State Department of Mental Hygiene
Albany, New York

**Howard H. Goldman, M.D., M.P.H., Ph.D.**
Assistant Professor of Psychiatry
Langley Porter Institute
University of California
San Francisco, California

**Lorraine V. Klerman, Dr.P.H.**
Associate Professor of Public Health
Florence Heller Graduate School for Advanced Studies
    in Social Welfare
Brandeis University
Waltham, Massachusetts

**and Associates**

**GRUNE & STRATTON**
*A Subsidiary of Harcourt Brace Jovanovich, Publishers*
New York   London   Toronto   Sydney   San Francisco

**Library of Congress Cataloging in Publication Data**

Morrissey, Joseph P.
   The enduring asylum.

   Includes index and bibliography
   1.  Mentally ill—Care and treatment—United
States.   2. Mental health policy—United States.   3.
Massachusetts State Hospital, Worcester.   I. Goldman,
Howard H., joint author.   II. Klerman, Lorraine V., joint
author.   III. Title.   [DNLM:   1. Hospitals, Psychiatric—
History—Massachusetts.   2. Deinstitutionaliza-
tion.   WM 28 AM4 W9S8M]
RC443.M68        362.2′1′097443        80-24875
ISBN 0-8089-1291-7

**Grune & Stratton, Inc.**
**111 Fifth Avenue**
**New York, New York 10003**


Distributed in the United Kingdom by
**Academic Press, Inc. (London) Ltd.**
**24/28 Oval Road, London NW 1**


Library of Congress Catalog Number   80-24875
International Standard Book Number   0-8089-1291-7


Printed in the United States of America

# Contents

## III.  PERSISTENCE AND CHANGE

# Preface

For more than a decade concerted efforts have been undertaken throughout the United States to dismantle state mental hospitals and to supplant them with community-based programs for the care and treatment of the mentally ill. Premised on the assumption that state mental hospitals are now obsolete, this policy of deinstitution-alization has been justified on the basis of humanitarian, clinical, fiscal, and civil libertarian considerations. Yet, despite a dramatic decline in the resident census of these institutions and the rapid growth of community mental health services, state mental hospitals continue to serve their historic functions of custody, control, and treatment for a substantial residue of the most disadvantaged and most disturbed patients. These realities challenge the exaggerated claims advanced in support of community mental health care; they prompt an assessment of the enduring functions of state mental hospitals; and they call for a series of fundamental reforms in the contemporary American mental health service delivery system.

This book addresses these concerns in the context of the insti-tutional history of Worcester State Hospital in Massachusetts, one of the oldest and most influential mental institutions in America. The social history of this hospital provides unique insights into the evolution of social policy in the mental health field during the 19th and early 20th centuries and into the cyclical reforms in the care of the mentally ill from community to institution and back again. Moreover, we believe that Worcester's experiences with deinstitu-tionalization in the 1970s provide a "window into the future" for viewing many of the unresolved problems of mental health care in the United States.

In many respects, this book represents the culmination of the Training Program in Social Research and Psychiatry jointly spon-sored by the Florence Heller Graduate School for Advanced Studies in Social Welfare at Brandeis University, Worcester State Hospital, and the Worcester Youth Guidance Center under a grant from the Social Sciences Training Branch of the National Institute of Mental

Health (NIMH-13154). The senior authors were affiliated with the Brandeis–Worcester program over its 7-year history from 1971–1978: Klerman as Project Director, Morrissey as Research Director during its later stages, and Goldman as the first graduate of the combined psychiatric residency training–doctoral studies program (see Klerman, Morrissey, and Goldman, 1978). Most of the contributing authors were affiliated with the hospital during the 1970s or served on the staff of the Brandeis–Worcester program. Our presence at Worcester under the auspices of this program provided a unique vantage point to identify the processes, problems, and prospects of deinstitutionalization and institutional endurance that are discussed in the book.

Although the idea for this book took shape in the final phases of this training program, its development and preparation were undertaken after the program's termination. Morrissey moved to the Bureau of Special Projects Research of the New York State Department of Mental Hygiene, Goldman to the Division of Biometry and Epidemiology at the National Institute of Mental Health, and Klerman took a leave from Brandeis to work at the U.S. Department of Health, Education, and Welfare. By broadening our perspectives on national and state-level developments in the mental health field and enhancing our understanding of the implications of deinstitutionalization at Worcester, these subsequent experiences were invaluable in shaping the final form of this book.

We owe a debt of gratitude to many persons and organizations whose assistance made this book possible. As the NIMH Project Officer throughout the life of the Brandeis–Worcester program, Kenneth G. Lutterman was a strong supporter of our efforts to sustain an innovative program during a period of retrenchment in federal support for such ventures; Fred Elmadjian and William Denham of the NIMH were also helpful in this regard. The directors and staff of the agencies that sponsored the Brandeis–Worcester program provided not only the financial support but also the advice and assistance that permitted our training and research activities to grow and mature. In particular, our thanks are extended to David Myerson, Edward Prunier, Conrad Nadeau, Andrew Murray, Harold Reiss, John Murray, and other personnel associated with Worcester State Hospital and its affiliated agencies; to Jack Scott, Lee Wylie, and the staff of the Worcester Youth Guidance Center; to Howard Freeman, who along with Jack Scott conceived the program; and to Arnold Gurin, Heller School Dean throughout most of the program's existence, and the faculty of the Heller School who instructed the resident-trainees during their four years of graduate study. Special thanks are also extended to the nine men and women who participated in the Brandeis–Worcester program and to John Morris, Milling Kinard, Linda Farrin, Bamby Philbin, and Leigh Maccini who served on its research and administrative staff.

We owe an intellectual debt to Gerald Grob, Sanbourne Bockoven, and David Shakow whose writings on the history of Worcester State Hospital provided the essential chronology and many of the analytical themes developed in the book. Our reconstruction of the history of the hospital from 1930 to 1978 and the developments in the Worcester community following its administrative disaggregation in the late 1970s was aided by extended conversations with a number of individuals. In particular, we would like to thank David Shakow, Fred Elmadjian, Walter Barton, David Myerson, Donald Broverman, David Higgins, Frank Karlon, John Ford, Tom Manning, Chris Healey, Cathy Schlater, and William Goldman. The assistance of Paul Foran and Virginia McSweeney in gaining access to the archives at Worcester State Hospital's medical library is also gratefully acknowledged. Most of the photographic reproductions included in the book were skillfully prepared by Ann Youngstrom.

The New York State Department of Mental Hygiene, through its Bureau of Special Projects Research, provided the research environment and technical support services that enabled us to transform this book from idea to reality. At every stage of manuscript development, our efforts were faciliated by the Bureau's commitment to the mental health research interests of its senior staff and encouragement of their collaborative work with investigators in extramural settings. Without this support, our efforts would not have reached fruition. We are especially indebeted to Theresa LaBarge, Leslie Long, Gail Bullis and the secretarial staff of the Bureau for their patience and good cheer in typing the seemingly endless chapter drafts and revisions.

Finally, we would like to thank our colleagues Henry Steadman, Richard Tessler, Ann Rosenfeld, and Carl Taube for their insightful comments and suggestions on early drafts of several of the chapters.

J.P.M.
H.H.G.
L.V.K.

# Associates

**Jeffrey L. Geller, M.D., M.P.H.**
Assistant Professor of Psychiatry
University of Massachusetts Medical School
Worcester, Massachusetts

**Gerald N. Grob, Ph.D.**
Professor of History
Douglass College
Rutgers University
New Brunswick, New Jersey

**Kevin J. Howley**
Assistant Director, Woodward Day School
Worcester State Hospital
Worcester, Massachusetts

**E. Milling Kinard, Ph.D.**
Research Associate
Florence Heller Graduate School for Advanced Studies in Social
    Welfare
Brandeis University
Waltham, Massachusetts

**Eric D. Lister, M.D.**
Clinical Instructor
Harvard Medical School and Beth Israel Hospital
Boston, Massachusetts

**Andrew E. Murray, M.S.W.**
Director, Woodward Day School
Worcester State Hospital
Worcester, Massachusetts

**David J. Myerson, M.D.**
Professor of Psychiatry
University of Massachusetts Medical School
Worcester, Massachusetts

**Wilfrid L. Pilette, M.D.**
Assistant Professor of Psychiatry
University of Massachusetts Medical School
Worcester, Massachusetts

**Claire M. Schmidt**
Head Teacher, Woodward Day School
Worcester State Hospital
Worcester, Massachusetts

**Barry Walsh, M.S.W.**
Director, Adolescent Treatment Complex
Worcester State Hospital
Worcester, Massachusetts

# List of Illustrations

Joseph P. Morrissey
Howard H. Goldman
Lorraine V. Klerman

# 1

# Approaches to the Study
# of Institutional Reform

There is at first a vague and general discontent and distress. Then a violent, confused, and disorderly, but enthusiastic and popular movement arises. Finally the
movement takes form; develops leadership, organization; formulates doctrines and
dogmas. Eventually it is accepted, established, legalized. The movement dies, but
the institution remains.

Robert E. Park and Ernest W. Burgess (1921:874)

The history of public intervention in America on behalf of the poor
and the mentally ill reveals a cyclic pattern of social policy initiatives spawned by economic or humanitarian motives. Sporadic exposés and demands for reform have led to programs designed to
provide an acceptable level of humane care. Although each wave of
reform improves the conditions of at least some of its beneficiaries,
it is frequently those with the least difficult problems who benefit
most. After each forward thrust there is a sliding back as the innovators realize the magnitude of unsolved problems and become dis-
couraged, or as other societal issues engage public interest. And for
those with the most serious problems, little progress is achieved.
Fortunately, another generation of reformers always appears and
the cycle begins again with some forward movement, but not

1

enough to overcome a continuing residual of unsolved problems. The history of public provision for the care and treatment of the mentally ill in America and the endurance of the asylum provide remarkable illustrations of this phenomenon.[1]

## CYCLES OF INSTITUTIONAL REFORM

The development of state mental hospitals in the early part of the 19th century represented the first formal system of public care for the mentally ill in this country (Caplan, 1969; Grob, 1973; Rothman, 1971). They were founded during an era of social reform in response to criticism of the inhumanity of "outdoor relief" and the practice of incarcerating the insane in local almhouses and jails. In contrast to the pattern of physical abuse, neglect, and ridicule that characterized these settings, the early mental hospitals were championed as repositories of hope and humane care for the mentally ill. Under the aegis of "moral treatment," the first state mental hospitals claimed high rates of recovery for persons brought under early care. Quick success fueled the reformist zeal of social activist groups whose lobbying efforts before state legislatures led to the proliferation of publicly supported mental hospitals throughout the country. These hospitals, however, were soon caught up in the throes of a rapidly industrializing and urbanizing society. Massive waves of European immigration and the growing belief in the incurability of insanity further accelerated the transformation of state hospitals from small, intimate, therapeutically oriented "asylums" to large, impersonal, custodially oriented "human warehouses."

For the last two decades, another major reform in public mental health services has held sway under the aegis of "community mental health." A central thrust of this reform movement has been *deinstitutionalization:* an effort to dismantle and close state mental hospitals and to supplant them by a network of community-based mental health services (Bachrach, 1976, 1978). These dual objectives were made plausible by changes in psychosocial treatment approaches, by the discovery and widespread use of psychotropic drugs, and by the growing availability of federally financed community mental health centers, of nursing homes, and of general hospital-based psychiatric services. The short-term accomplishments of this movement rival the success claimed for the early mental hospitals. Between 1955 and 1975, for example, the resident population of state mental hospitals was reduced by more than 365,000 persons and, since the mid-1960s, over 600 community mental health centers were created serving catchment areas representing 40 percent of the American population.

Already there are unmistakable signs that the "bold new approach" embodied in this reform has created new problems and left many old ones unsolved.[2] Thousands of "deinstitutionalized" patients have been returned to communities only to encounter hostility and rejection by citizens and the new community centers alike. Many severely and chronically disabled patients have been "dumped" in the rooming houses and decaying hotels of innercity areas while other tens of thousands have been "reinstitutionalized" in nursing homes and chronic care facilities. Still others who remained in state hospitals have suffered and even died because the resources essential to maintain adequate care have been shifted to community-based agencies. Just as the mature state mental hospital in the latter half of the 19th century bore little resemblance to the humanitarian ideals espoused by their founders, so the deinstitutionalized mental health system has not achieved the optimistic goals advanced by many early community mental health advocates.

In both instances, the sweeping new reforms which captured the imagination of both professional and lay groups proved to be flawed in a number of fundamental respects. Each intervention was launched with little or no experimentation. Nor was there sufficient appreciation of the practical limits to which the core ideas could be pushed. In the case of the early public mental hospitals, "moral treatment" proved to be viable only in a special set of circumstances. The therapeutic orientation of these hospitals persisted only to the extent that their patients and staff shared a common religious, ethnic, and cultural value system; their caseloads were held to a relatively small size so that intimate personal relationships could be developed and sustained; their admissions consisted of relatively acute as opposed to long-term, chronic cases; their institutional mission and legitimacy was protected by influential members of their local communities; and their state and local governments were willing to appropriate adequate funds for their operation. Even then, the idea of a "moral asylum" proved to be only a partial approach to the problems of mental illness. The social reality upon which moral treatment and its associated practices were predicated did not allow for chronicity and its promise was viable only for the relatively mild and acute forms of mental disorder (Grob, 1973).

While the practice of moral therapy managed to survive in a number of elite private mental hospitals where social supports were more ample, it began to disappear from state mental hospitals

during the 1850s. The forces that led to its demise were wholly unanticipated by the humanitarian reformers and medical superintendents a generation earlier. As a consequence, safeguards to insure
the curative orientation of state hospitals were never firmly established and it was supplanted by a custodial approach.

During the late 1840s and early 1850s, with the advent of industrialization and the influx of impoverished immigrant groups,
pauperism or public dependency for the first time became a major
social problem in America. State legislatures, responsive to the
growing ethnic and class prejudices of the native born who were
the original constituency of state hospitals, established laws for the
easy and indefinite commitment of the indigent insane who were
being disproportionately drawn from the ranks of immigrant
groups. The purpose of hospitalization began to be stated in social
control and community protection terms and emphasis was placed
on the custody of the largest number of patients at the lowest possible cost. Control over admissions rested ultimately with the
courts, which encouraged the imposition of legal as opposed to
medical criteria for hospitalization. The state-supported mental
hospitals began to be inundated with ever-increasing numbers of
chronic cases that overcrowded existing facilities and undermined
therapeutic practices. Under these circumstances, cure rates
dropped off precipitously and, increasingly, in both the public and
the professional views, insanity became associated with pauperism
and incurability.

What began as a limited-purpose, noble experiment had been
transformed into a general purpose solution to the welfare burdens
of a society undergoing rapid industrialization and stratification
along social class and ethnic lines. With the death or retirement of
the early moral therapists, the new generation of psychiatrists passively accepted the social role of these hospitals while actively attending to their own professionalization. In time, both hospital staff
and local communities came to believe that the majority of patients
committed to state hospitals were destined to reside there for many
years. With overcrowding and staff shortages, the hospitals imposed a uniform routine on all patients which ultimately led to an
insidious process of "institutionalization," or total dependency on
the hospital. The rate of retrogression was uneven during the last
half of the 19th century with no clear point of demarcation between
moral treatment, which was practiced in some form in a few hospitals until the 1880s, and custodial care. During the 1860s and later
in the 1890s, a number of imaginative proposals for reforming institutional practice—several of which contained elements remarkably

similar to contemporary community mental health ideals—were developed but they failed to gain wide or lasting acceptance (Caplan, 1969). The character of these hospitals as large, understaffed, and otherwise deprived custodial institutions was firmly established by the close of the 19th century, and these conditions persisted in essential detail for the next several decades.

In the mid-20th century, the idea of deinstitutionalization became a practical consideration due to the resurgence of interest in psychosocial treatment approaches, the advent of psychotropic drugs, and the growth of nursing homes for the care of the aged and senile. While these innovations allowed for the initial reversal of the state hospital's custodial image, they failed to provide a firm foundation for the complete changeover of public mental health services from an institutionally based to a community-based delivery system. By the early 1970s, despite the rapid development of community mental health centers, the practical limits of this policy were becoming apparent. There were two key tactical flaws in the implementation of the deinstitutionalization policy. First, it was assumed that the new community mental health programs would accept responsibility for the aftercare needs of former state hospital patients and would ultimately also prevent institutionalization. Second, it was assumed that citizens would accept such individuals as neighbors and almost without exception would be in favor of state hospital closings. Both assumptions proved erroneous.

The rapid depopulation of state hospitals was undertaken without careful planning with community agencies to develop the support services needed for the maintenance of large numbers of disabled patients outside institutional settings. The new Community Mental Health Centers had grown up largely as a separate system without formal linkages to state hospitals (Chu and Trotter, 1974; Windle and Scully, 1976; Bassuk and Gerson, 1978). These centers were oriented primarily toward new or "underserved" constituencies in their local communities. Many were still on the drawing boards at the time of the initial influx of deinstitutionalized patients. With the phase-out of federal staffing grants, many of these centers encountered severe financial crises of their own and the claims that community care would be more cost-efficient than institutional care proved exaggerated. Although federal guidelines now mandate 12 essential services, few of these centers had the well-developed spectrum of services required for the care of chronic patients such as half-way houses, group homes, foster-care programs, and other residential centers. As a consequence, many ex-patients "fell through the cracks" of the fragmented and incomplete community health and welfare system and then often gravitated back to state hospitals or led isolated existences in inner-city areas (Reich and Segal, 1973; Koenig, 1978).

With regard to community acceptance, similar miscalculations became evident. For years, the latent social function of state hospitals was to serve as a "dumping ground" for residual social problem cases that were unwanted by families, rejected by other health and welfare agencies, or otherwise regarded as "public nuisances" in their local communities (Belknap, 1956). The prospect that they would now be "returned home," or less euphemistically, released en masse, stimulated the social prejudices and economic worries of community groups rather than their humanitarian ideals. Outraged citizens began to lobby for the restrictive zoning of residential areas while actively blocking the creation of community residences. Stereotypic fears of "madmen on the loose" also heightened concerns for neighborhood safety and public decency.

While the public was vaguely aware of the possible long-term financial benefits to states of closing mental hospitals, it was acutely concerned about the probable short-term economic losses individual communities might experience. They realized not only that real estate values in certain neighborhoods might be jeopardized by an influx of former mental patients, but also that institutional closing could result in financial deprivation. In many parts of the country, state hospitals represented major sources of employment and a prime market for locally produced goods and services. The closing of these hospitals meant severe economic burdens to local communities, both in terms of lost income and in expansion of welfare rolls. Civil service unions also actively lobbied against any hint of job cutbacks or employee transfers that would be necessitated by state hospital phase-downs (AFSCME, 1975).

Thus, in a number of respects, history has seemingly repeated itself. Deinstitutionalization has followed the cycle of earlier reform movements that started with great aspirations but ended in disillusionment and disarray. "Unhappily," as Etzioni (1975:12) has noted,

> collective amnesia seems to be at work, insuring that each new generation of policymakers learns little from past mistakes and is as ready as the last to be lured by a new fashion's flashy promise and untested payoff.

Even a casual reading of the history of mental hospitals in America suggests that, while putative ameliorations are often received with great enthusiasm, there is a danger in accepting them without a critical assessment of the resources necessary to sustain them. Complex, multidimensional, recalcitrant social problems such as mental illness require complex, multifaceted solutions. Public policy in the mental health field—whether in support of centralized asylums or of community-based programs—has been overly concerned with the *locus* of care rather than its modus. Consequently, many severely disordered and chronically disabled patients have been transferred to communities which did not have the formal network of community mental health and social welfare agencies necessary to meet their aftercare needs. The transfer of these patients from the "back wards to the back alleys," as Borus (1978) poignantly described it, may well constitute abdication of responsibility rather than the embodiment of a noble humanitarian ideal.

Today, the deinstitutionalization movement is in a transitional phase. Some public officials and mental health professionals now question the claim that state hospitals have outlived their utility. Others, however, proclaim the "death of the asylum" (Talbott, 1978) and call for the outright closure of these hospitals. The "problem" of the state mental hospital, therefore, is back in the forefront of public policy debate. Although considerable information now exists on the prospects and pitfalls of deinstitutionalization, there is a lack of detailed case studies that focus on the state hospital as an organization caught up in the throes of institutional change. Yet, it is often only through such in-depth analyses that we are able to grasp the full meaning and significance of *why* these hospitals endure, for *whom*, and for *what* purpose.

The present volume seeks to meet this need by providing a comprehensive description and assessment of the processes and outcomes associated with the deinstitutionalization of Worcester State Hospital (WSH) in Massachusetts. This pioneering hospital has served as a model for the rest of the nation since its founding in 1830 (Bockoven, 1972; Grob, 1966; Shakow, 1972). Its well-documented social history provides a telling record of the best and worst features of the institutional care of the mentally ill in America and illustrates the cyclical patterns of institutional reform during the past 150 years. In the early 1970s, WSH embarked on a concerted program intended to supplant its predominantly custodial and social control functions with an active therapeutic role in the mental health service network of central Massachusetts. Although initially successful, the transformation of WSH into a network of institutional and community-based services was ultimately halted in the late 1970s. The administrative, political, and economic forces that led to the demise of this organizational arrangement parallel the conditions that undermined its role as a therapeutic asylum over a century ago. Today, WSH serves more as the "floor" rather than the "hub" of the mental health service system in Worcester. It continues to perform its historical treatment, custody, and social control functions for a sizeable residue of the most-disadvantaged and most-disturbed patients. Other local service agencies, created in part with staff and resources formerly assigned to WSH, are thereby able to deal selectively with more-advantaged and less-disturbed clients. In effect, WSH endures as an institution of last resort and it continues to anchor a two-class system of mental health care.

In this work, the contributing authors—participants in, as well as observers of, WSH's deinstitutionalization—assess these experiences from sociological, clinical, and administrative perspectives. We believe that our analyses help to identify, in "microcosm", the overarching policy and programmatic issues that must be considered in the ongoing debates about the future role of state mental hospitals in this country.

## ANALYTICAL THEMES

Three interrelated themes guide the presentations offered in this book. These will be previewed here to provide our readers with a schematic understanding of the guiding framework that informs each of the following chapters. First, we have relied upon a social institutional perspective to examine the manifest and latent roles of state hospitals and to overcome the overly narrow approach to deinstitutionalization that has dominated the current literature in the field. Second, we have employed an organizational perspective to highlight the changes that have occurred in the mental health services arena and to evaluate the extent to which functions once performed almost exclusively by state mental hospitals have now been reallocated to other community service agencies. And third, we have grounded our approach in a model of social policy analysis that specifies the nature and scope of the fundamental changes that are required if policy makers are to accomplish the elusive goal of phasing-out state mental hospitals.

### Social Institutions

The first perspective developed in this volume emphasizes the sociological as opposed to the clinical aspects of deinstitutionalization. Viewed in clinical terms, deinstitutionalization is intended as a remedy for "institutionalism," the social–psychiatric syndrome associated with prolonged exposure to a debilitating custodial environment (Wing, 1962; Barton, 1966; Gruenberg, 1974). In sociological terms, "institution" refers to a distinctive type of social organization that develops over time as an adaptation to the opportunities and pressures of its external societal environment and the strivings and inhibitions of its internal interest groups (Selznick, 1957). As social "institutionalization" progresses, organizations begin to embody the values of their community environment and they come to serve a multiplicity of roles that often bear little resemblance to their original or manifest organizational purpose. These mostly unplanned adaptations shape the special character of the organization—its distinctive aims, methods, and role in the community. This special character, in turn, determines the organization's competence (or incompetence) to do a particular kind of work. The multiplicity of competing and often contradictory functions that are served for diverse interest groups inside and outside of the organization make mature social institutions particularly resistant to change.[3]

"The study of institutions", according to Selznick (1957:141), "is in some ways comparable to the clinical study of personality. It requires a genetic and developmental approach, an emphasis on historical origins and growth stages. There is a need to see the enterprise as a whole and to see how it is transformed as new ways of dealing with a changing environment evolve. As in the case of personality, effective diagnosis depends upon locating the special problems that go along with a particular character structure; and we can understand character better when we see it as the product of self-preserving efforts to deal with inner impulses and external demands."

This sociological interpretation of "institutionalization" has two important implications when applied to contemporary state mental hospitals. First, it implies that a policy oriented simply to the depopulation and closure of these hospitals will not effectively "deinstitutionalize" the mental health delivery system. Institutionalization involves an intricate web of social relations and value premises that transcend the physical boundaries of any single organization. State hospitals may be closed and their patients may be dispersed to other settings, but without alterations in the values and structural conditions underlying the current mental health systems, these locational shifts may only lead to "transinstitutionalization" in the community (Schmidt et al., 1977; Talbott, 1979b). Second, by emphasizing that social institutions persist in response to extraorganizational as well as intraorganizational needs and expectations, the sociological perspective implies that plans for effective "deinstitutionalization" must incorporate strategies for changing the larger mental health service system as well as the internal structures and processes of state mental hospitals.

## Organizational Change

Next, an emphasis on organizational boundaries—their establishment, maintenance, constriction, expansion, and dissolution—is the second theme that guides our presentations and analyses. The interface between an organization and its environment can be conceptualized as a "boundary" across which there is a reciprocal flow of people, products, raw materials, money, information, and legal sanctions (Aldrich and Herker, 1977). Organizations are boundary-maintaining systems, and a minimal defining characteristic of formal organizations is the distinction made between members and nonmembers: some persons are admitted to participate in the organization, whereas others are excluded (Aldrich, 1979). The ability to control entries and exits is critical for the maintenance of organizational autonomy and the accomplishment of organizational objectives.[4] Some organizations, however, lack control over these processes and are dependent on other organizations and agents in their external environment.

The organizational autonomy of health and welfare agencies—especially their discretionary power to accept or reject clients—has been a major topic of social science research in the past few decades.[5] A prominent finding of these studies is the tendency for human service agencies to disassociate themselves in a variety of ways from the client groups which the organization was primarily established to assist. One aspect of these organization–client encounters is the process of "creaming," whereby "inappropriate" applicants, "undesireable" cases, and in general, those persons most likely to jeopardize the realization of certain professional or organizational goals are selectively eliminated from further attention (McKinlay, 1975). The ability to accept or reject clients, however, varies in quantity and quality for different agencies in a community service network. Agencies with "high applicant boundary control" (typically those in the private sector) are able to acquire selectively their clientele while passing on to agencies with "lower applicant boundary control" (typically those in the public sector) clients who, for whatever reasons, are deemed unsuitable for their services (Greenley and Kirk, 1973).

Historically, state mental hospitals have been among the most dependent types of human service organizations in this regard. Admissions boundary control resided in the hands of external agents (local courts, policy authorities, and community physicians) and hospital personnel had to accept passively whomsoever was presented for care and custody. The absence of staff control over patient admissions led to the *internalization* of boundary control in the social structure and ward ecology of these institutions (Morrissey, 1976). Confronted with an unselected and heterogenous case mix and a deficit of organizational resources, the staff of these hospitals resorted to a variety of practices designed to allocate scarce manpower in the face of nearly overwhelming patient caseloads (Belknap, 1956). These practices included the preferential allocation of treatment personnel to "front" or acute care wards and the segregation of chronic cases to a mosaic of "back" or continued care wards where minimal custodial attention was the rule. Over time, the internal selection process operated as a "downward escalator system" (Bucher and Schatzman, 1962): patients were moved from "front to back wards" as a function of their level of deterioration, their deportment, and their usefulness in the work life of the institution. While these internal adaptations enabled state hospitals to survive and meet the multiple and contradictory functions they were expected to perform, they ultimately became grounds for the widespread criticism of these hospitals and demands for their reform.

The environmental and technological changes of the past few decades gradually altered the historic constraints on the boundary control of state mental hospitals. In the 1950s and 1960s, these institutions were able to "open their back doors" for the release of many long-stay patients who could be managed at home or in alternative settings with psychotropic medication and supportive services. Control over exit boundaries also led to sharp reductions in the length of stay of new admissions and the resurgence of active treatment programs. It was not until the early 1970s, however, that many state hospital authorities were able to "close their front doors" on the basis of the legal and administrative changes associated with deinstitutionalization movement. In so doing, they were able to exercise some degree of control over their entry boundaries.

This organizational boundary control perspective provides a framework for analyzing the efforts to transform WSH from a custodial to a therapeutic institution in the late 1960s and 1970s. Our presentations focus on WSH's efforts to alter its inputs (patient admissions), throughputs (manifest and latent functions of hospitalization), and outputs (patient discharges). From the outset, its top administrators realized that, if this "institution-building" mission was to succeed, new organizational boundaries would have to be drawn.

In some instances the boundaries of the hospital were narrowed. This was done by establishing treatment-oriented admission criteria and restricting the services to those that could be uniquely provided by the hospital. In other instances, however, the hospital expanded its boundaries. Community health and social service agencies were encouraged to develop the capacity to serve the needs of the alcoholics, drug abusers, and senile individuals who were not admissible under the new criteria. New programs were organized for children and adolescents whose special needs could be uniquely served by the secure environment of WSH, but these programs involved greater interaction with community-based organizations than previously had been experienced. In effect, while contracting its boundaries and responsibilities for certain functions historically performed by state hospitals, WSH began to extend its responsibilities for new functions in collaboration with community groups by internal reorganization of services and redeployment of staff to community-based programs. The assessment of these organizational processes and impacts constitutes the core of the materials presented in this volume.

Moreover, issues of boundary creation and boundary control remained as unresolved problems for the mental health service organizations that grew up in the wake of WSH's administrative disaggregation. Many of the resource problems and conflicts that plagued the old institutional system were displaced into the community, where a new generation of organizations in the private and public sectors were attempting to establish distinctive service domains and legitimation for their programs. In this sense, the organizational boundary control theme serves both as a framework for analyzing WSH's deinstitutionalization experiences and as a template for understanding the functional ecology within which WSH's institutional successors now operate.

## Social Policy

A concern with social policy is the third theme which informs the presentations and evaluations offered in this book. Our overarching policy framework is drawn from Gil (1973), who argues that three interrelated societal processes—resource development, division of labor (task or status allocation), and rights distribution—are the key mechanisms that shape a society's posture or policy toward its members. This model serves as a heuristic device for analyzing the means–ends relationships involved in any social policy and the extent to which its implementation can result in fundamental as opposed to *ad hoc* administrative changes in the problems to which it is addressed.

Based upon WSH's experiences, this model will be used in the final chapter to highlight the historical antecedents of the two-class system of mental health care in this country, as well as the key sources of diversity and segmentation in the current mental health services delivery system. Just as the social history of WSH provides a "window into the past" for reviewing the successes and failures of prior efforts at institutional reform, its recent experiences prefigure many of the problems and challenges that will remain unresolved under current deinstitutionalization policies. Many of the administrative changes advocated under these policies have already been implemented in the Worcester area and WSH is now in a situation that other hospitals may not realize for several years. Thus, a critical assessment of Worcester's enduring mental health service problems—"après deinstitutionalization"—can shed light on the policy dilemmas that will condition public debates on the future role of state mental hospitals.

In particular, our analyses suggest that a policy oriented simply to the closure of state mental hospitals will not end the two-class system of mental health care. If an equitable and truly human system of care is to emerge in this country, then policymakers must focus on the fundamental tasks of altering the resource base, division of labor, and rights distribution upon which the current system rests.

## PLAN OF THE BOOK

The remainder of the book is organized into three parts. Part I, *Cycles of Institutional Reform*, contains three chapters presenting sociohistorical analyses of the founding and institutional development of WSH through the late 1970s. In Chapter 2, Grob explores the social, intellectual, and economic currents that led to the founding of WSH in 1830 and the forces that shaped its early transformation from a therapeutic hospital to a custodial institution.

In Chapter 3, Morrissey and Goldman review the evolution of

WSH from 1856 to 1968. This chapter highlights the efforts of WSH's medical superintendents to adapt the structure and functions of the hospital to changing social conditions and the ever-increasing demands of its patient caseload. Their efforts to resolve the hospital's ambiguous legacy—created by the widening gulf between its original therapeutic ideals and the realities of its custodial practices—led to periods of innovation during which WSH regained the national prominence it held during its formative years. But it was not until the 1950s and 1960s that environmental and technological conditions gradually made it possible for the hospital to shed its custodial image and practices.

In Chapter 4, Myerson reflects on his tenure as WSH's last medical superintendent from 1969 through 1977 and the organizational innovations that led to the hospital's transformation into the hub of a network of community mental health services. The chapter's central theme is the tension between institutional and community-based services that was reflected in his dual role as superintendent and as area director of community mental health services.

Part 2, *Changing Organizational Boundaries,* contains six chapters that analyze various aspects of WSH's deinstitutionalization experience and the consequences of the efforts to realign its functional boundaries in relationships to community agencies.

In Chapter 5, Goldman presents a socioecological analysis of the tensions and conflicts within and between the boundaries of institutional and community-based care systems. From this perspective the segmentation and differentation of the mental health system is viewed as an adaptation to conflict and competition for scarce resources. The chapter suggests that the ecological conditions which gave rise to conflict within the state hospital have now been displaced into the community by the process of deinstitutionalization.

In Chapter 6, Lister and Geller examine the interface between WSH and the courts following the 1971 change in the commitment laws in Massachusetts. Their research indicates that, while this legal reform did lead to the "voluntarization" of WSH's admissions process, it failed to reduce the flow of involuntary commitments from the courts, and it perpetuated the hospital's social control functions.

In Chapter 7, Klerman and her co-authors describe an educational program for emotionally disturbed and aggressive adolescents co-sponsored by WSH, the Worcester Youth Guidance Center, and the Worcester Public Schools. The evolution of this program illustrates the problems faced by WSH in expanding its boundaries into the community. Alternatively praised and criticized by its source of actual and potential support, the Woodward Day School, like WSH, remains a last resort for the outcasts of society.

In Chapter 8, Walsh explores the origins and maturation of an institutional program for adolescents which developed strong ties with a community agency and slowly separated from WSH. The evolution of the Adolescent Treatment Complex suggests that, while client boundary control may enhance the distinctiveness and quality of a treatment program, it can lead to a precarious existence for organizations seeking an independent role in the community.

In Chapter 9, Goldman analyzes the relationships between WSH and The Memorial Hospital, an interface between the public and the private sector. This chapter highlights the problems of cooperative relationships across the boundaries of organizations and explores the interdependencies and mutual benefits which initiate and sustain them. It also identifies some of the limitations of the psychiatric unit in the general hospital as a functional substitute for the state mental hospital.

In Chapter 10, Kinard presents data from a follow-up study of discharged mental hospital patients. The findings suggest that WSH's boundaries must remain fluid to accomodate patients whose treatment needs are not met by community-based services.

Part III, *Persistence and Change*, consists of two chapters. In Chapter 11, Morrissey and Goldman present an assessment of the environmental and policy changes in the mid-1970s that led to the demedicalization and disaggregation of WSH. These administrative changes represented the culmination of the century-old trend toward evolution of control away from the hospital. The aftermath of these changes led to the growth of a number of new public and private mental health service organizations in the Worcester area, but many of the boundary problems and conflicts of the old institutional order remained unresolved.

In Chapter 12, Morrissey, Goldman, and Klerman analyze the broader implications of the "Worcester experience" for the mental health field. Deinstitutionalization was an attempt at major institutional reform, but its administrative changes failed to alter completely the historic functions of the state mental hospital. Moreover, the fundamental determinants of social policy—division of labor, resource development, and rights distribution—remained largely unchanged. As a result, the asylum endures.

## Notes

1. In the public welfare field, Piven and Cloward (1971) have shown the same cyclic pattern.

2. In his message to Congress proposing the Community Mental Health Act of 1963, President Kennedy hailed the legislation as a "bold new approach" to mental health care. An overview of the problems that have surfaced in the implementation of this legislation during the past fifteen years can be found in Bassuk and Gerson (1978).

3. Although Philip Selznick (1957) is credited with developing the institutional perspective into a distinctive approach to organizational analysis (c.f. Perrow, 1972:177–204), its intellectual roots can be traced to the Chicago School of Sociology of the 1920s and 1930s (Park, 1939). Everett C. Hughes (1939) and his many students at Chicago (c.f. Becker et al., 1968) championed this perspective as a general sociological frame of reference. Harvey L. Smith (1955, 1957, 1958, 1968) and Anselm Strauss and his colleagues (Bucher and Strauss, 1961; Strauss et al., 1964; Schatzman and Strauss, 1966) are responsible for much of the early seminal work on psychiatry as a social institution.

4. According to Miller and Rice (1970:262) boundary regulation is an essential managerial function in any enterprise, industrial or nonindustrial: "The need for boundary controls (is) to protect the conversion process from interference from the environment and to adjust both intake and output to environmental demands . . . In its 'purest' form, boundary control permits only those transactions between the system and its environment that are essential to performance of the primary task. It admits the necessary intakes, releases the outputs, and maintains and replinishes the resources of the task system."

5. Studies of client selection processes have been conducted on psychiatric clinics, family agencies, child guidance clinics, blindness agencies, social service departments, child welfare agencies, and emergency rooms in general hospitals. For a review and discussion of this literature see Greenley and Kirk (1973), Nagi (1974), Kirk and Greeley (1974), and McKinlay (1975). The policy and research implications of the client selection perspective for state mental hospitals is discussed in Morrissey and Tessler (1980).

# PART I

# Cycles of Institutional Reform at Worcester State Hospital

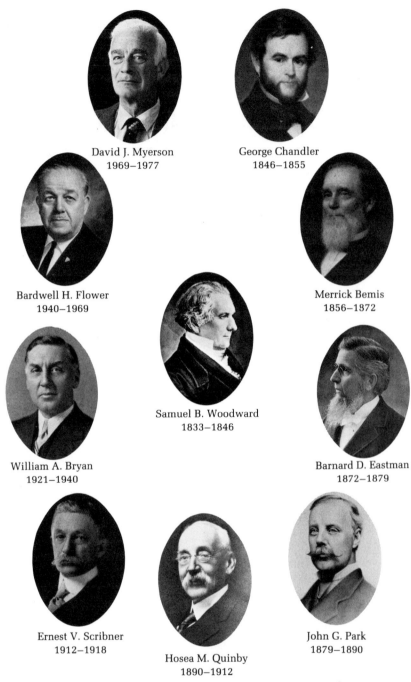

David J. Myerson
1969–1977

George Chandler
1846–1855

Bardwell H. Flower
1940–1969

Merrick Bemis
1856–1872

Samuel B. Woodward
1833–1846

William A. Bryan
1921–1940

Barnard D. Eastman
1872–1879

Ernest V. Scribner
1912–1918

Hosea M. Quinby
1890–1912

John G. Park
1879–1890

Fig. 1.   Medical Superintendents of Worcester State Hospital, 1833–1977.
Sources: John Curwen, The Original Thirteen Members of the Association
of Medical Superintendents of American Institutions for the Insane (Warren, PA, 1885); Medical Library, Worcester State Hospital.

Gerald N. Grob

# 2

# Institutional Origins and Early Transformation: 1830–1855*

*Webster's Dictionary* (1949:400) defines a hospital as an "institution in which patients or injured persons are given medical or surgical care." Thus a mental hospital is ostensibly an institution treating persons suffering from various forms of mental illness. In this sense there is little difference between a general and a mental hospital: the latter is simply a specialized version of the former. Similarly, the function of the psychiatrist is precisely the same as that of the general physician or specialist; namely, to diagnose the nature of the illness and to prescribe appropriate remedies.

In reality, of course, a mental hospital is *not* like any other hospital, nor is mental illness like other illnesses. Although the psychiatrist historically regarded himself as a medical specialist dealing with a physical illness in the conventional sense of the word, he always had difficulty in presenting convincing evidence to corroborate this assumption. Thus the belief that mental disease was somatic in nature—a natural consequence of psychiatry's medical origins—remained largely unproven for much of the nineteenth and twentieth centuries. With the exception of syphilis, no disease entity down to 1920 was identified in terms of its etiology and symp-

---

*Reprinted with minor editorial changes by permission of the author and publisher from "The state mental hospital in mid-nineteenth century America: A social analysis," Am Psych 21:510–523, 1966. ©1966 by the American Psychological Association. All rights reserved.

tomological manifestations and then correlated with structural lesions and changes. Psychiatric research was in most cases a nosological catalogue of disease classifications based on outward behavioral symptoms—a catalogue that tended to change rapidly from time to time.

Yet a mental hospital is a functioning institution. It separates patients by various criteria; it treats some patients and offers custodial care to others; it has all of the characteristics of a complex social organization, including a hierarchy of authority, specialization, and the like. But if its identity is not always determined by medical and scientific factors, what does determine it? In dealing with this question, the development of Worcester State Hospital in the quarter century following its opening in 1833 is instructive. The reason for focusing on this particular hospital is not difficult to understand, for Massachusetts was the pioneer in establishing a comprehensive system of public mental hospitals; its experiences served as a model for the rest of the nation. Worcester State Hospital, being the first of its kind in Massachusetts as well as the prototype of the modern American state mental hospital, was one of the most influential public institutions in the nation; its example was emulated by many other states when the movement for public responsibility and care for mental illness became widespread.

## ORIGINS

Like most institutions that arise in response to the needs of society, the mental hospital grew out of a specific cultural milieu and reflected the unique characteristics of its indigenous environment. The history of Worcester State Hospital is particularly revealing in this respect. The institution was a logical outgrowth of a number of historical trends and ideas current in 1830, the year in which it was established by an act of the Massachusetts legislature. What factors, therefore, were responsible for its founding?

First, the urbanization of Massachusetts had caused the informal mechanisms for the care of mentally ill persons to break down. The concentration of population in relatively small areas also led to a greater public awareness of "queer" or deviant behavior. Consequently, there were demands that special provision be made for the mentally ill not only to protect the general public but to provide as well for the care and welfare of such persons.

Second, the changing intellectual climate during the eighteenth century was to prove a decisive factor not only in softening popular antipathy toward the insane,[1] but also in reforming the custodial and prisonlike institutions of that period. The rise of experimental science and the emphasis on empiricism led to demands that mental disease be approached from a more naturalistic point of view. A prevailing sense of optimism, which grew out of the conviction that science had provided the means of understanding and dealing with human problems, resulted in an almost messianic sense of humanitarian concern. Not only did the feeling become widespread that the conquest of disease was momentarily pending, but also that mental illness was no longer an object of pessimistic despair. Thus faith in science, belief in progress, and a warm humanitarianism converged by the 18th century to set in motion the long-deferred improvement of the human race.

Third, a vigorous reform movement had been set in motion in the United States by the resurgence of Christianity about 1800 in an event known to historians as the "Second Great Awakening." The Awakening had the immediate effect of weakening the Calvinistic emphasis on the essential depravity of human nature and the inability of men to save themselves. In place of such pessimistic tenets, Protestant leaders substituted the idea of a loving and benevolent God whose first concern was the happiness of his creatures. The twin themes of their liberalized theology were the doctrine of the free individual and the belief in a moral universe. When the belief in the free individual was fused with the millenial vision of a society performing a divine mission and eradicating all evidences of evil, Evangelical Protestantism was transformed into a radical social force seeking the abolition of the restraints that bound the individual and hindered his self-development. Thus, many ministers and laymen began to work actively to destroy the evil institutional restraints that imprisoned the individual. All persons, they maintained, were under a moral law that gave them a responsibility for the welfare of their fellow man. As a result of the teachings of Evangelical Protestantism, virtually dozens of reform movements sprang forth during the first half of the 19th century, including movements to better the condition of the insane, the inebriate, the blind, the deaf, the slave, the convict, and other less fortunate members of society.

Finally, the traditional interpretation of mental disease—that it was a demoniacal possession resulting from a compact with Satan or a punishment inflicted upon the individual for his sins—was being modified as a result of the work of Philippe Pinel in France,

William Tuke in England, as well as many others. The work of Pinel was of particular importance, since it provided reformers with ammunition to support their contention that mental illness was neither of supernatural origins, nor was it incurable. While Pinel's contributions to psychiatric theory were not of critical importance, his contributions to therapy easily made up for his theoretical deficiencies. Because he rejected the idea that insanity could occur only in conjunction with physical lesions, he made room for a psychologically oriented therapy, which heretofore had been a theoretical impossibility.

Kindness was the fundamental ingredient in Pinel's therapeutic approach. Seeking to gain the patient's confidence and instill in him a sense of hope, he developed what became known as "moral treatment" (which in contemporary psychiatry corresponds to milieu therapy). Moral treatment involved the creation of a total therapeutic environment: social, psychological, physical. It assumed that insanity was a curable disease, given understanding, patience, kindness, and proper treatment. While moral treatment included all of the known nonmedical techniques, it more specifically referred to therapeutic efforts which affected the patient's psychology. "Moral treatment," Esquirol (1960:519), one of Pinel's most famous students, wrote, "is the application of the faculty of intelligence and of emotions in the treatment of mental alienation." Implied in this new therapy was the more active participation of the patient in the therapeutic process prescribed by the physician. Thus each individual could be considered separately in terms of his unique needs. Advocates of moral treatment also placed great emphasis on providing mentally ill persons with a new environment in order to break patterns associated with the patient's past history. Such an emphasis was quite natural, since most physicians were influenced by associationist or sensationalist psychology, as well as faculty psychology and phrenology (which at this time was a scientific psychology that combined a theory of localized brain functions with a behavioristic faculty psychology)—all of which, directly or indirectly, involved the influence of the physical environment over the individual's mental state.

Surprisingly enough, much of the leadership in the movement to reform the condition of the insane in the early 19th century was provided by middle- and upper-class laymen. The establishment of the Worcester hospital, for example, resulted from the work of Horace Mann, who later achieved a national reputation as a great educational reformer. Indeed, many of the early mental hospitals were run by laymen rather than physicians. Perhaps the unspecialized nature of society made it easier for laymen to assume such positions of leadership. Most of these laymen were broadly educated and thoroughly versed in the scientific knowledge of their day. Having also been influenced by the optimistic and humanitarian currents that had grown out of the Enlightenment, they sought to eradicate the evil remnants still existing within society.

### THE THERAPEUTIC HOSPITAL

The opening of the Worcester hospital in 1830, then, represented a new chapter in the history of the care and treatment of mental illness in the United States. At this time the establishment of a comprehensive hospital system based on rational therapeutic principles, and open to all regardless of social or economic class, lay in the future. Most insane persons were confined to jails, houses of correction, and poorhouses, living amidst conditions that almost defy the imagination. A number of private and public institutions had been founded after the War of 1812, but all were small and catered largely to upper- and middle-class patients able to pay for their upkeep.

Like so many institutions, the initial success of the Worcester hospital was due largely to the efforts of its leader. Samuel Bayard Woodward, the first superintendent, was a man of unusual ability. His achievements at Worcester were of such high order that his professional colleagues elected him in 1844 as the first president of what is today the American Psychiatric Association.

At the time of his appointment as superintendent, Woodward already enjoyed a distinguished reputation as a physician and social reformer. He had been born in Connecticut in 1787 and had studied medicine under the tutelage of his physician father. As a young boy he had been influenced by the Second Great Awakening that swept through Connecticut. Influenced by a liberalized Congregationalism stripped somewhat of its Calvinistic pessimism, Woodward developed a strong sense of social idealism and warm humanitarian concerns that led him to accept a religious obligation to improve the condition of his fellow man; he consistently rejected a life devoted merely to the pursuit of material goods. Consequently, he was active in reform movements throughout his career. Given his strong religious convictions and belief in the eventual perfectibility of man, it is not surprising that Woodward's entire personality and character was marked by an irrepressible optimism. No evil was so extreme as to be ineradicable; no person was so sinful as to be unredeemable; no illness was so severe as to be incurable; no situation was so far gone as to be beyond control.

During his 13 years as superintendent, Woodward undertook to mold the hospital in accordance with his own ideas regarding the nature and causes of insanity. If Woodward had few original thoughts on such matters, he managed at one time or another to become at least partly acquainted with some of the major writers on mental disease and to incorporate into his own thinking those ideas which seemed most appealing.

Rejecting a supernatural interpretation of mental disease, Woodward began with the assumption that it was a somatic disease, not unlike other diseases. That he took such a view is not surprising, for psychiatry, being a branch of medicine rather than of philosophy or psychology, had traditionally interpreted disease in physical terms. Most of Woodward's contemporaries believed that mental illness was always a consequence of physical damage or malfunctioning. The general direction of medical thought in the nineteenth century, leading to a localized pathology that identified specific disease entities by correlating lesions with symptoms, also influenced psychiatry by tending to discourage a psychological approach in favor of a somatic one.

Although holding to a somatic pathology, Woodward accepted modifications that permitted a psychologically oriented therapy. For example, he adhered to a form of Lockean psychology, for he believed that knowledge came to the mind only through the senses. If the senses (which were physical organs) became diseased, then false impressions would be conveyed to the mind, leading in turn to faulty thinking and abnormal behavior. Such a psychology was eminently suited to therapy, both physical and psychological. If insanity resulted from impaired sensory mechanisms, medical treatment of the diseased organ was all that was required to cure the patient. At the same time, sensationalist and associationist psychology was also conducive to psychological or moral therapy. If the physician could manipulate the environment, he could thereby provide the patient with new and different stimuli. Thus older and undesirable patterns and associations would be broken or modified and new and more desirable ones substituted in their place.

Finally, Woodward found in phrenology a means of connecting mind with matter. Phrenology in the early nineteenth century represented a significant advance over previous psychological systems. Its supporters believed that anatomical and physiological characteristics directly influenced behavior. The mind was not unitary, but was composed of independent and identifiable faculties, which were localized in different "organs" or regions of the brain. To this theory phrenologists added the postulates of a behavioristic psychology and a belief that individuals could deliberately and consciously cultivate different faculties by following the natural laws that governed physiological development and therefore human behavior. From phrenology Woodward took the idea that the normal and abnormal functioning of the mind was dependent on the physical condition of the brain.

Woodward's theories concerning the etiology of insanity followed directly from his somatic definition of mental disease. Mankind, he felt, was governed by certain immutable natural laws that provided a guide to proper living. If an individual followed these laws, a healthy mind and body would result. If these laws were violated, however, the physical organs would not function normally. In other words, insanity, though a somatic illness, could have psychological as well as physical causes. Thus it was the abnormal behavior of the individual (who possessed free will) that was the primary cause of insanity, leading as it did to the impairment of the brain (the organ of the mind). Insanity, therefore, was in some respects self-inflicted; by ignoring the laws governing human behavior the individual placed himself on the road to mental illness.

The causes of insanity, Woodward believed, included intemperance, ill health, religious excitement, masturbation, domestic affliction, loss of property, fear of poverty, personal disappointment, as well as the pressures of an industrial and commercial civilization (which he regarded as unnatural) upon the individual. In general, his etiological theories were derived from the experiences of his own background. Having grown to maturity in a staunch New England middle-class Protestant home, he tended to make the standards of his own class applicable to all of society.

Conceiving of insanity in predominantly naturalistic and somatic terms, it is not surprising, given his faith in progress and generally optimistic outlook, that Woodward believed the disease to be as curable as, if not more curable than, other somatic illnesses. If derangements of the brain and nervous system produced the various types of insanity, it followed that the removal of such causal abnormalities would result in the disappearance of the symptoms and therefore the disease. The prognosis for insanity thus was quite hopeful. Woodward, however, did add one important qualification to his theory; namely, that the sooner the mentally ill were brought to the hospital for treatment, the better the chances for recovery.

In caring for his charges, Woodward relied on various forms of therapy; in this sense he was a pragmatic eclectic. But above all, he was a confirmed believer in moral therapy. While susceptible to many interpretations, moral therapy meant kind, individualized care in a small hospital with occupational therapy, religious exercises, amusements and games, kind treatment, and in large measure a repudiation of all threats of physical violence and an infrequent resort to mechanical restraint. In brief, the new therapy implied the creation of a healthy psychological environment for the individual patient as well as the group.

On the other hand, Woodward never neglected medical treatment. He was concerned about the general health and well being of the patient as well. Thus he used medication for specific symptoms as well as tonics to improve the general condition of the individual. He also relied extensively on narcotics such as morphine and opium; their purpose was to quiet the patient and thus make him amenable to moral treatment.

After the patient's health had been cared for, Woodward then brought moral treatment into play. He insisted on a regular living regime, a substantial though simple diet, emphasis on personal cleanliness, occupational therapy, religious exercises, amusements, and sports. The staff was required to treat all patients with kindness and respect. Rejecting the idea of confining patients, Woodward permitted a high proportion of them complete freedom to walk about the grounds or go into the city without supervision.

In its early days the hospital had about 120 patients, all of whom were on an intimate basis with the superintendent. There seems little doubt that Woodward, working with a relatively homogeneous group of patients—many of whom were Protestant and literate—developed extraordinarily close relationships with many of them. Not all patients, on the other hand, received the same or equal treatment. To a certain extent middle- and upper-class patients or those with more formal education were accorded special privileges. Similarly, the method of classifying patients and wards served indirectly to differentiate patients on the basis of class. By refusing to force patients to associate with persons whom they found distasteful, Woodward implicitly permitted a homogeneous grouping whereby persons of the same social, economic, and educational status tended to come together. Finally, advanced and violent cases of insanity, which occurred with a high frequency among lowerclass inmates who had previously been confined in jails and almshouses for long periods of time, received the least attention. Undoubtedly the wide social and educational differences between such patients and the physician contributed to their partial inability to communicate in a meaningful manner with each other.

How successful was Woodward in treating patients in this way? *"In recent cases of insanity* [persons ill for 1 year or less],*"* Woodward remarked, *"under judicious treatment, as large a proportion of recoveries will take place, as from any other acute disease of equal severity* (Woodward, quoted in *Worcester State Lunatic Hospital Annual Report*, 1835:35).*"* According to Woodward's figures, 2,583 cases were admitted to the hospital between 1833 and 1846. During this same period 2,215 were discharged, of which 1,192 were listed as recovered. When the fact is taken into consideration that those who were discharged as stationary represented largely old and chronic cases, Woodward's figures regarding the chances of recovery of new and recent cases become even more imposing, particularly by contemporary standards.

Were Woodward's claims valid, or was he guilty of a form of unconscious self-deception? Fortunately, one of Woodward's successors in the late 19th century decided to undertake a follow-up study of persons discharged from the hospital as recovered on their only admission or on their last admission. This study, which took nearly 20 years to complete, traced the history of over 1,000 individuals throughout their lives. The results proved highly informative. By 1893 no less than 1,157 persons had been included in the study. Complete information had been gathered on 984, of whom 317 were alive and well at the time of reply, while 251 had remained well until their death and had never again entered a mental hospital. In other words, nearly 58 percent of those discharged as recovered had not had a relapse. The results are even more impressive when the fact is taken into consideration that the survey included friends, relatives, ministers, and employers of former patients, all of whom were asked to give their impression of the individual concerned. It is therefore possible to infer that the familial atmosphere of the hospital, coupled with the kind, humane, and

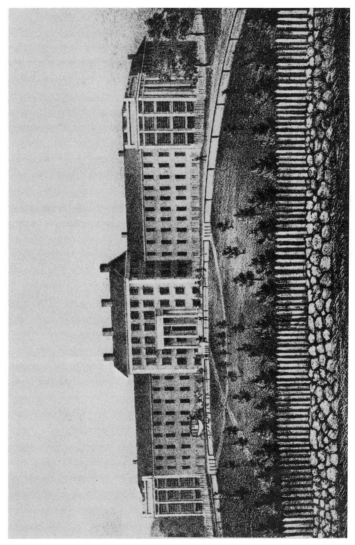

Fig. 2. State Lunatic Hospital at Worcester, 1837. During the decade following its opening in 1833, the Worcester hospital served as the programmatic and architectural prototype of the public mental hospital in America. Source: Worcester State Lunatic Hospital, Annual Report V (1837).

optimistic attitude of Woodward toward his charges, produced a psychological climate within the hospital which had a beneficial effect upon its inmates.

## FROM THE THERAPEUTIC
## TO THE CUSTODIAL HOSPITAL

At this point an obvious question emerges. If the Worcester, along with other early 19th century mental hospitals, were so successful in treating patients, what was responsible for the regression that clearly took place in the second half of the century as well as in the 20th century, when most state hospitals were transformed into custodial rather than therapeutic institutions? While the answer to this question is extremely complex and must include attention to psychiatric theory and practice, it is also clear that part of the answer lies in the rapidly changing social, intellectual, and economic environment of mid-19th century America. An examination of the post-Woodward era from 1846 to 1855 illustrates this latter point.

When Woodward retired from the superintendency, the trustees of the hospital selected as his successor George Chandler, a former assistant to Woodward who had become head of the Asylum for the Insane at Concord, New Hampshire. While the trustees may not have realized it at the time, they had set an important precedent; for the next several decades—with only a single exception—the superintendency was occupied by individuals who had spent most of their professional careers at the hospital, and who had been elevated to the position by virtue of the seniority they had acquired. Indirectly this practice of inbreeding was to prove a potent factor in the hospital's history. Since superintendents came up from the ranks and were often isolated from external influences, they often had difficulty in viewing the needs facing the hospital dispassionately and at a distance. By and large, they tended to follow along paths that had been laid out by their predecessors. Consequently, many problems faced by the hospital were intensified, for older routines and practices often proved ill adapted to new situations.

Although Chandler was probably groomed by Woodward as his heir apparent, there were marked personal and professional differences between the two men. Woodward was a person of catholic tastes who was driven by his faith in religion and science, both of which, he believed, would help mankind to create a better world. Never focusing on a single object to the exclusion of all others, he could support many worthy causes. While superintendent, for example, he found time to advocate institutional treatment of alcoholics, to publish a guide to mental and physical health for young people, and to aid various other reform movements.

Chandler was a quite different person. Lacking Woodward's enthusiasm and faith in the inevitable improvement of the human race, he was more the prototype of future superintendents at the hospital. Basically he was an administrator who ran things competently though unimaginatively. While aware of institutional shortcomings, he did not fight for remedial measures nor did he conceive of himself as a crusader and missionary on behalf of the insane.

Under Chandler the role of the superintendent underwent a subtle transformation. Woodward, for example, was devoted to the welfare of the individual patient. His understanding of moral therapy was that a physician could influence behavior by manipulating the individual's environment. The part played by the psychiatrist was in some ways comparable to that of a father looking after the welfare of his children and teaching them proper and ethical habits. As long as the number of patients remained relatively small, Woodward was able to supervise personally the care of his patients and to administer the general affairs of the hospital as well; there was no inherent conflict between these tasks.

Chandler's primary interests, on the other hand, lay in standards and routines of hospital management. These interests, however, did not spring from any defects in character or callousness to suffering. Like most persons attracted to a career in psychiatry at this time, he too was motivated by a desire to help the mentally ill. But the situation that he found himself in by the late 1840s and 1850s was unlike that of the 1830s. By Chandler's time the hospital was facing a crisis as a result of the pressure of rising admissions, a pressure that it could not resist because of the legal system under which it functioned.[2] The internal growth of the hospital, a response to these external factors, created an entirely new set of circumstances. No longer was Chandler able to run the hospital in a loose and informal manner as Woodward had done. With 400 to 500 patients the problems of social organization and adjustment were much more complex. The theory of moral treatment provided few answers or guidelines, for it was based (according to Chandler) on a direct and personal relationship between doctor and patient.

Since no theoretical framework existed that could harmonize or rationalize an individualistic therapy with a collective social system having different objectives, the tendency was for the demands of the social system to outweigh the requirements of therapy. Thus Chandler found himself in an unenviable dilemma; his concern for the welfare of his patients was conflicting with the larger goal of maintaining order in a complex social institution.

Chandler's difficulties were compounded even further by outside pressures. The hospital, for example, played a dual role, one therapeutic, the other custodial. As long as it remained small, it was relatively easy for the superintendent to combine both of these roles. The hospital's growth, however, made this more difficult. Increasingly the superintendent found himself confronted with the responsibility of having to sacrifice one of these goals in order to achieve the other. Given a choice, therapeutic considerations might well have been dominant. But the superintendent could not only be concerned with the welfare of his patient; he had to take into account the demands of society for protection against those who ostensibly menaced the community. As more and more lower-class patients entered the hospital, the public clamor for adequate protection increased sharply. Consequently, therapeutic considerations receded into the background.

Under this set of circumstances Chandler's immersion in administrative problems was hardly surprising. An intricate social institution like a mental hospital required formal mechanisms to ensure order and efficiency; formal mechanisms, in turn, often defeated the aims of moral treatment, which was based on the ability of the physician to manipulate the environment of the individual and group as the need arose. Custodial considerations merely reinforced administrative concerns, for custody required a tight and efficiently run institution governed by rational and clearly defined procedures.

Chandler's immersion in administrative psychiatry was by no means atypical. By the middle of the 19th century, American psychiatry had become identified with hospital management. Leading psychiatrists, with a few exceptions, were concerned with problems of administration, organization, architectural standards, occupational therapy, efficient heating and ventilating systems, and the like. Few undertook, as did their European counterparts, any basic research; the pages of the *American Journal of Insanity*, the outstanding psychiatric periodical of this period, are notable only for the lack of articles embodying the results of original research.

While French, German, and to a lesser extent, British physicians were performing autopsies, correlating symptoms with pathological anatomy, studying the nervous system, and trying to observe the course and development of identifiable disease entities, their brethren across the Atlantic remained aloof from such concerns. In this respect American physicians were representative of their milieu, for during the 19th century there was little basic research in either science or medicine in the United States. Americans were an intensely practical breed; they were most interested in concrete results. American doctors, for example, excelled in applied research of immediate utility, such as surgery. There were practically no studies that combined clinical–pathological approaches, and as late as 1860 Oliver Wendell Holmes could ridicule science as having no value for actual medical practice.

The development of administrative psychiatry was accompanied by other internal changes in the profession. The emphasis on management techniques fostered a narrow specialization that made alienists less receptive to outside criticism, help, or advice. The ensuing professionalization of psychiatry opened a chasm between lay reformers and physicians. The greater their sense of professionalism, the less were psychiatrists willing to listen to others or to take advantage of advances in related fields. The coalition of reformers and physicians that had been so influential in founding mental hospitals, developing a more humane therapy, and modifying public attitudes, had been broken.

The transformation of the psychiatrist into an administrator also had a subtle effect upon psychiatric theory and practice. A comparison of Woodward's views on etiology with those of Chandler's, for example, offers a good case in point. Ostensibly Chandler's ideas of etiology were approximately the same as those of his predecessor. Yet Woodward's psychiatric theories had been developed within a broad religious framework that emphasized above all the responsibility of the individual for the welfare of those less fortunate than himself. Thus feelings of sympathy and compassion tempered and softened his attitudes. Although he frequently warned that immoral acts (masturbation, intemperance, etc.) played a part in etiology, he never condemned or treated harshly patients whose illness had resulted from improper acts. On the contrary, such persons were worthy of the aid and sympathy of any true Christian.

Chandler, however, lacked Woodward's religious commitment. While emphasizing the role of the individual in causing mental disease, he did not temper his views by overarching humanitarian and religious beliefs. When large numbers of Irish paupers entered the hospital, he was unable to accept them in the way that he accepted natives. His awareness of class and cultural differences was more distinct because of the absence of the religious fervor that had universalized rather than particularized humanity. Thus in discussing etiology, he began by dividing the causes of insanity into two general classes, the moral or psychological and the physical. Both were usually involved in bringing on mental disease. The leading causes of insanity involved behavior that deviated from the standards of the average middle-class New Englander. Thus intemperance, which by this time was often associated with the alien Irishman as contrasted with the sober and upright native citizen, was singled out as a major cause of mental disease.

Like Woodward, Chandler was probably influenced by phrenological thought, for he placed considerable emphasis upon the inculcation of proper living habits as early in life as possible, so as to permit the brain to develop in a normal manner. In Chandler's eyes the prevention of insanity was just as important as its cure. This could be accomplished by having each individual obey "the laws of health, which include those that regulate the passions and emotions of the mind as well as those that govern the physical system (Chandler, quoted in *Worcester State Lunatic Hospital Annual Report*, 1849:47)." What were the laws of health? They included, among other things, avoidance of certain behavior patterns that would lead hereditary predispositions to become operative, and a regime that was balanced between physical and mental labor. Chandler was also influenced by an incipient anti-intellectualism. He felt that overcultivation of bookish or intellectual qualities was wrong; hence long confinement in school or among books was dangerous to mental health. Not surprisingly, he argued that farmers and mechanics had provided New England with its healthiest individuals; urban areas were indebted to these groups for their active and successful population. Finally, Chandler maintained that the ambitions of many children were being overstimulated by the allurements of success in the free and open competition of the marketplace, and insanity resulted when their hopes were not fulfilled. His norm, in other words, was an individual who was neither poor nor rich, who did not overvalue physical or mental labor, who knew his place in life and did not overstep its boundaries, who avoided excesses in either drinking or religion—an individual, to put it another way, who came from a middle-class, Protestant background. In large measure Chandler's views on the etiology of insanity were derived principally from his own moral, ethical, religious, and philosophical ideas.

The dissimilarities between Chandler and Woodward had significant implications for therapy at the hospital. Under Woodward moral treatment was administered with enthusiasm and optimism. Probably few patients remained completely immune to the charged and dynamic atmosphere at the hospital in its early days. Chandler, on the other hand, was dealing with a more heterogeneous and much larger group of patients. Considerations of order and efficiency could not be ignored; they tended to limit the degree of innovation and the flexibility that moral treatment required. What happened was not that moral treatment was abandoned; rather it was institutionalized and forced into a regular and predictable pattern, with a consequent loss of its inner spirit and drive.

Chandler was by no means unaware of what was happening at the hospital. When queried by a legislative investigating committee in the late 1840s, he made known his preferences for a small rather than a large hospital in no uncertain terms. His ideal of a small hospital—an ideal shared by most persons at that time—however, was becoming obsolete because of the continuous pressure of new admissions. By 1852 the average number of patients exceeded 500, and the strain upon the hospital's facilities became almost unbearable. At this time the medical staff still consisted of the three physicians that it had nearly a decade before: the superintendent and two assistant physicians. The former spent most of his time on administrative duties; responsibility for caring for the patients fell upon the latter. Since the two assistants were responsible for a number of tasks, including the preparation of all medical prescriptions, they were unable to devote their undivided energies to the care and treatment of patients.

The growth of the hospital had other effects as well. First, the increase in the size of the patient population forced the superintendent to place greater reliance upon attendants and nurses. At that time no formal training was available for nonprofessional personnel; as a result inexperienced persons were normally hired. Since salaries were low, there was a high turnover rate, averaging close to about 40 percent per year.

The inexperience of nurses and attendants, however, was not the critical variable in explaining the declining success of moral treatment. Much more important was the intangible change in atmosphere at the hospital. The transfer of many of the psychiatrist's functions to a low-paid, inexperienced, nonprofessional staff with low morale had an adverse effect upon inmates. By and large, nurses and attendants were not motivated by altruistic concerns (as the high turnover rate indicates), nor did they view their occupation in terms of a calling to help those less fortunate than themselves. Outwardly moral treatment remained constant; inwardly there was a shift in its complexion and spirit, leading to a deterioration of its effectiveness.

Although Chandler and others were aware of the problem, the thought of training attendants and nurses and giving them greater responsibility for the welfare of the patient was never seriously considered. In this respect Chandler reflected the growing belief of his profession that treatment was the sole prerogative of the physician; at best laymen were useful auxiliaries. Since mental illness, like smallpox and other organic diseases, was something that a patient had, responsibility for his care and treatment had to remain within the hands of the psychiatrist. The doctor–patient relationship was an inviolate one that precluded the intrusion of a third party. Although psychological factors entered into etiology and therapy, the patient was still viewed as a passive agent who was active only in the sense that he followed or complied with the directions of the physician; his status was not that of an equal partner. Given such a medical model, it is easy to understand the failure to employ attendants and nurses in a deliberate and meaningful manner—a failure that remained constant for most of the 19th as well as the 20th century.

Second, the growth of the hospital led to greater reliance upon physical restraint. With more patients, the need for formal mechanisms of ensuring order became greater. Under such conditions, the easiest way of ensuring order was to keep violent or hard-to-manage patients under some form of restraint. Such restraint usually took one of two forms. Extremely difficult patients were confined in solitary rooms, where they required little or no attention. Other patients were confined by straps and waistbands.

There is little doubt that the use of restraints eased the burdens of the staff and permitted the hospital to maintain a high degree of order. In this respect the goals of restraint had changed sharply since the 1830s. To Woodward restraint was partly therapeutic; it was intended to protect and quiet violent and dangerous patients, who could then be brought within the range of moral treatment. Under Chandler the institutional setting had so changed that his use of restraint also undermined moral treatment. Neglected and ignored, restrained patients at best remained in a stationary condition; at worst they became even further demented. Furthermore, the hostility of physicians toward patients who upset the hospital's routine contributed to the deterioration in the condition of such inmates. It does not require much imagination to conceive of a patient's reaction when a physician could describe the case in the following words, which were not at all unusual: "No improvement in this degraded woman—is wholly lost to shame and has no more regard to exposing herself than a dumb beast."[3]

By the 1850s restraint at the hospital was quite common. In this respect Chandler was following practices that were sanctioned by the overwhelming majority of American superintendents. Generally speaking, restraint was more common in the United States than in England or on the continent. In England its use had been severely restricted by the work of John Conolly and others. In the Pinelian tradition of humanistic psychiatry, Conolly advocated a therapeutic system that involved attitudes of respect, kindness, patience, understanding, and truthfulness on the part of the staff toward the inmates, and an almost total elimination of restraint. The nonrestraint system, however, never made very much progress in the United States, largely because a burgeoning population so taxed hospital facilities that superintendents used it as an administrative device to maintain order. "Restraints and neglect may be considered synonymous," Conolly (quoted in Deutsch, 1937:221) had written in perceptive words, "for restraints are merely a general substitute for the thousand attentions required by troublesome patients."

In the third place, the character of therapy, both medical and moral, was transformed as the Worcester hospital grew in size. Between 1834 and 1853 the doctor–patient ratio rose from 1:58 to 1:140. Consequently, physicians devoted less time to each case. The manuscript case histories offer striking corroboration of this generalization. During Chandler's years in office the case histories became more fragmentary and uninformative than they had been under Woodward. Sometimes the physician in charge would not enter any statements about his patient for a 3- to 5-year period, and when he did so his remarks tended to be cursory and superficial.

Other aspects of patient care also deteriorated. Since the hospital authorities were handling larger numbers of patients, they found Woodward's precedent of relying on drugs a useful one. The practice of ensuring a manageable patient population, however, tended to become an end in itself. Unlike his predecessor, Chandler did not regard it primarily as a prelude to other forms of therapy. Drugs were useful and necessary because they facilitated the management of a large patient body with a minimum of trouble. Thus while the use of drugs, including morphine and opium, remained more or less constant between 1833 and 1855, the underlying rationale changed considerably. Similarly, occupational therapy became more haphazard during the later period. As the hospital increased in size, work was assigned more to meet the needs of the hospital than the needs of the patient. In 1853 the trustees estimated that only one-quarter of the patients were employed in the summer and one-fifth in the winter. The hospital, in other words, was custodial for more than three-quarters of its patients.

Finally, the hospital's growth increased the influence of ethnic, religious, and class factors in determining care and treatment. During the 1840s and 1850s the rise in the number of patients had resulted partially from an influx of immigrants into Massachusetts, especially from Ireland. Quite naturally, the Irish began to constitute a higher proportion of the population at the hospital. In 1846 only 12 Irish patients had been admitted; by 1854 this figure had risen to 96. Chandler considered this to be an important development, and in 1855 he included in his annual report a table that specifically singled out the Irish at the hospital in the previous decade.

Chandler's action in identifying the Irish was hardly unusual. The overwhelming majority of them were Catholic, and Massachusetts since its founding had been a center of no-Popery sentiment. In the 17th century the General Court had actually passed a number of laws intended to prevent the migration of Catholics into the province and to make impossible the propagation of their religion. As long as the number of Catholics had remained insignificant, the strong feelings against them were quiescent. But as the impact of Irish immigration became more pronounced, public hostility increased in virulence. After 1830 anti-Catholicism became a movement of national significance.

But antipathies toward the Irish were not solely a result of religious friction. On the contrary, their economic condition also played a role in arousing hostility. Prior to their arrival in large numbers, the economy of the Bay State was oriented toward small-scale skilled enterprises rather than large-scale unskilled ones. Generally speaking, poverty and pauperism were of no great importance, for broad occupational diversity minimized the impact of changes within a particular trade or occupation. By the 1840s, on the other hand, the economy of Massachusetts was beginning to change as the movement toward industrialism accelerated. In this development the Irish played a crucial role, for they contributed the necessary cheap and unskilled surplus labor without which in-industrialization would have been impossible.

The economic transformation of Massachusetts soon created problems that had few precedents. For the first time in their history Bay Staters were confronted with the problems of slums, poverty, and pauperism that accompanied industrialization. Since the Irish—more than any other group—were associated with these developments, they bore the major share of the blame. To middle-class natives the abject poverty of the Irish—exemplified by the slum areas in which they congregated—was destroying the beauty and homogeneity of American society and burdening the more thrifty and prosperous classes with a rising tax bill to care for the impoverished and improvident. Still others feared the competition of Irish laborers willing to work for low wages. Above all—especially as the newcomers developed a sense of group consciousness—native citizens became aware of the differences that separated the two groups. Slowly but surely the older tradition of anti-Catholicism merged with the more recent fear of the changes that were transforming the Bay State, giving rise to strong feelings of distrust and even hatred.

The ethnic, social, and economic tensions that divided Massachusetts society had an important influence over conditions among the mentally ill, for they exacerbated existing class differences in institutional care and treatment. Increasingly the argument was heard that the public burden of supporting foreign-born paupers, including insane persons, was fast becoming an unbearable strain. "This is only the beginning of troubles," commented the influential *Boston Medical and Surgical Journal,* one of the leading medical journals in the United States, upon the subject of the foreign insane:

> for the new hospital that is to be reared will soon be in their possession also. Never was a sovereign State so grieviously burdened. The people bear the growing evil without a murmur, and it is therefore taken for granted that taxation for the support of the cast-off humanity of Europe is an agreeable exercise of their charity (Editorial, 1852:537).

The charge that foreign paupers, including the insane, were the single largest group supported by the state was quite true. The state auditor estimated that during the 10 years ending in 1851 nearly 2,500 out of a total of 3,722 insane state paupers were Irish. Since most Irish immigrants came from lower-class backgrounds—indeed, many were nearly destitute upon their arrival on American shores—it was not surprising that when mental illness struck they were completely dependent upon public charity.

As the proportion of Irish patients at the hospital increased, public attitudes toward the mentally ill began to undergo a subtle transformation. Many Americans began to draw invidious distinctions between the native insane and the Irish insane. The former were still treated with compassion and sympathy; but the latter were the objects of a growing hostility. The older and still dominant New England natives not only were reluctant to extend their hopeful attitudes toward insanity to include lower-class Irish immigrants, but they actually believed that the Irish constituted a separate race whose members were not as responsive as native Americans to therapy when afflicted with mental disease.

The hostile feelings toward foreigners in general and the Irish in particular had a considerable impact over their treatment within the hospital. Most staff physicians reflected to some extent the popular anti-Catholic feelings then prevalent, and undoubtedly these feelings influenced their relationships with patients. Equally if not more significant was the fact that the Irish were drawn almost exclusively from lower-class backgrounds. They worked at unskilled jobs; they received low wages; they congregated in slums; they provided a disproportionate share of paupers; they had little if any formal education; and they tended to band together and to develop a strong sense of group consciousness and cohesion. To the physicians—most of whom came from middle-class homes and had been reared in a Protestant-dominated culture—the Irish, by virtue of their lower-class character, appeared as social undesirables who were responsible for many of the evils that afflicted American society. Rather than being the victims of an impersonal system, the Irish were the cause of all problems. Thus they were poor not because they came from an impoverished environment, but because they were unable to assimilate and adjust to the demands of American ideals.

Chandler's attitude toward the Irish is a case in point. Although he claimed that he made no distinctions between patients who came from different ethnic and economic backgrounds, there is evidence to show that care and treatment were partly dependent upon social and economic status and ethnic origin, both of which were closely related. Chandler, for example, admitted that he was more successful in dealing with native-born patients than with foreign ones, although he laid responsibility for this situation at the latter's doors. As he reported in 1847:

> Most of the foreigners are Irish. The want of forethought in them to save their earnings for the day of sickness, the indulgence of their appetites for stimulating drinks, which are too easily obtained among us, and their strong love for their native land, which is characteristic with them, are the fruitful causes of insanity among them. As a class, we are not so successful in our treatment of them as with the native population of New England. It is difficult to obtain their confidence, for they seem to be jeal-

ous of our motives; and the embarrassment they are under, from not clearly comprehending our language, is another obstacle in the way of their recovery (Chandler, quoted in *Worcester State Lunatic Hospital Annual Report*, 1847:33).

There is little doubt that the ethnic and social backgrounds of the professional staff indirectly played an important role in determining patient care at the hospital. Though physicians may not have been aware of their hostile attitudes, it is quite probable that patients toward whom this antipathy was directed would be suspicious and uncommunicative. The mutual distrust hardly could have been conducive to successful therapy, which usually required a close and trusting relationship between doctor and patient. Chandler's observation that he had trouble in communicating with foreign patients was quite true, but not for the reasons he gave. Since he and others usually approached foreign pauper patients with an air of condescension and dislike, patients tended to reciprocate in kind. A superficial perusal of the case histories proves this point. Most of the descriptions of foreign paupers at the hospital are marked by feelings of revulsion on the part of the physician. One Irish female, to cite only one example out of many, was described in 1854 in the following terms: "This girl is much of the time noisy and troublesome. Has nymphomania and exposes her person . . . Is vulgar and obscene." A month later there is a similar description: "There has been no perceptible change in her condition or habits. Is noisy destructive violent and vulgar. Almost constantly excited. Screaming and tearing her clothes."[4] Middle-class native patients, on the other hand, received considerably more attention and sympathy.

### CONCLUSION

The experiences of Massachusetts during the first half of the nineteenth century[5] in establishing a system of public mental hospitals was fairly typical of the rest of the nation, if only for the reason that most other states followed its lead. Thus the forces that were operative in the Bay State were also operative elsewhere. The result was that by the end the century the custodial as opposed to the therapeutic hospital had become the norm rather than the exception.

Looking in retrospect at the development of the state mental hospital, it is possible to make some broad generalizations. Because a "scientific psychiatry" often proved more of a dream than a reality, the development of the mental hospital was often determined—perhaps unconsciously—by external and internal social, psychological, economic, and intellectual influences. Moral treatment, for example, which had enjoyed great success during the first half of the nineteenth century, was not based on a systematic theory nor had it grown out of controlled experimentation. On the contrary, it developed out of the humanitarian and religious concerns of the period. Moral treatment was based on the assumption that there would be a close relationship between the therapist and patient—a relationship made possible by the fact that both probably came from the same ethnic, economic, and religious backgrounds and environment, and shared a common cultural heritage.

After 1850, as patients from diverse ethnic, religious, and economic backgrounds entered the hospital, moral treatment became less and less successful. Because psychiatrists were never fully aware of the important part that their own attitudes played in their professional rationale and ideology, they were unprepared to cope with the heterogeneous patient population that accompanied the new urban and industrial society. Consequently, they were prone to place responsibility for their declining successes elsewhere. Some psychiatrists attributed their inability to help patients coming from low socioeconomic backgrounds to the fact that such individuals had inherent character defects that not only explained their impoverished straits, but also their lack of response to therapy. Others accused the legislature of not appropriating sufficient funds, thus implying that inadequate financial resources were blocking further progress in treating mental disease. But whatever the reasons offered, it was evident that most psychiatrists no longer adhered to the belief that mental disease, irrespective of a patient's background, was a largely curable malady.

The internal transformation of the mental hospital into a custodial institution also influenced psychiatric thought. When psychiatrists were confronted with the decline in the effectiveness of moral treatment, they began to adjust their theoretical approach in the light of their experiences. Up to the middle of the 19th century they had accepted the role of psychological factors in etiology and treatment. After this time, however, they began to revert to an outright and explicit somaticism. But a strictly somatic approach—which was reinforced by the direction taken by nineteenth century scientific and medical theory—usually led to therapeutic nihilism.[6]

After all, if the basis of insanity was physical, of what use would be a psychological therapy? Lacking any visible means of therapy, psychiatrists tended to engage in a vast holding operation by confining mentally ill patients until that distant day when specific cures for specific disease entities would become available.

The rise of the custodial hospital was related to other influences as well. One such influence was the growing sense of professionalism among psychiatrists. Although professionalism is often defined in terms of a set of special skills and knowledge required for complex functions beyond the reach of ordinary untrained individuals, it also had far broader implications in a historical sense. Specifically, professionalism involved not only a monopoly of special skills, but the creation of a subculture that gave members of a specialty both a common experience which facilitated communication within the group and excluded all nonspecialists, including, of course, laymen. The establishment of a professional psychiatric subculture—with its explicit and implicit system of values and norms—resulted in the erection of a barrier between psychiatrists and other groups. The founding of the present-day American Psychiatric Association in 1844 was one indication of this development, since one of the major purposes of this organization was to define standards that would govern therapy, administration, and management. By insisting that special skills and knowledge were required for treating mental illness, psychiatrists were able to justify the exclusion of all other persons having formal training and instruction in this specialty.[7]

Undoubtedly the creation of a psychiatric community and the establishment of minimum standards permitted the adoption of more rigorous guidelines to govern care and treatment of the mentally ill. On the other hand, professionalism had adverse effects as well. Indeed, professionalism resulted in the exclusion of those laymen whose work had been responsible for much of the élan and drive—to say nothing of the material success—that had characterized the early efforts to aid the mentally ill in the first half of the 19th century. Professionalism also tended to isolate psychiatrists from those social and humanitarian influences that might have tempered the pessimistic outlook of late nineteenth and early 20th century psychiatry. Having rejected as subjective and unscientific such affective sentiments as humanity, love, compassion, psychiatrists found their own supposedly objective and scientific approach barren because of the ambiguities that marked their efforts to define and identify the essential attributes and nature of mental disease.

Last, professionalism, when combined with intellectual isolation, deprived psychiatry of some of the insights of other disciplines and approaches that might have been useful in dealing with some of the philosophical and scientific problems growing out of mental illness.

Other forces contributed to the custodial-like nature of the mental hospital. If the hospital's existence could not be justified by the number of patients that it cured, then its *raison d'être* had to be rationalized in custodial terms. Indeed, much of the support that the mental hospital received was predicated on the assumption that it provided protection against groups that menaced the safety and security of society. The easiest way to get appropriations was to appeal to the legislature for funds with which to provide accommodations to care for the growing number of chronically deranged individuals.

The emergence and transformation of the mental hospital, therefore, was related to a variety of factors—social, intellectual, economic. Despite the use of the term "hospital," it is clear that the character of mental hospitals was not related solely to psychiatric theory, but to many other determinants as well. Oliver Wendell Holmes, the noted physician and man of letters, understood this fact very well. Writing over a century ago, he noted in perceptive words that

> The truth is that medicine, professedly founded on observation, is as sensitive to outside influence, political, religious, philosophical, imaginative, as is the barometer to the changes of atmospheric density. Theoretically it ought to go on its own straightforward inductive path, without regard to changes of government or to fluctuations of public opinion. But . . . [actually there is] a closer relation between the Medical Sciences and the conditions of Society and the general thought of the time, than would at first be suspected (Holmes, 1891:177).

Far from merely reflecting certain scientific and medical currents, the mental hospital as well as psychiatry both emerged out of the interaction of complex social, intellectual, and economic forces.

**NOTES**

1. No doubt some readers will be offended at the constant use of the terms "insane" and "insanity" as opposed to "mentally ill" and "mental illness." Although the former two have acquired an odious connotation, they were perfectly

good terms in the past. This usage, therefore, is a historical one and is not intended to imply any derogatory connotation. After all, it is probable that the phrase "mental illness" itself will in the future be looked down upon with the same disfavor as "insanity" is at present.

2. The increasing pressure on the hospital resulted from a variety of influences. First, the existence of a mental hospital meant that jails and almshouses were not the only places for the confinement of insane persons. Families that had once been reluctant to send loved ones to substandard institutions were now more willing to consider the possibility of institutionalization. Second, the growing urbanization made it more and more difficult to care for the mentally ill in the community. Deviant behavior in densely populated areas not only posed greater problems than in rural areas, but it was also less likely to be tolerated. Third, the establishment of a mental hospital increased societal awareness of mental disease, and undoubtedly some who had been considered quaint or odd were now looked upon as insane. Finally, the rapid growth in population, which was partly associated with industrialization and partly with the tremendous increase in immigration from Ireland, was accompanied by a proportionate increase in the number of mentally ill persons.

3. Entry of November 3, 1851, Case No. 3260, Case Book No. 24, p. 105, Record Storage Section, Worcester State Hospital, Worcester, Massachusetts.

4. Entires of October 3, November 3, 1854, Case No. 4710, Case Book No. 28, p. 240, Record Storage Section, Worcester State Hospital, Worcester Massachusetts.

5. Beginning in the early 1850s Massachusetts began the practice of establishing new state hospitals as the need arose; by the 1860s it had also created a centralized administrative framework within which the individual institutions operated. These practices and others made the Commonwealth the leader in the United States insofar as the care and treatment of the mentally ill were concerned.

6. This statement is a historical one and is not intended or prove or to disprove the thesis that mental illness is or is not somatic or psychological in nature. It is only to state that for the 19th century, as well as for a good part of the 20th, somaticism ran hand in hand with pessimism. A psychological approach, however, often—though not always—implied optimism and therefore therapy.

7. It should be noted that the increasing professionalization of psychiatry was matched and paralleled by professionalization in other specialities in medicine as well as in virtually every field of the sciences and arts. Indeed, the growth of professionalism was closely related to other societal determinants such as urbanization, industrialization, the rise of the mass communication media, rationalization, the availability of organizational techniques, and the development of accreditation procedures, particularly in the universities and professional schools.

Joseph P. Morrissey
Howard H. Goldman

# 3
# The Ambiguous Legacy: 1856–1968

The opening in 1833 of Massachusetts' Worcester State Hospital marked the inception of an extensive asylum-building program throughout the United States. Yet, new doors hardly opened before facilities were jammed with inmates drawn from the almshouses and jails of small towns and cities. Efforts of the early asylum superintendents—the psychiatric leaders of their time—to avoid this swamping of a medical institution by a miscellaneous and often untreatable avalanche of indigent, deviant, and mentally deficient people were frustrated. And during this period, the character of the state hospital in the United States, with its growing static population and contradictions in its functions, became set. The public, in general, having achieved a comfortable disposition of its local responsibilities by sending its mentally ill citizens to a large, centralized, and somewhat isolated institution, now found it easy to forget them, and settled into an indifference which . . . persisted well into the twentieth century.

Ivan Belknap (1956:17)

The initial success of the early public mental hospitals in meeting the therapeutic ideals of their founders fueled the humanitarian zeal of a new generation of social reformers. Dorothea Lynde Dix, who was attracted to the cause of the insane poor in the 1840s, became the principal spokesperson and lobbyist for the construction of public asylums throughout America.[1] Ironically, even as this new wave of asylum building got underway, the social reality that supported the idea of a "moral asylum" was rapidly fading.

The therapeutic ideals of these hospitals remained viable only

45

to the extent that their patients and staff shared common religious, ethnic, and cultural values; their caseloads were held to a relatively small size so that intimate staff–patient relationships could be developed and sustained; their admissions consisted of recent as opposed to long-term or chronic cases; their sense of purpose was championed by charismatic superintendents and influential laymen; and their governmental sponsors were willing to appropriate adequate funds for their operation. During the mid-19th century, each of these supports was undermined by social, economic, and intellectual forces beyond the control of hospital superintendents. Slowly but inexorably, public mental hospitals were transformed from small, therapeutic asylums into large, custodial institutions.

In the process, public mental hospitals acquired an ambiguous organizational character: while retaining the ideals and architectural form of therapeutic institutions, their functions and practices increasingly came to be defined in terms of custody and social control. Not only were they entrusted with the function of caring for mentally disordered individuals, but they also became central repositories for aged, infirm, and indigent members of minority groups as well as for persons who were deemed socially disruptive by the community.[2] In time, their structure and functions resembled those of welfare institutions rather than the private asylums upon which they were modeled.

In the Commonwealth of Massachusetts, the social and intellectual currents that led to this transformation were present, in incipient form, by the 1850s. However, their convergence into an explicit public policy for dealing with the problem of mental illness in a rapidly industrializing and urbanizing society did not occur until the 1870s. The intervening years were a period of reassessment and exploration for alternatives to large custodial institutions. The decisions made during these years laid the groundwork for the Commonwealth to assume responsibility for the care and confinement of the mentally ill, established the precedent of building new custodial facilities as the need arose, and led to the growth of a centralized administrative structure to govern the ever-growing number of facilities. By the late 1870s, the new system was well established in Massachusetts, and its approach was soon emulated by other states.

This centralized administrative structure sustained public mental health care in the United States for the next several decades. Sporadic reforms attempted to resolve the ambiguous character of the state mental hospitals, but the pessimism and therapeutic nihil-

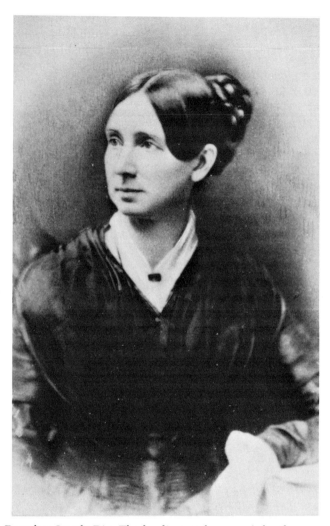

Fig. 3. Dorothea Lynde Dix. The leading spokesperson for the cause of the insane poor in mid-19th-century America, Dix's memorial before the Massachusetts legislature led to the expansion of the Worcester hospital in 1844. Before her death in 1887, she helped in the creation or expansion of more than 30 state mental institutions throughout the United States. *Source:* Houghton Library, Harvard University.

ism which enveloped psychiatry and the public concern for cheap custodial care inhibited fundamental alterations in the state hospital system.

Gradually, the mental hygiene movement in the early 20th century led to the growth of community-based alternatives to custodial institutions in the form of dispensaries, child guidance clinics, psychopathic hospitals, and psychiatric units in general hospitals. Eventually, in the 1950s and early 1960s, the community mental health movement ushered in a new wave of institutional reform that dramatically altered public policy toward the care of the mentally ill and challenged the foundations upon which the state hospital system had been erected. In many respects, these policy and programmatic developments have brought the public mental hospital system full circle to the issues of community responsibility for the mentally ill, a set of issues that initially led to the founding of state mental hospitals in this country.

This chapter will trace out these cycles of reform as they shaped the ambiguous legacy and institutional development of Worcester State Hospital from 1856 to 1968.[3]


## THE END OF MORAL THERAPY

The administrative, legal, and financial structure established by the Massachusetts legislature in 1832 prior to the opening of the State Lunatic Hospital at Worcester had a profound, although largely unanticipated, impact on its internal development. At the time, it was assumed that the new hospital would serve a transitory population. As patients recovered after brief periods of hospitalization, their discharge would make room for new admissions. Annual turnover would thus allow the hospital to care for 2–3 times its capacity of 120 patients. In practice, these assumptions proved to be unrealistic. Within a very few years, the hospital was incapable of meeting the demands placed on its facilities.

Under the law of 1832, all dangerous lunatics already confined in jails and houses of correction throughout the state had to be transferred to Worcester. Moreover, hospital authorities had no effective control over admission policies since they were given no discretion about accepting or rejecting persons committed by the courts. Many of these persons constituted the oldest and most advanced cases of mental illness and they had the least chance of recovery. Such patients, although unresponsive to moral therapy, could not be discharged because the law provided for their release only when the original cause of commitment ceased to exist. In combination with the natural accumulation of other patients who failed to recover for a variety of reasons, the hospital became filled with an increasingly static population of chronic cases. As a result of expansions in its physical plant in 1836 and 1844, the average number of resident patients rose from 107 in 1833 to 359 in 1846.

These legal constraints were compounded by the fiscal structure under which the hospital was forced to operate. Under the law, the hospital had to be a self-supporting institution; legislative appropriations were authorized only for capital expenditures. Localities were financially responsible for all judicial commitments and for the pauper insane sent to Worcester but their charges could not exceed cost. Families sending private patients, on the other hand, were liable for whatever charges were set by hospital authorities. In 1844, in response to growing complaints by local officials, the legislature set a specific per capita figure for the care of the indigent insane. As costs exceeded income, hospital authorities were forced to raise charges for private patients in order to maintain the hospital. This policy tended to exclude some persons who could not afford the cost of hospitalization and to reinforce the influence of social class in securing preferential treatment and living accommodations.

Problems of overcrowding and shrinking fiscal resources at the Worcester hospital were exacerbated in the 1840s with the rapid influx of European immigrants and the reluctance of localities to meet their financial obligations for foreign paupers. In 1848, a joint legislative committee was formed to review the need for a further expansion of the Worcester hospital. The committee acknowledged that a single state hospital could not meet the needs of an ever-expanding population of indigent insane and, in lieu of expanding facilities at Worcester, it recommended the construction of a second hospital. In 1854, when the new hospital opened in Taunton, it took over 200 patients from Worcester. Although these transfers reduced the census at Worcester from 559 to 345, the relief was only temporary. That same year the Worcester trustees petitioned the legislature for authorization to erect a new physical plant and described the hospital as "one of the poorest, if not the very poorest, in the country" (Grob, 1973:369).

When informed of the substandard conditions at Worcester, the legislative Committee on Public Charitable Institutions decided that the problems growing out of mental illness were so complex that an

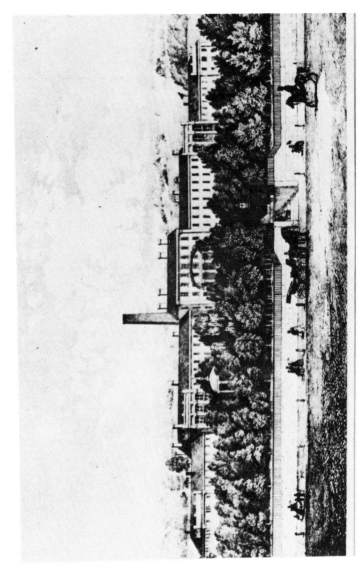

Fig. 4. State Lunatic Hospital at Worcester, 1857. By the mid-1850s, the Worcester hospital had acquired an increasingly chronic and static patient population. As its facilities and active treatment programs deteriorated, the hospital lost its position of national prominence. Source: Medical Library, Worcester State Hospital.

impartial and exhaustive analysis was required that would provide the basis for a more intelligent and enlightened policy. The result was the influential *Report on Insanity and Idiocy in Massachusetts* by Edward Jarvis (1854), which constituted the most important and comprehensive investigation of the problems of mental illness in 19th-century America. On the basis of a detailed enumeration of all known cases of insanity in the Commonwealth, Jarvis was able to demonstrate that the scope of the problem was much larger than had been realized and that, despite overcrowding at the Worcester hospital, it cared for only a minority of the insane. Moreover, he concluded that pauperism and insanity were intimately related, especially among immigrant groups. Although his findings contributed to a growing pessimism about the curability of insanity, Jarvis strenuously argued for the benefits of early therapeutic treatment to prevent chronicity and a long-term burden on the state. He also called for the creation of numerous small hospitals geographically dispersed throughout the state to increase patient access to the benefits of early hospitalization. The one concrete impact of Jarvis' proposals was the creation in 1858 of a third hospital at Northampton in the western part of the state. However, his report was to play a continuing role in public debates over the next two decades both in Massachusetts and in the rest of the country.

The person who guided the Worcester hospital during these difficult years was Merrick Bemis, who originally came to Worcester in 1848 as a temporary physician. Soon afterwards he became Superintendent Chandler's assistant. Bemis, like Chandler, lacked the leadership and missionary zeal that Woodward brought to Worcester in 1830. When he assumed the superintendency in 1856 at the age of 36, however, he inherited a vastly more complex set of problems than Woodward had faced. While sharing his predecessor's advocacy of moral treatment, Bemis faced the formidable task of adapting these principles to a new social reality. His inability to do so, largely because of social forces beyond the hospital's control, made the achievement of therapeutic goals impossible. In the process, the functions of the hospital became attuned to societal and professional concerns and its patients languished.

Bemis' early years as superintendent were devoted to the hospital's management and fiscal problems as much as to the care of its ever-growing patient population. By the 1860s, there was a critical need for additional beds and a continued demand for economizing because of minimal state funding and the reluctance of the towns to pay for the care of their indigent patients. In 1865, under the strain of these seemingly irreconcilable and intensifying problems, Bemis became so depressed that he could not perform his duties. He was granted a leave of absence and spent four months at the Pennsylvania Hospital for the Insane under the care of Thomas Kirkbride, one of the foremost psychiatrists in America. Upon returning to Worcester he began to push for the adoption of some fundamental changes at the hospital. Gradually, he came to accept the fact that the large hospital had become a permanent fixture in American psychiatry, but he was convinced that its basic flaw was the indiscriminant grouping of all patients under the same roof regardless of their social circumstances and stages of illness.

Over the next few years, Bemis utilized the Annual Reports of the Worcester hospital (widely distributed since the days of Woodward) as a forum for advancing his proposals. Still troubled by ill health, he was granted another leave of absence in the summer of 1868. He traveled extensively in Europe, visiting many of the mental hospitals in England and the continent. He was deeply impressed with the renowned colony for the insane in the Belgian town of Gheel where the cottage-type institution had reached its highest state of development. At Gheel, the insane were boarded in the homes of local townsfolk, where they worked alongside the cottagers in a familial atmosphere that permitted considerable personal freedom. Bemis returned to Worcester certain that the large state hospital was an inappropriate place for the insane.

With enthusiastic support from the trustees, he set out to secure legislative approval for a proposal to rebuild the Worcester facility along the lines of a decentralized cottage hospital, loosely modeled on the Gheel system. His plans called for a main building surrounded by a number of smaller houses. The main structure would be a two-story building with two attached but functionally self-contained wings. This building would be used to care for acutely ill patients (including the violent, suicidal, and troublesome) who would constitute no more than one-third of the total patient population. All others would live under the supervision of married couples (attendants) in small houses accommodating from 12 to 15 persons. Some of these cottages would house convalescent patients, others would be used for harmless and industrious incurable cases, and still others would be reserved for more difficult private patients able to afford individualized care. As patients improved, they would be moved to houses further and further away from the central hospital building so as to facilitate their reintegration into society. In his Annual Report for 1865, Bemis described his aspirations for the new hospital in the following terms:

One great benefit to accrue from all this is a near approach to the family system, and the kindly influences of home treatment. Could this system be adopted and carried into operation, the insane would have all the benefits they now have, with the added advantage of the family circle, to such as could be admitted to its privileges, homely surroundings, and the enjoyment of many of the social comforts which make life pleasant. They would have also the advantage of well trained nurses and attendants, whose business for life it would be to care for and sympathize with them. They would enjoy a more free and generous style of amusement and exercise, and more frequently, and with less restraint mingle in the society of friends and relatives—in a word, all the enjoyments of life would be multiplied, and all the social endearments, to a great extent, preserved, without diminishing in any degree the prospect of recovery, or increasing in any way the labors of the institution. (WSH, 1865:60–63).

By the end of 1869, Bemis' proposals had gained wide support. He had already received the strong backing of Samuel Gridley Howe (a former Trustee at Worcester) who was chairman of the Board of State Charities which oversaw the operation of the state asylums and welfare institutions in Massachusetts. The hospital trustees authorized him to take an option on a new site for the proposed hospital, and the Board of State Charities petitioned the legislature for permission to purchase land and build a new hospital. The governor, after a site visit in late 1869, had also offered his strong endorsement.

The petition for a new hospital was favorably acted upon by the legislature, and in May 1870, the governor signed into law a bill that authorized the Worcester trustees to acquire land and erect a hospital for 400 patients. This legislation also called for the sale of the land and physical plant of the original hospital with the proceeds paying most of the costs of the new facilities. Shortly thereafter, the trustees purchased a 300-acre estate in the eastern part of the city. The estate contained a number of homes and, rather than waiting for the completion of the new hospital, Bemis renovated four houses for immediate occupancy. In the spring of 1871, 36 female and 25 male patients were living in them and plans were underway to transfer small groups of patients to the other vacant homes.

For a moment, it seemed as though Bemis was about to usher in a new era. In some respects, his plans were to recreate a hospital where a modified form of moral treatment could be practiced. By segregating and subclassifying patients according to their social status (nativity and ability to pay) as well as their clinical condition (recent versus advanced cases), he firmly believed that the hospital's therapeutic functions could be restored to a position of paramount importance. Rather than being confined in a stifling custodial environment, patients would live and work in intimate familiar surroundings with a minimum of restraint. Furthermore, by providing a series of graduated placements for its patients, Bemis maintained that the very structure and layout of the new hospital would promote rehabilitation.

In other respects, however, Bemis' plans represented an unconscious adaptation to the class and ethnic prejudices of the larger society in which the hospital now operated. By this time, nearly half of the patients at Worcester were Irish immigrants and many of the others were native paupers. Under these conditions, the image of the hospital was rapidly becoming cast as an institution catering to undesirable elements. The fear that paying patients would go elsewhere for their care led to concerns among the trustees about the fiscal viability of the hospital. Moreover, private patients were seen as the group most amenable to moral treatment. Bemis hoped that by providing them with separate accommodations, the therapeutic functions of the hospital would be sustained.

Despite the initial support for Bemis' plans, opposition quickly developed from several sources. Proponents of governmental economy argued that the new hospital would be much more costly to build, operate, and maintain than a centralized or congregate institution. Others were fearful that the plan did not make adequate provisions to prevent patient escapes, and thus would compromise the hospital's community-protection functions. Vigorous criticisms from many of Bemis' professional colleagues also undermined the early support for his proposals.

Pliny Earle was Bemis' chief opponent within the American psychiatric community. By 1870, Earle had become one of the nation's leading psychiatrists (Bockoven, 1972:43–54). He was inspired to enter the field of psychiatry by Woodward and he had observed the latter's work at Worcester on numerous occassions. After spending several years in private practice, he held positions at the Friends' Asylum in Pennsylvania and the Bloomingdale Asylum in New York City—two of the foremost private mental hospitals in the country. As the first medical superintendent of the latter hospital, he was one of the founders of the Association of Medical

Superintendents of American Institutions for the Insane (AMSAII), the predecessor of the American Psychiatric Association. He had also traveled extensively in Europe and America and was intimate ly familiar with the major public and private asylums of the time, including the colony at Gheel. At the time of the controversy over Bemis' plans for the new Worcester hospital, Earle was super-intendent of the Northampton State Lunatic Hospital in Massachu-setts where he had established a reputation for efficient and economical management.

In 1871 and 1872 Earle used the Annual Reports of the North-amptom hospital to make known his opposition to Bemis. He indi-cated that the decentralized hospital had advantages as well as disadvantages. Smaller residences were more easily ventilated and permitted a wider separation of the different classes of patients. But Earle claimed that these modest gains would be offset by excessive costs and the need for more employees because of the greater dis-tances involved. Moreover, he noted that the plans departed from the standards of the profession. In 1851, the AMSAII had adopted Thomas Kirkbride's guidelines for centralized asylums of not more than 250 patients. This standard was also affirmed in Jarvis' in-fluential report. Based on the precepts of moral treatment, one of the major purposes of the centralized layout was to permit the su-perintendent to supervise directly all activities at the hospital. Earle's fear was that a decentralized layout would require much greater delegation of power and responsibility to nonmedical staff and that, in time, it would erode the authority of the superinten-dent. Earle also challenged Bemis' claims that the new system would diminish the use of restraints, and argued that more rather than less control was often essential for the proper management of an insane asylum. Furthermore, he emphasized that occupational activities for patients and many of the social amenities of the cot-tage plan could be incorporated into small, centralized institutions.

Earle's criticisms did much to rally the profession against Be-mis' proposals and the general idea of a decentralized hospital. Others joined the growing debate. In 1870, the Board of State Char-ities disavowed ever having advocated the introduction of a modi-fied Gheel system into Massachussetts. The following year the Board repudiated its approval of Bemis' plans and recommended instead that the Commonwealth maintain the existing closed asy-lum system while gradually boarding out harmless chronic pa-tients.

In the spring of 1872, while the debate was still unfolding, Bemis and the Worcester trustees became embroiled in an internal conflict. Charges were brought against Bemis that reflected upon his management of the hospital. During April and May the trustees held several meetings to hear witnesses and take testimony. In late April, Bemis' wife resigned as matron, a position which she had held since 1856. A few weeks later Bemis sent the trustees a brief letter of resignation. They accepted it and, within a few months, they had hired a new superintendent. Concurrent with Bemis' resignation, the trustees decided to abandon the proposed cottage hospital in favor of a more conventional one. Although the trustees' deliberations were never made public, the plans for the new hospital rather than charges of mismanagement appear to have been the key issue. Throughout Bemis' 16-year tenure, there had been no hint of scandal and the trustees had been unanimous in support of his administrative abilities.

The cottage hospital was a source of public and professional controversy throughout the country at this time, and the debate in Massachusetts was being watched closely. It was clear to all that the issues transcended the new hospital at Worcester. At stake was the redefinition of the purpose and organizational form of the public asylum. Given the Commonwealth of Massachusetts' recognized leadership role in these matters, the decision made at Worcester would set a precedent for the future direction of state policy across the country. The whole debate, however, took place within a pessimistic atmosphere, for both sides were agreed that a large proportion of the insane were incurable and therefore ought to be separated from curable cases. Many of those who supported the cottage hospital did so because it was well suited to differential treatment of the insane. Defenders of the centralized congregate-care hospital, in turn, suggested that separate facilities for the curable and the incurable insane could accomplish the same ends at less cost. The Willard Asylum For The Chronic Insane in New York, established in 1865 for 1500 patients, offered the first example of a congregate hospital devoted exclusively to incurable cases.

The defeat of the cottage plan in 1872 had important implications for the care and treatment of the insane in Massachusetts. The continued existence of the large congregate custodial hospital was assured and the precedent was established that it would be replicated as the need arose. Ironically, a century later, in the aftermath of the state hospital deinstitutionalization movement, the Gheel system would again be advocated as a "natural therapeutic community" capable of caring for chronic mental patients in a noninstitutional environment (Srole, 1977).

## THE ERA OF PESSIMISM

By the 1870s the functions of state mental hospitals in Massachusetts and the nation as a whole had been clearly delineated. Their central purpose was defined in terms of custodial care and community protection; treatment was of secondary importance. This institutional transformation was reinforced by the growing pessimism and therapeutic nihilism that began to envelop psychiatric theory and practice. Since its early days, American psychiatry held to an eclectic model viewing insanity as both psychological and somatic in origin. Therapy, to a large extent, was pragmatic and its efficacy was judged by the results obtained. After 1850, when the changing character of state asylums lessened the success of moral or psychological treatment, most psychiatrists reverted to an outright and explicit somaticism. The rise of scientific medicine also provided a strong impetus for viewing insanity as a specific disease entity. These influences led to a diminution of interest in the psychological aspects of insanity and a widespread belief in its incurability. The posture of most practitioners was that until identifiable lesions could be correlated with abnormal behavior, no therapy—physical or otherwise—would be possible.

This prevailing ethos had a profound effect on developments at Worcester. When the trustees reversed their approval of Bemis' plans for a decentralized cottage hospital, they broke with tradition by not seeking his replacement from within the existing staff. Instead they selected Barnard Douglas Eastman as the new medical superintendent. Eastman had served as an assistant physician at the New Hampshire Asylum for the Insane and then spent several years at the Government Hospital for the Insane in Washington, D.C. before coming to Worcester. With Eastman's approval, the trustees authorized the construction of a conventional centralized hospital and increased its planned capacity from 400 to 500 patients. The new facility conformed to the architectural layout prescribed in Thomas Kirkbride's influential treatise, On the Construction, Organization, and General Arrangements of Hospitals for the Insane (1854). Completed in 1877, the new hospital consisted of a four-story central administration building with 500-foot-long wings on either side. Each wing was divided into separate and distinct wards having dining and dressing rooms, a bath, a lavatory, and an exercise corridor. Suites of rooms were also available for well-to-do patients. Directly to the rear was a second building containing a chapel and matron's quarters and beyond that was the kitchen building. To the north and east of these buildings was 150 acres of farm land. All windows in the ward areas were heavily barred, giving the overall appearance of a large jail. These arrangements conformed not only to the prevailing psychiatric ideology but also to the overall objectives of society which increasingly were stated in protective terms.

When the new facility opened, its caseload consisted of 325 patients. Only 100 were from the original hospital; the others were transfers from the state hospitals at Taunton and Northhampton. Contrary to its earlier plans, the Board of State Charities authorized the continued use of the original hospital while changing its name (and purpose) to the Temporary Asylum for the Chronic Insane. It soon became a permanent part of the burgeoning state system, and in the 1890s it was administratively merged with the new Worcester hospital.

Despite new quarters, all the old and familiar problems of the Worcester hospital—overcrowding, lack of occupational facilities for patients, turnover among the nonprofessional staff—continued unabated. In 1877 the average census was 496; by 1890 it was 811. The burden on the superintendent was partially relieved by the expansion of medical staff; during the 1880s the number of assistant physicians increased from 3 to 5–6. For most patients, however, hospitalization continued to be dreary and monotonous. There was little emphasis on moral treatment, drugs to quiet violent patients were used regularly, and restraint and seclusion were common. In these respects, the Worcester hospital mirrored the conditions at most state hospitals throughout the country.

In the 1870s the Board of State Charities attempted to centralize control over the individual institutions. Since insanity was believed incurable, attention could be focused on a uniform and cost-efficient system of custodial care. The Board's efforts to achieve greater standardization of policies and operating procedures were strongly resisted by the medical superintendents, who fully realized that such proposals, if enacted, would undermine their authority and power. Ultimately, the issue was resolved in favor of centralized state control, but this would not occur fully in Massachusetts until the early 1900s.

The 1870s were also a period of considerable friction between the superintendents and trustees at Worcester. The split between Bemis and the trustees that led to his resignation in the spring of 1872 promoted internal dissensions that continued unabated during Eastman's tenure. In February 1879 events reached a crisis stage, and Eastman resigned. [He subsequently became superinten-

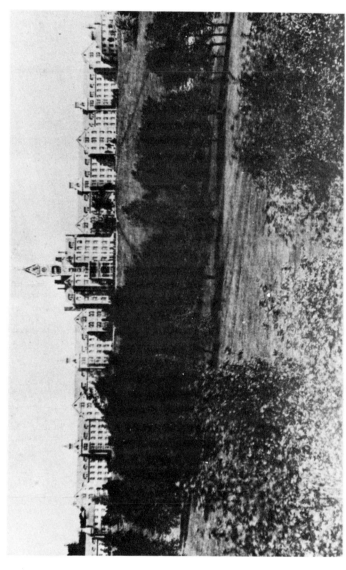

Fig. 5. State Lunatic Hospital at Worcester, 1892. The monolithic and prison-like architecture of the new Worcester hospital completed in 1877 reflected the growing therapeutic nihilism that engulfed American psychiatry in the late 19th century. *Source: Medical Library, Worcester State Hospital.*

dent at the Topeka (Kansas) state hospital]. As his replacement, the trustees selected John G. Park, who had served as Eastman's assistant superintendent for five years. At the time of his appointment, Park was director of the Worcester Asylum for the Chronic Insane. During Park's tenure (which lasted until 1890), internal dissension subsided. The new superintendent, an efficient administrator, continued to oversee a custodially oriented institution within the framework of prevailing state policies.

The most noteworthy event in Park's superintendency was the completion of a series of statistical studies which were used to explode the older belief in the curability of insanity (Bockover, 1956, 1972; Grob, 1966). The number of recoveries reflected in the annual statistics of the Worcester hospital had been falling steadily since the 1840s. During the Woodward era over 51 percent of those discharged were listed as recovered; under Chandler the figure was 45 percent, under Bemis it was 40 percent, and under Eastman and Park it had dropped sharply to about 24 percent. In 1872, Pliny Earle had persuaded Eastman to undertake a detailed analysis of all cases treated at Worcester since its opening in 1833 in order to reassess the early rates of recovery. The study was completed by Park in 1879. The results revealed that while the Annual Reports of the Worcester hospital purported to show 11,000 *cases* over this 46-year period, only 8,204 *persons* had actually been admitted. Thus 2,796 readmissions had been counted as new cases. Of those admitted for the first time only 3,191 (39 percent) had been discharged as recovered; of the readmissions, the recovered figure was 1,191 (43 percent). In the Annual Report of the Worcester hospital for 1879, Park argued that the most important inference to be derived from these data was that recovery rates in earlier years were fallacious in that they conveyed the idea of a permanent restoration to health:

It is a sad and almost cruel blow to the worth of the earlier tables of this Hospital, which gave 70, 80, and even 90 per cent of recoveries, to know that deaths occurring within a few days of admission were not taken into account at all, but stricken entirely from the reports; that many a patient who helped to swell the tables of recoveries to the large per cent mentioned, returned again and again to this Hospital, and finally died here; that many more, after repeated admissions to this and other hospitals, died in the town or city almshouse, having been, to take the cold, utilitarian view which is the fashion of this world, "a burden on their own property, on that of their friends, or upon the public treasury," from the time of their first admission to the Hospital to their death. (WSH, 1879:14–15).

In 1881, in an effort to secure further data, Park began one of the most detailed follow-up studies in the annals of American psychiatry. He set out to discover what actually happened to a large group of patients discharged from Worcester as recovered on their only admission or on their last admission.[4] His starting assumption was that if he could demonstrate that a substantial proportion of those who were listed as recovered actually had relapses at a later date, it would disprove the claim that insanity, like other diseases, was amenable to therapy in most instances. To obtain the necessary information, he sent questionnaires to relatives, "overseers of the poor of the different towns," physicians, and others presumed to be knowledgeable about former patients (Bockoven, 1972:60).

Although the study was not completed until 1893, Park reported interim findings in the Annual Reports of the Worcester Hospital beginning in 1881. His first report was based on 94 (45 percent) of 211 inquiries concerning patients discharged prior to 1840 during Woodward's superintendency. To Park's satisfaction, the results indicated that 46 patients (49 percent) relapsed, while 48 (51 percent) remained well. He noted that

> . . . there can be no doubt that the public have been hitherto widely misled as to the meaning of "recovery," as used in the hospital reports, and as to the permanency of cures from insanity. Not a small number of patients who were discharged as recovered in the earlier reports of this hospital have many times since became a burden to the public or private purse by reason of a return of the malady" (WSH,1881:12–13).

By the following year, 798 (68 percent) of the 1,171 inqi res sent out had been returned. Satisfactory information was avail le for 669 of the patients. Of this number, 319 patients (48 percent) had relapsed, while 350 (52 percent) had remained well. In the Annual Report of 1883, Park noted:

> Information as to the subsequent history of persons who have been discharged from this hospital . . . confirms the results shown . . . last year . . . About 50 percent suffered no relapse, but as no answers were received to one-third of the circulars sent, and taking into account the liability of relapse of those now reported well, I am inclined to believe that this percentage should be reduced one-half. (WSH, 1883:20).

These figures were interpreted by Park and his contemporaries as providing strong evidence that Woodward and his generation had falsified curability figures, and that insanity was much more incurable than had been supposed. Pliny Earle, for example, reviewed the work of Eastman and Park in his widely read volume, *The Curability of Insanity* (1887), and drew similar conclusions.

Ironically, at the time it was conducted, the most striking finding in Park's study never received the attention it deserved. When the study was completed in 1893, *the results showed that 58 percent of the patients never had a relapse following discharge* from the Worcester hospital.[5] Thus, in contrast to Park's interpretation, the study offered impressive evidence that the majority of these patients did recover from their illness, and that the overall recovery rate was substantially the same as Woodward and his generation had claimed. However, these data remained buried in the Annual Reports of the hospital for 60 years until they were discovered and reanalyzed by Bockoven (1956). Subsequently, the Joint Commission on Mental Health and Illness (1961:24, 32–33) would view these findings as evidence that mental patients " . . . can be helped to lead useful, satisfying lives if treated in a humane and rational manner" and as support for its recommendations on community-based mental health services.

In the 1870s and 1880s, however, the mind-set of the psychiatric profession was so wedded to the incurability thesis that contrary evidence was largely ignored (Bockoven, 1972: 61–68). The biased reporting of the Worcester studies did much to reinforce and justify the custodial orientation of state policy in Massachusetts and elsewhere. In so doing, these reports helped to condone the therapeutic pessimism that predominated during the late 19th century.

## THE PROMISE OF INSTITUTIONAL REFORM

Despite the seemingly irreversible course that state policies and institutional programs had followed, the voices calling for institutional reform had not been completely silenced. In the early 1870s, American psychiatrists had come under attack from their British counterparts for the deteriorating conditions in state asylums, the overreliance on physical restraint to maintain order, and the general stagnation of the profession. These criticisms were met by denial and counter charges from the medical superintendents. Gradually, however, these essentially intraprofessional disputes were transformed into a progressive social reform movement with a broad base outside of psychiatry. Neurologists, social workers, and lay reformers began to publicize some of the shortcomings that characterized American psychiatry in an effort to break the stranglehold of medical superintendents over the care of the insane.

By 1875, members of the rising speciality of neurology had formed their own society and begun to challenge the exclusive authority of medical superintendents to speak on matters of mental illness. In 1879, William Hammond offered a direct attack on asylums and their medical officers in an address before the Medical Society of New York:

> It is the commonly received opinion among physicians and the public generally that as soon as possible after an individual becomes insane, he or she must be placed under the restraint of a lunatic asylum. No matter what the type of mental aberration, no matter what the facilities for receiving care and attention at home, the asylum is regarded as the necessary destination of the one so unfortunate as to be deprived wholly, or in part, of the light of reason. For this state of affairs the medical officers of insane asylums are mainly responsible, for they have very diligently inculcated the idea that they alone by education, by experience and by general aptitude, are qualified to take the medical superintendence of the unfortunate class of patients in question, and that restraint and separation from friends and acquaintances are measures in themselves which are specially curative in their influence (Hammond, 1879).

The most blistering and far-reaching criticism of state asylums was offered by S. Weir Mitchell, a renowned neurologist, before the 1894 convention of the American Medico-Psychological Association (formerly, the Association of Medical Superintendents of American Institutions for the Insane). In no uncertain terms, Mitchell accused his audience of complacency and lectured them about their shortcomings—a lack of interest in research, haphazard management practices, unwillingness to train and employ qualified medical personnel, and their isolation from the rapidly developing field of scientific medicine.

> You look back with just pride as alienists on the merciful changes made for the better in the management of the chronic insane. It is to be feared that you also have cause to recall the fact that as compared with the splendid advance in surgery, in the medicine of the eye and the steady approach to precision all along our ardent line, the alienist has won in proportion little . . . It is easy to see how this came about. You soon began to live apart, and you still do so. Your hospitals are not our hospitals; your ways are not our ways. You live out of range of critical shot; you are not preceded and followed in your ward work by clever rivals, or watched by able residents fresh with the learning of the school (Mitchell, 1894: 101).

Mitchell went on to acknowledge that some of the problems facing the superintendents arose from circumstances beyond their control, but he stressed that, as a group, they had to bear a large measure of responsibility for the existing state of affairs.

Although there was little consensus on specific ameliorative programs, the emergent reform outlook of the 1890s was characterized by a renewed optimism and the belief that the individual could be changed by altering his social environment. Many reformers combined traditional religious values with the ardent belief that scientific inquiry would solve many of the complex social and technological problems confronting American society at the turn of the century (Hofstadter, 1955). Psychiatry itself was not wholly immune from these developments. A few alienists began to reexamine some of the traditional assumptions of the profession and the relative failure of somaticism rekindled an interest in the psychological. The Worcester hospital once again was to be involved in these currents of change.

Park resigned in 1890. Following tradition, the trustees filled the vacancy from within by choosing Hosea M. Quinby as the Worcester hospital's sixth medical superintendent. At the time of his appointment, Quinby had worked at Worcester for nearly 20 years. He had joined the staff as an assistant physician in the early 1870s after graduating from the Harvard Medical School, and when Park succeeded Eastman as superintendent in 1879, Quinby took over responsibilities for the Worcester Asylum for the Chronic Insane. Quinby assumed his new office without controversy and the hospital continued to function as it had for the past decade.

In 1894, in the wake of Mitchell's criticism of mental hospitals, the State Board of Lunacy and Charity (the successor to the Board of State Charities) offered a number of proposals for improving the staffing and professional orientation of state hospitals in Massachusetts. These included the development of more precise medical records, the creation of medical societies to disseminate advances in scientific and therapeutic knowledge within the institutions, and the organization of nurse training schools at all state hospitals. The recommendation that was to have the greatest impact in the next few decades, however, was the appointment of a state pathologist to conduct scientific research on a full-time basis. The Board saw clearly that medical superintendents had already acquired a multiplicity of competing roles—they were held accountable as farmers, stewards, caterers, treasurers, business managers, and physicians. They could not be expected to be scientists as well. If institutional psychiatry was to develop a research base, a well-trained specialist who could devote full time to this work was needed.

Shortly after these recommendations were publicized, Quinby persuaded the Board and his own trustees that Worcester was the most favorable site of operation for the new pathologist. To fill the position, he sought the advice of Edward Cowles, superintendent of McLean Hospital, one of the few centers of psychiatric research in the country at that time. Cowles recommended a young Swiss neurologist by the name of Adolf Meyer, who had come to the United States in 1892. Quinby and Meyer entered negotiations that were rapidly and successfully completed. Although few realized it at the time, Meyer was destined to become one of the most influential American psychiatrists of the first half of the 20th century. His tenure at Worcester, although brief, was to leave an enduring mark on the internal structure and operations of the hospital.

Meyer had superb credentials for his new position at Worcester. He had been trained in medicine and neurology in Zurich and, after immigrating to the United States at the age of 21, he served for three years as pathologist at the Illinois Eastern Hospital for the Insane at Kankakee. During this period, he was actively involved with the scientific community at the University of Chicago, where he taught a course on the comparative anatomy of the nervous system. One of the factors that attracted him to Worcester was the opportunity to become affiliated with Clark University, a new graduate center headed by G. Stanley Hall (one of the leading psychologists in America) that was becoming world renowned for its work in psychology and biology.

Upon arriving at the Worcester hospital in 1896, Meyer began to initiate a series of far-reaching reforms. His goal was the transformation of the hospital into an institution modeled on the few great clinical and research hospitals then in existence. Underlying his reforms was a multidimensional psychobiological conception of mental illness that rejected a purely somatic or a purely psychological approach to psychiatric phenomena (Meyer, 1896). Mental disease in Meyer's view was both a physiological and a psychological disorder, and, although evidence to support his position was incomplete, he insisted that psychiatry's most basic need was to collect empirical data that would serve as the raw material for a deeper analysis of these interconnections. Such research, however, had to be integrated into the administrative and clinical structure of the hospital; it could not exist apart from patients and staff. The fundamental task that he faced at Worcester was to reorient the staff and

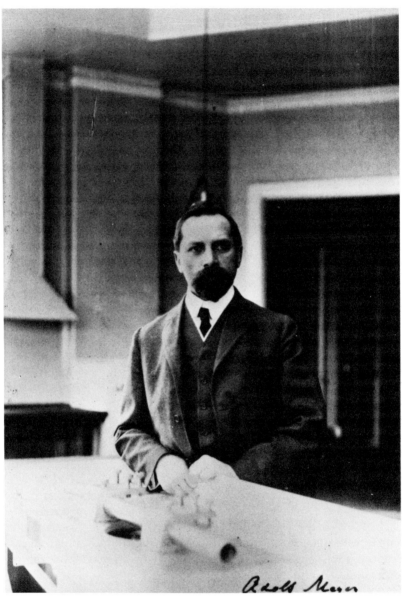

Fig. 6. Adolf Meyer. As Director of Clinics and Pathologist from 1896 to 1902, Meyer was responsible for transforming the Worcester hospital into one of the nation's foremost centers of scientific research and training in psychiatry. *Source:* Institute of the History of Medicine, Johns Hopkins University.

organizational structure of the hospital so that this clinical research agenda could be fruitfully pursued.

Quinby was quite receptive to Meyer's plans and he began to provide the resources that the young pathologist deemed necessary for his work. Space was made available for laboratories, a reference library, and clinical examination rooms. In addition, funds were provided to recruit four assistants. From this base, Meyer proceeded to introduce a number of radical changes in hospital routines. He completely revamped the format and content of the medical record system which had remained largely unaltered since Woodward's era; initiated the first use of Kraepelin's psychiatric nosology in an American mental hospital; changed the method of ward assignment so that all recent cases would be located on the first two floors of the hospital where they could be observed more closely; and reorganized staff responsibilities to promote the integration of clinical and research work.

Meyer's official position was Director of Clinics and Pathologist, but he persuaded Quinby to give him authority over all medical concerns. Although the superintendent remained legally responsible for both administrative and medical matters, Quinby thereafter confined his activities to administration. While this arrangement allowed Meyer to institute the changes in hospital organization and procedures that he desired, it had an unanticipated consequence. The separation of duties soon led to a compartmentalized social structure within the hospital. Removed from direct patient contact, the superintendent became concerned exclusively with the goals of economic and efficient management; practicing psychiatrists, in contrast, judged hospital performance in relation to therapeutic ideals. In time, these divergent orientations would undermine Meyer's program at Worcester.

During his first year at Worcester, Meyer developed a close relationship with Hall and the psychology and biology faculties at Clark. Meyer was appointed a Docent and he offered a series of clinics at the hospital for Hall's students on neurological and psychiatric problems. The success of this initial program led to a regular series of course offerings during the period 1897–1902. Meyer also initiated a formal psychiatric training program at the hospital so that young physicians could study under experienced physicians and be exposed to research. Exacting standards of recruitment and training of assistant physicians and interns led to a sharp rise in the caliber of the hospital's professional staff.

In addition to his teaching and clinical duties, Meyer published more than a dozen research articles on special neurological

and anatomical topics during his Worcester years along with several major theoretical and programmatic statements advancing his
psychobiological conception of psychiatry (Meyer, 1912). His assistant physicians also undertook original studies on the biological
and chemical aspects of mental illness which resulted in a large
number of additional publications. In a very short time, the work of
Meyer and his students gave the Worcester hospital a national reputation as a major teaching and research center.[6]

Although Meyer, with the help of his colleagues, made a significant start toward creating his concept of an ideal hospital, he
soon encountered obstacles that proved difficult to overcome. The
size of the hospital was not conducive to the intensive type of
work that he had in mind. In 1896 (his first year at Worcester), the
average census at the hospital was 956; by 1901 it had risen to
1,088. By 1899, most of the time and energy of the staff were going
into clinical work, and important components of the research program were deliberately being neglected because of the amount of
routine work. The staff had grown under Meyer's direction and
Quinby was unwilling to pressure state authorities for the additional staff positions that Meyer sought.

By 1900, Meyer began to recognize that clinical research opportunities for the future were being restricted by the institutional
framework within which he had to work. Meyer and Quinby also
began to develop irreconcilable differences about the role of research at the hospital. When Meyer first arrived at Worcester,
Quinby wanted him to concentrate his attention on "the more interesting and acute cases." Meyer succeeded in persuading Quinby of
the fallacy of this position, arguing that all cases had to be studied
equally well if a research base for psychiatric practice was to be established. Subsequently, their relations were quite harmonious.
However, Quinby never fully understood or accepted Meyer's insistence on an integrated clinical research program. As the volume of
research work began to exceed the available laboratory facilities, for
example, Quinby wanted to erect a separate laboratory building removed from the main hospital and central offices. As long as he remained at Worcester, Meyer managed to block these plans. He
realized that they would diminish his contacts with patients and
that separation of clinical and laboratory work would defeat the
very ends he was seeking.

Meyer also became dissatisfied with his Clark ties. Although he
got along well with Hall, his relationships with the University had
never gone beyond the offering of courses and clinics. Moreover, although his psychobiological teachings sought to identify the com-

mon ground between psychology and psychiatry, the two still remained distinct and specialized disciplines separated by a different approach and philosophy. The prospects for drawing a psychol ogist into the research orbit of the hospital were dim, and Meyer's visions of multidisciplinary collaboration had not been realized.

When the opportunity arose in 1901 to continue his work in a more favorable setting, Meyer was quick to seize it. He accepted the position of director of the Pathological Institute in New York City which had been created by the State Commission on Lunacy in 1895. Meyer was to achieve much greater fame, first at the Pathological Institute and then at the Henry Phipps Psychiatric Clinic at the Johns Hopkins University in Baltimore. However, he looked favorably on his years at Worcester and the base that they had provided for his subsequent accomplishments. Twenty years later, Meyer (1921:80) wrote

> As I look back over my psychiatric career I cannot help considering my Worcester period as one of the soundest, and in a way the most solidly useful phase of my work—since I see in it the period during which I collected the most lastingly valuable and most substantial material for work.

Meyer's experiences at Worcester contributed significantly not only to his own professional growth and development (as well as to that of a new generation of psychiatric researchers), but also to the radical reorientation of the hospital. Routines had been sharply altered, case histories had taken on a new look and a new meaning, high standards had been established for the staff, research had been partially integrated with clinical work, and a spirit of optimistic inquiry had replaced the pessimistic outlook which had enveloped the hospital for decades. Although the neurological and chemical research of Meyer and his students had few immediate effects on patient care and therapy, Meyer's innovations had shattered the complacent outlook that marked insitutional psychiatry in the United States. When Meyer left Worcester the concept of what a mental hospital was and what it ought to do had been completely altered. He had reintroduced in somewhat different form an attitude of hope reminiscent of his early 19th-century predecessors.

Unfortunately, after Meyer's departure the Worcester hospital reverted to a number of older patterns. No one of comparable stature replaced him and the institutional barriers that impeded Meyer's work became even more pronounced and unyielding. The lack of forceful and positive leadership from Quinby and Ernest Scribner (who succeeded to the superintendency in 1912) allowed the destiny of the hospital to be shaped by external forces and events. Both men were concerned primarily with efficient management and the expansion of the physical plant to keep pace with the rising volume of admissions. Many of the structural reforms Meyer had introduced were retained, but without appreciation of their inner purpose. Shortly after Meyer left, for example, Quinby proceeded to erect a new laboratory building that resulted in the relative isolation of research work from patient care.

During the next two decades, the twin forces of governmental economies and psychiatric professionalism led to the centralization of control for the entire complex of mental hospitals under state government. In 1898, a new State Board of Insanity was created which separated the problem of insanity from the larger social welfare context in which it had been addressed since the 1850s. At least two of its five members were to be "experts in insanity"; its chief executive officer was also to be a physician who was expert in the field. When directed by the governor, its members could exercise the powers held by individual boards of trustees. All plans for new buildings had to meet its approval, and it was also invested with broad investigatory and visitation powers. In effect, the creation of the Board of Insanity had formalized the definition of insanity as a distinct social problem, solidified the claims of psychiatry for exclusive jurisdiction over the insane, and centralized control over all state mental institutions.

The Board's influence grew considerably in 1904 when the legislature passed the State Care Act which established a "state monopoly" in the public care of the mentally ill (Marden, 1968:348). Chapter 123, Section 2 of the Massachusetts General Laws was amended so that

> The Commonwealth shall have the care, control and treatment of all mentally ill, epileptic and mentally deficient persons, . . . the care of whom is vested in it by law. No county, city or town shall establish or maintain any institution for the care, control and treatment of mentally ill, epileptic or mentally deficient persons or be liable for the board, care, treatment or act of any inmate thereof.

The new legislation invested the Board of Insanity with executive powers to carry out the state's exclusive responsibility for the treatment of the mentally ill in Massachusetts.

In 1914, the Board was superseded by the Commission on Mental Diseases, which adopted policies that further eroded the autonomy of the superintendents and restricted hospital trustees to an advisory capacity. Finally, following the constitutional convention of 1919, the Department of Mental Diseases was created as part of the executive branch of state government with fiscal as well as policy control over the 13 state mental hospitals and 2 institutions for feebleminded children in Massachusetts.

In the course of these administrative changes, the state hospitals began to respond to other ideological and socioenvironmental developments. In 1907 Clifford Beers, a former mental patient, wrote of his experiences in his widely read volume, *A Mind That Found Itself*. Beers became the symbol of the progressive reform movement much as Dorothea Dix had been in an earlier era. In 1909, the movement took on a definite programmatic character when Beers founded the National Committee for Mental Hygiene with the help of Harvard professor William James and Adolf Meyer (then at the Phipps Psychiatric Clinic). The Committee's interest in psychological factors and prevention was reinforced by European developments in psychotherapy which were gradually becoming accepted in the United States. This interest was heightened in 1909 when Sigmund Freud (along with Carl Jung and Sandor Ferenczi) visited Worcester at Hall's invitation on the occasion of Clark University's 20th anniversary. At Clark, Freud delivered a series of lectures on psychoanalysis (Freud, 1957) before many of the leading psychologists, educators, and behavioral scientists in America. This was Freud's first recognition by an academic institution and his only appearance at an American university. His visit, and Hall's backing, did much to popularize his theories in this country.

These forces soon would move psychiatry away from the stranglehold of the medical superintendents and a focal concern with the mental hospital. Increasing emphasis was to be placed on clinical practice based in university medical centers, general hospitals, child guidance clinics, and private medical offices. Proposals to reform the structure and functions of the state hospitals and bring them into line with these new developments continued to be advanced. Meyer, for example, called for integrating the operations of mental hospitals into a network of community-based medical and welfare services to serve the population in their immediate geographical areas (c.f. Caplan, 1969:306–309).

These currents of change led to the creation of a new type of mental hospital in several states. In Massachusetts, the Boston Psychopathic Hospital was opened in 1912 to serve as a small observation or receiving institution for the screening of early cases of mental illness, research, and training. Under the direction of Elmer Ernest Southard, it soon became one of the leading mental hospitals in the United States. However, Southard's work continued to emphasize a somatic approach to mental illness and the ongoing research had little impact on patient care or treatment.

While the Worcester hospital remained largely custodial in na-

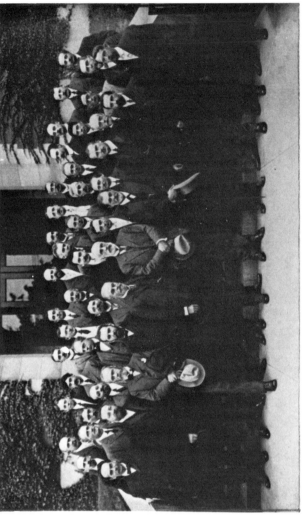

Fig. 7. Clark University 20th Anniversary Convocation Group, 1909. *Beginning with first row, left to right:* Franz Boas, E.B. Titchener, William James, William Stern, Leo Burgerstein, G. Stanley Hall, Sigmund Freud, Carl G. Jung, Adolf Meyer, H.S. Jennings *Second row:* C.F. Seashore, Joseph Jastrow, J. McK. Cattell, F.F. Buchner, F. Katzenellenbogen, Ernest Jones, A.A. Brill, Wm. H. Burnham, A.F. Chamberlain *Third row:* Albert Schinz, J.A. Magni, B.T. Baldwin, F. Lyman Wells, G.M. Forbes, E.A. Kirkpatrick, Sandor Ferenczi, F.C. Sanford, J.P. Porter, Sakyo Kanda, Hikoso Kakise. *Fourth row:* G.E. Dawson, S.P. Hayes, E.B. Holt, C.S. Berry, G.M. Whipple, Frank Drew, J.W.A. Young, I.N. Wilson, K.J. Karlson, H.H. Goddard, H.J. Klopp, Solomon Carter Fuller. *Source:* Medical Library, Worcester State Hospital.

ture, it was unable to remain immune to or isolated from some of the social forces that were creating pressure for improving the care and treatment of the mentally ill. Upon succeeding to the superintendency in 1912, Ernest Scribner made a determined effort to alter the image and practices at the hospital. He succeeded in reducing the use of mechanical restraints and increasing patient activity programs. Two occupational instructors were added to the staff in 1913 and the position of director of industrial therapeutics was created in 1915. By the following year, the Worcester hospital had the highest percentage (over 91 percent) of patients engaged in industrial work of all state institutions. He also began to implement liberal discharge and visiting policies that coincided with the Board of Insanity's mandate for each institution to develop outpatient clinics to provide aftercare, family care, and mental hygiene services in the local community. The growth of these services led to development of a social service department within the hospital and the recruitment of trained social workers.

Although the Worcester hospital's functions expanded greatly during these years, it was in an ad hoc manner largely as a response to external pressures rather than to an inner sense of purpose. By this time, the hospital had become a part of a large bureaucratic structure and its superintendents had settled into the pattern of adapting to the goals and needs of the system in a passive or reactive manner. The varied functions that the hospital was called upon to perform had given it an ambiguous organizational character; these included societal protection, custodial and therapeutic care of 2000 patients, the training of personnel, research on mental illness, and community-oriented prevention services. To a large extent, as the hospital entered the 1920s, these functions remained highly compartmentalized and antagonistic and the institutional leadership necessary for their integration was lacking.

## ADMINISTRATIVE CONSOLIDATION AND
## THERAPEUTIC REJUVENATION

When Scribner died in 1918, the medical superintendency of Worcester State Hospital (as it was then known) remained vacant for nearly three years. The delay in filling the position was symptomatic of the impotent role of the trustees under the new Department of Mental Diseases and the reluctance of Commissioner George M. Kline (a psychiatrist who trained at Worcester under Meyer) to fill the position from within the hospital. In order to consolidate the Department's newly acquired control over the individual state institutions and to bring a fresh outlook to the hospital, Kline wanted the next superintendent to be an outsider with broad experience in other institutional settings. The man finally selected to serve as the hospital's eighth medical superintendent was William A. Bryan.

Bryan was the prototype superintendent that Kline was seeking to develop. A graduate of the George Washington University Medical School, he completed a medical internship at the U.S. Public Health Service Hospital in Chelsea (Massachusetts) in 1909, and then served for six years as an assistant physician at the Clarinda and Cherokee (Iowa) State Hospitals. After a year as a senior assistant physician under Southard at the Boston Psychopathic Hospital, he became assistant superintendent at the Danvers (Massachusetts) State Hospital until he was recruited by Kline to serve as assistant commissioner of the new Department of Mental Diseases. After ten months in that position, he was appointed to the superintendency at Worcester.

Shortly after his arrival in Worcester, the trustees offered a prophetic assessment of their new superintendent in their Annual Report (1921:2).

> His keen mentality, united with his love for humanity, his common sense backed by willingness to work, his vision and command of others are qualities which will make the Worcester State Hospital most progressive.

Indeed, during his tenure at Worcester (which lasted until 1940), Bryan was to become the foremost superintendent in the United States and to return Worcester State Hospital to the position of national prominence it held a century earlier.

Bryan brought to the position of the superintendent a point of view and a management style that had been lacking in his predecessors. In his view, the administration of the hospital was itself a major therapeutic instrument when carried out according to the precepts of participatory democracy. His book *Administrative Psychiatry* (Bryan, 1936), the first volume devoted to mental hospital management in the United States, codified many of his innovative principles and practices. In the conclusion to a chapter on staff development, Bryan (1936:71) summarized his point of view in the following words:

> Active leadership is essential in the administration of psychiatric hospitals. Such leadership will demand much from a staff. It will set up an atmosphere of intellectual freedom where each individual may think as he likes but will be tolerant of the opinion of others. The goal of the mental

hospital must be psychiatric rather than economic if the institution is to be a real, living, breathing hospital. Every administrative process must be made subservient to that end. The autocratic executive will eventually be superseded by the creative leader. Partnership of executive and personnel is one of the aims of mental hospital management. The administrator achieves this by group planning rather than by authority flowing from the top. Committees and group conferences are important factors in attaining this result. They weld groups and departments into a harmonious whole.

In 1921, Bryan began to reorganize the hospital in keeping with his philosophy that it was an institution whose inner social structure and environment were related to the efficacy of its therapeutic functions. At the time of his appointment, the hospital had an average daily resident census of nearly 2000 patients with another 300 patients on "visit" status in the community. Of the resident patients, approximately 1500 were located at the "Main Hospital" campus constructed in 1877 on the eastern edge of the city and another 500 chronic patients were housed a few miles away at the "Summer Street Division" on the site of the original hospital in downtown Worcester.

One of Bryan's first innovations was the creation of a consultant staff of internists from general hospitals in the Worcester area to oversee the medical and surgical service at the hospital. This soon led to a major reorganization of the medical service with the consultant staff assuming complete responsibility for physical and surgical care of the patients so that the staff psychiatrists could devote themselves full time to psychiatric care.

Bryan also began to develop a number of community outreach clinics during these early years. The original outpatient clinic, established by Scribner at the Summer Street Division of the hospital, had never gained much community acceptance due to its location at a facility long recognized as "a place for the incurable insane." In 1923, Bryan closed this unit and replaced it with three new clinics: a Mental Hygiene Clinic for children in the Outpatient Dispensary at the Memorial Hospital, a clinic for unwed mothers located at the Girls Welfare Society Home, and a Habit Clinic for children at the Temporary Home and Day Nursery operated by a private charitable agency. Each of the clinics was conducted by hospital staff on a one-afternoon-per-week basis with clients referred by social workers from local charitable and welfare agencies.

In 1925, a new adult outpatient clinic was established at the Worcester City Hospital and the Mental Hygiene Clinic at the Memorial Hospital was reorganized into one of the first Child Guidance Clinics in the country.[7] In addition, the hospital began to

develop traveling teams for the diagnosis and evaluation of mentally retarded children in the schools of the 59 towns located in its
service region. By 1928, these clinics were recording in excess of
1250 visits and consultations per year (WSH Annual Report, 1928).

In the mid-1920s, Bryan also began to upgrade and expand the
teaching functions of the hospital. When he became superintendent
in 1921, the hospital typically had one or two medical and surgical
interns for a 12-month period. Bryan expanded and formalized this
training function to 8–10 positions and he began to attract students
from leading medical schools. In 1923, a school for training occupational therapists was started which was subsequently merged with
the Boston School for Occupational Therapy. An affiliation with
the Smith College School of Social Work also led to a 9-month
practicum for social work students at the hospital. In addition, Bryan expanded the inservice nurse training program and arranged for
undergraduate nurses from five local general hospitals to spend 3-
month rotations at the hospital for special training in psychiatric
nursing care.

With the appointment of Rev. Anton Boisen as Protestant
Chaplain in 1924 (one of the first such appointments at a state hospital in the United States), the Worcester hospital embarked on an
unprecedented experiment in paraprofessional training. Boisen,
after serving several years in the ministry, was hospitalized for 15
months with an acute schizophrenic condition at the Boston Psychopathic and Westboro (Massachusetts) State Hospitals (Boisen,
1960). During his recovery, he began to take courses in psychology
at Harvard and the Boston Psychopathic Hospital where he developed a keen interest in the relationship of religious experience to
mental illness. At Worcester, Boisen developed the first clinical
pastoral training program in the United States. In 1925, four theological students employed as attendants were enrolled in the training program and, by 1928, 12 students were in training.[8] Boisen
was also actively involved in research on the parallels between
schizophrenic thought processes and religious experience.

The program that was to draw the greatest attention to Worcester State Hospital, however, was the creation of a schizophrenia research service in 1927 (Shakow, 1972). For the next 20 years, the
hospital sponsored one of the largest multidisciplinary research
programs ever undertaken on the biological, psychological, and sociological aspects of dementia praecox (schizophrenia). The research program was carried out in collaboration with the Memorial
Foundation for Neuro-Endrocrine Research, the Worcester Foundation for Experimental Biology, and several universities in the

Worcester and Boston area (Harvard Medical School, Boston University, and Clark University).

The research program had its embryonic beginnings between 1925 and 1927, when two staff psychiatrists (Lewis B. Hill and Francis H. Sleeper) undertook a limited study of the physiological aspects of schizophrenia. The systemic development of the Research Service began in 1927 when the Worcester hospital was selected as a field site by the Memorial Foundation for Neuro-Endocrine Research. The Foundation had been created by Katherine Dexter McCormick whose husband (son of the inventor of the reaper) suffered from schizophrenia prior to his death. In setting up the Foundation, Mrs. McCormick imposed stringent limitations on the use of estate funds, directing that money be allotted only to organic, mainly endocrinological, research on schizophrenia. Her strongly antipsychological and antipsychiatric attitude purportedly was due to her preception that her husband's prolonged and extensive treatment by a leading psychoanalyst was ineffectual (Shakow, 1972:69–70). Roy C. Hoskins, one of the leading endocrinologists in the country, was recruited as Director of the Foundation. Hoskins selected Worcester as the field site for the Foundation because of Bryan's enthusiastic support for the venture and Hill and Sleeper's research in these areas.

Additional sources of support soon became available to broaden the scope of studies beyond psychoendocrinology. Bryan realized that an active research program was essential for the recruitment of high-caliber staff to the hospital's teaching and treatment programs. He began to mount a campaign to persuade the legislature that support for research into the causes of mental illness would have long-range benefits for the state. "In my opinion," Bryan noted in the Worcester State Hospital Annual Report (1929:24), "the time has arrived when some other method of meeting the increasing demands upon the State for more housing facilities should be carefully scrutinized with the idea of making an attempt to solve the problem in some other way. It would seem that some money could be diverted for research into the causes and prevention of mental disease, and it is my earnest recommendation that this program be pursued for a sufficient length of time to enable us to ascertain if more patients cannot be returned into the community."

Bryan's plea was echoed by the trustees in their Annual Report (1930:3) the following year:

The Board wishes to again express its complete accord with the policy of carrying on extensive research into the cause and treatment of mental disorders. The Board believes that the research work being done in the hospital and in the Child Guidance Clinic will bring immeasurably greater results at the end of a period of years than will the policy of neglecting such research and community work, and putting the available money into additions to the hospital.

In 1930, after Bryan presented his case before the Ways and Means Committee of the Massachusetts Legislature, a special appropriation was made to support Worcester's research in dementia praecox. This was the first direct grant by the state to a designated hospital in Massachusetts. It provided funding for several research positions and related expenses that allowed for the expansion of psychological studies of schizophrenia. (The Dementia Praecox Fund continued to be appropriated until the mid-1970s). The other major source of funding for the Research Service was a 10-year grant (1934–1944) from the Rockefeller Foundation which enabled the hospital to acquire research equipment and additional personnel.

The accomplishments of the Research Service were prodigious. During its peak period of activity (1930–1946), over 400 publications—literary, scholarly, and encyclopedia articles as well as several monographs and books—resulted from work carried out at Worcester (Shakow, 1972). The range of studies included the endocrinological, metabolic, physiological, biochemical, and psychological aspects of schizophrenia. In its later years, the Research Service also undertook therapeutic studies (including some of the first clinical trials on insulin coma and electroconvulsive therapy in the United States) and investigations of the socioenvironmental and prognostic features of schizophrenia.[9] Throughout these years, members of the Research Staff held important positions in national professional organizations and on the editorial boards of leading scientific journals.[10] A large number of students were trained at Worcester and many went on to distinguished careers in psychiatry, psychology, and related disciplines.

The larger societal context in which the Worcester hospital was imbedded, however, continued to shape its internal activities. The principal external influences were the bureaucratic structure of the Department of Mental Diseases within which the hospital operated and the socioeconomic climate engendered by the Great Depression of the 1930s.

The Department of Mental Diseases had developed a complex set of standardized procedures governing the operation of state institutions. Although the Worcester hospital under Bryan's leadership had evolved an internal organization and atmosphere akin to

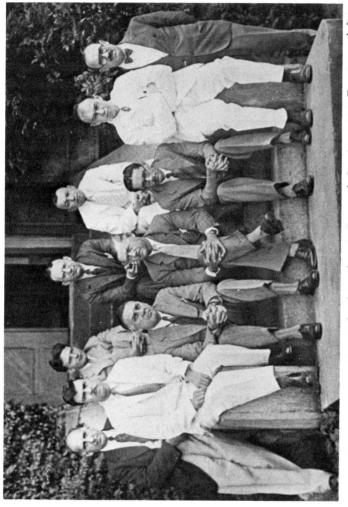

Fig. 8.    Worcester State Hospital Schizophrenia Research Service, 1930. *Front row, left to right:* Anton Boisen, Milton H. Erickson, William A. Bryan, Roy G. Hoskins, Francis H. Sleeper, James R. Linton, Vladimir Dimitroff. *Second row:* David Shakow, Morris Yorshis, Harry Freeman. *Source:* Medical Library, Worcester State Hospital.

a university, it was a maverick institution in an otherwise tightly knit state system. A constant struggle was necessary to sustain the innovative programs that had been developed over the considerable resistance of state officials and others oriented toward custodial care. Although state appropriations for research and training had mitigated many of the resource problems encountered in the 1920s, these funds came with "strings attached" in the form of uniform salary schedules, Civil Service requirements for filling positions, and strict employee time reporting (Shakow, 1972:82; Shakow, 1968). The Worcester staff viewed these requirements as "petty" external constraints that had to be circumvented in order to accomplish the goals of research, training, community service, and high-quality patient care.

The economic depression of the 1930s also shaped the internal character of the Worcester hospital. Few teaching and research institutions competed for personnel and prospects for employment or further schooling of graduate students were dismal. Thus, the Worcester hospital was able to attract many staff and students who would otherwise have refused employment in a state institution.

During these years the quality and stability of the attendant staff also changed dramatically. Due to low wages and difficult working conditions, Worcester and most state hospitals had experienced high turnover rates among nursing and attendant personnel for decades. In the 1920s, for example, the average stay was only 3.7 months (Shakow, 1972:78). Aside from a small core group of competent and highly motivated attendants, the hospital was forced to employ whoever would accept the position, regardless of his/her qualifications. In the 1930s, however, many unemployed mechanics and other workers from Worcester's machine-tool factories were recruited as attendants. This helped to enhance the quality and job stability of ward staff, and contributed to the viability of the training and research program as well. Many of the new attendants preferred to live at home with their families rather than in hospital dormitories as was the traditional practice. The maintenance portion of the attendants' salaries was used as modest stipends to support students during their hospital residency (Shakow, 1972:80).

The Depression also had more insidious effects. Patient labor, originally developed as a therapeutic measure, became vital for institutional maintenance. With the tightening of budgetary allocations, patients operated the farms and assisted the buildings and grounds staff. This economic dependence on patient labor prolonged hospital stay.

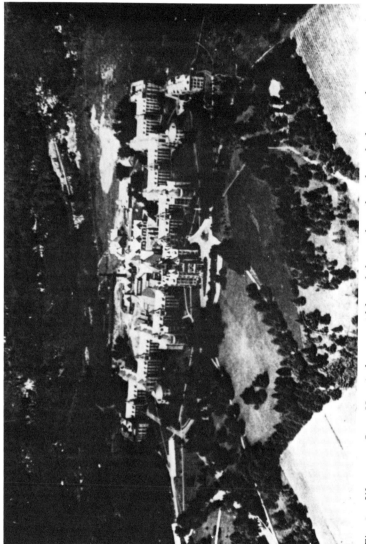

Fig. 9. Worcester State Hospital, 1933. Although located on the edge of a large urban community, the Worcester Hospital in the 1930s functioned as a minature "city-state" surrounded by sprawling grounds and farmland. *Source:* Medical Library, Worcester State Hospital.

Another depression-related phenomenon was the pressure on the hospital to relieve family economic burdens by admitting aged, senile, and medically infirm patients. Political patronage and the employment of workers displaced from their regular jobs were other ways in which the hospital was expected to meet community needs.

As a result of these forces, Worcester State Hospital functioned as a miniature "city state" or small society. Most of the professional and patient-care staff lived on the grounds of the hospital and, despite a regular annual turnover of perhaps 30 percent, the majority of its patients were long-term residents of the hospital. As Shakow (1972:80) relates: "The geographic isolation and the structures imposed by the Depression, with its pittance of salaries and limitations on movement, emphasized the primacy of the Hospital as a center of social life as well." The hospital was located on a 350-acre tract of land on the eastern edge of the city, removed from the major residential areas. It had its own radio station; 200 acres of farm land with facilities for processing and canning the produce; prize herds of cattle and swine; a security force; staff dormitories and recreational facilities; medical–surgical services for staff as well as patients; a chapel; and libraries for staff and for patients.

Despite the hospital's multiple functions, Bryan constantly challenged his staff to remember that its ultimate purpose was therapy, and its basic goal the return of patients to a useful life in the community. The reality, of course, was that no effective psychiatric treatment (whether psychological or somatic) was available. Bryan and his senior staff clearly recognized that psychiatry was still in its infancy, thus their commitment to Worcester's extensive training and research program. Yet, the other reality that constantly intruded on the future-oriented, scientific approach to the cause and cure of mental illness was the hospital's caseload of over 2,000 patients needing humane care. These dual commitments created a continuing tension and creative dynamic within the hospital during Bryan's superintendency.

Bryan developed elaborate procedures based on industrial management principles to insure that all patients were regularly bathed, fed, examined, and exercised (Bryan, 1936). He was constantly trying to improve the quality of care and encouraged the staff to do everything and anything to interrupt the isolation of the patients and their inability to do things for themselves. Beginning in the early 1930s, for example, L. Cody Marsh (1932, 1933) carried out extensive programs of group activity and remotivation for patients on the hospital's continued treatment wards. These programs ranged from small group therapy sessions to large "pep" rallies designed to prevent the deterioration of patients during prolonged hospital stays. In many respects Marsh's work anticipated the "total push" approach later made famous by Abraham Myerson (1938).

Marsh (1935) also extended his group work to community clincs where he developed family therapy programs for the parents of disturbed patients as well. These efforts were complemented by John Watson (1939) who developed one of the first state–city cooperative clinics in Massachusetts to provide mental hygiene services to the poor as an outreach program of the Worcester hospital.

In 1940, when the hospital was at the height of its program development, Bryan resigned to accept the superintendency of Norwich (Connecticut) State Hospital. His decision, in part, was motivated by a basic precept of his administrative philosophy which held that executives would lose their creativity and adversely affect the organization if they stayed too long. Despite the breadth of his administrative talents, Bryan saw himself primarily as an institution-builder and innovator. Over a period spanning nearly two decades, he had guided Worcester to a preeminent position among state mental hospitals in the United States. Connecticut was a progressive state and the newly completed Norwich hospital offered challenges and opportunities for innovative work. Indeed, prior to his death in 1944, Bryan was able to replicate at Norwich many of his Worcester programmatic and staff development accomplishments.

Other considerations influenced his decision to leave Worcester. He was deeply disappointed in not being named Commissioner of the newly constituted Department of Mental Health in 1938. These feelings were further aggravated when Clifton Perkins was selected as the Commissioner. Perkins had worked on Bryan's staff at Worcester since 1928 and, when appointed Commissioner, he was Bryan's Assistant Superintendent. Over the next five years, Bryan had innumerable disagreements with Perkins and other members of the state bureaucracy over the operation of the Worcester hospital. George Kline, the former Commissioner of the Department of Mental Diseases, had been a strong supporter of Bryan and, on a number of occasions, had suspended rules and regulations that would have blocked Bryan's efforts to enhance the quality of patient care at Worcester. Perkins, in contrast, continuously frustrated these efforts by his lack of aggressiveness in articulating the needs of the Department and his acquiesence to the politicization of the state hospitals and to the increasing control being asserted by other state agencies over hospital operations. The declining autonomy of the superintendency and its transformation into a managerial position under elaborate and increasingly inflexible rules undoubtedly influenced Bryan's decision to move to a setting more favorable to innovation and quality care.

Bryan's legacy to the Worcester hospital and to his successors was reflected not only in the quality of the treatment and educational programs he had put in place but also in the infrastructure of strong department heads and a highly articulated and coordinated organization. During his tenure, the promise of reform engendered under Adolf Myer's tutelage had been realized in a fuller and more comprehensive way than could have been expected at the time of his appointment in 1921. His accomplishments at Worcester had demonstrated that a state mental hospital was not inherently antitherapeutic. Indeed, under committed leadership it could become the vanguard of a new era of humane care for the mentally ill. In his volume on *Administrative Psychiatry* (1936:337), Bryan offered a vision made credible by his Worcester experience:

> I see the state mental hospital of the future as a powerful and leading factor in the public health of the community, its interest broad and far-reaching and its leadership unquestioned by those whom it serves. It will control the community clinics which I believe will be dotted all over the country, it will represent the finest type of medical service, and it will be the coordinating agency which ties up all activities dealing with human beings. The hospital will have the complete confidence and respect of society and it will be free from the domination of partisan politics and the manipulation of its work by unscrupulous politicians.

When Bryan resigned, his responsibilities were assumed by Assistant Superintendent Walter Barton on an interim basis. Barton had spent all of his professional life at Worcester, beginning with an internship in 1931 and rapidly moving up the professional hierarchy under Bryan's tutelage. He was held in high regard by the staff who believed he was Bryan's protégé and the logical choice to be his successor.[11] However, under Kline, the Department had developed the policy that all new superintendents had to have spent some time working at the state level prior to their appointment. Perkins insisted that this was an inflexible rule and that it disqualified Barton, despite his unanimous endorsement by the hospital's trustees. After serving as acting superintendent for over a year, Barton withdrew his name from consideration, indicating that " . . . a long period of temporary tenure would exert an adverse effect upon the affairs of the hospital" (WSH Messenger January 15, 1941:1).

In March 1941, H. Bardwell Flower was appointed superintendent. Flower was well known to the Worcester staff. After graduating from the Harvard Medical School in 1928, he interned at Worcester City Hospital, and then completed his residency training at Worcester State Hospital in the early 1930s. During this period, Flower served as chief of the hospital's medical and surgical service where he worked closely with Barton. His subsequent experience conformed closely to the Department's superintendent development model. After leaving Worcester, Flower served as Assistant Superintendent of the Grafton (Massachusetts) State Hospital (1934–1938) and then as Assistant Commissioner under Perkins (1938–1941).

With the sudden entry of the United States into World War II in December 1941, the Worcester hospital began to undergo a period of retrenchment. Mobilization led to the induction or enlistment of a large proportion of the senior medical staff as well as many nurses and attendants. The resurgence of employment opportunities in local defense-related industries also led to declines in attendant and support personnel. Community clinic activities and other "nonessential" programs were curtailed so that available staff could be redeployed to cover the inpatient services. At the same time, the hospital's region was expanded and the volume of admissions began to rise. Once again, under the impact of forces operating in the larger social environment, conditions at Worcester reverted to a "holding operation." However, the postwar years would soon usher in another wave of institutional reform that would dramatically affect the character of Worcester State Hospital.

## THE ERA OF COMMUNITY MENTAL HEALTH

The late 1940s and early 1950s were a period of significant activity in national mental health policy. Public awareness of the problems of mental illness was heightened by the numerous reports of psychiatric casualties among returning service personnel and the large number of selective service rejections due to psychiatric disorders (Mechanic, 1969). At the same time, the apparent success of military psychiatrists in dealing with combat neuroses and other psychiatric conditions led to a renewed optimism about the prevention and treatment of mental disorders. The shortage of trained professionals to deal with psychiatric problems and the paucity of services outside of the large state mental hospitals led to increasing Congressional concern about the federal government's role in the provision of mental health services. In 1946, Congress passed the National Mental Health Act which established the National Institute of Mental Health for the purpose of having "the traditional public health approach applied to the mental health field" (Mechanic, 1969). Over the next decade, developments at Worcester State Hospital would make a significant contribution to the national movement toward community-based care for the mentally ill.

The postwar years at Worcester were a period of gradual recovery from the overcrowding, staff shortages, and other hardships that the hospital was forced to endure.[12] In the late 1940s, there were still 300 staff vacancies (including 14 physician positions) and the average daily resident population had increased to over 2,800 patients, or 600 more than 1940 (Bockoven, 1972:120). In 1949, the Massachusetts legislature upgraded the state salary system which enhanced the hospital's competitive position to attract desperately needed personnel. With the help of the extensive network of Worcester "alumni" throughout the country, Flower mounted an intensive recruitment effort to fill the vacancies and he succeeded in hiring a number of people who had been trained at Worcester. Bockoven (1972:121) indicates that

> . . . the psychiatrists returning to the hospital from the military were a spirited, enthusiastic group, interested in getting the hospital back on its feet as a therapeutic institution. The spirit of activism was strengthened by the return of the hospital's former clinical leader, Dr. David Rothschild. The staff members began in earnest to "dig out from under"; like Dr. Flower, they were disturbed by the excess of patients and by the negative effects on them of overcrowding and substandard living conditions.

Over the next few years, Flower and Rothschild developed a program aimed at reducing the hospital's resident census.[13] Teams composed of psychiatrists, nurses, and social workers conducted systematic mental and physical evaluations of every patient on the hospital's Continued Treatment (Chronic) Service. On the basis of these evaluations, the wards were reorganized into different levels of nursing care and patients were regrouped according to their level of care needs. This experience made it clear to the staff that many of the elderly chronic patients could be returned to the community if alternative facilities could be found. Nurses were then assigned the tasks of developing discharge plans for these patients and conducting a search for suitable placements in the community.

As a result of these efforts, Worcester was one of the first state mental hospitals in the United States to experience a decline in its resident patient census (Bockoven, 1972:116). Between 1950 and 1955, the average daily resident patient census gradually declined from 2,858 to 2,693 ( −6 percent) despite a continued increase in its annual number of admissions from 770 to 880 (+13 percent) over the same interval.

This downward trend was accelerated in the late 1950s due to the increasing use of the new psychoactive drugs as well as a number of other factors.[14] In 1957, a new admission building was opened on the main campus of Worcester State Hospital. This led to the closing of the Summer Street Division and the relocation of its back-ward patients to the new building. These patients began to receive increased attention and improved environmental care. In a short period of time, many of them were ready for community placement. When federal funds became available for the support of elderly patients in nursing homes, Flower persuaded nursing homes in the communities served by the hospital to accept discharged patients. As the patient population steadily decreased, nurses previously involved in caring for elderly patients were reassigned to other duties. In addition to discharge planning, they were trained in individual, group, and milieu therapy. These efforts led to more intensive treatment, shorter lengths of stay, and increased discharge rates.

These administrative and treatment interventions continued the dramatic rate of decline in the hospital's census. In 1955 the resident census was 2,693; by 1963 it was 1,357. Concurrently, there was a marked alteration in the pattern of admissions at Worcester. In 1955 there were 880 admissions to the hospital; by 1963 there were 1,215. Whereas the number of first admissions remained relatively constant during this period (at about 618 per year), the annual number of *readmissions* had more than doubled (from 241 to 568).

When Flower and his staff embarked on this large-scale effort at census reduction and community placement, the prevailing assumption was that most patients were destined to reside in the hospital for life. Flower's plan to reduce the hospital's census was based on pragmatic considerations. Staff shortages and overcrowded wards made reduction of the chronic caseload the only way the hospital could begin to offer a semblance of humane care and active treatment. No precedents existed for this plan and the staff had no assurance that it would work. In a short time, however, it became clear that the climate of opinion in the community was becoming more tolerant. The initial successes fueled the zeal of the

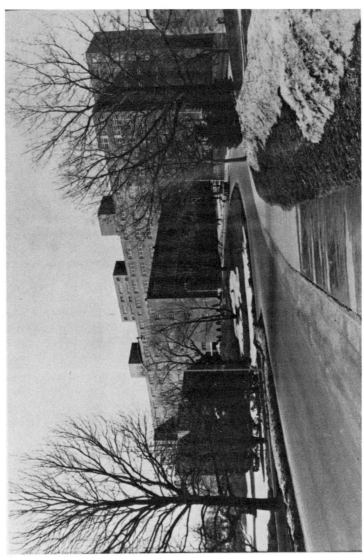

Fig. 10. Bryan Treatment Center, 1957. Named in honor of the Worcester hospital's eighth medical superintendent, the William A. Bryan Treatment Center was opened in 1957 with new facilities for inpatient treatment, day and night hospitalization, and outpatient care. *Source: Medical Library, Worcester State Hospital.*

staff and the release program was stepped up as fast as family and other placements could be found.

As the patterns of hospital utilization began to change in the 1950s, other programmatic reforms were introduced. With the exception of the Youth Guidance Center, all of the community clinics developed under Bryan's administration were disbanded during the war years. Faced with a paucity of services in the community, Flower and his staff developed outpatient and aftercare programs for the growing number of discharged patients residing in the local area. In the early 1960s, the hospital was reorganized into four separate sections or intensive treatment units which replaced the traditional Reception (acute) and Continued Treatment (chronic) Services (Hyde, 1962:34). New admissions were assigned to each section on a rotation basis and the same staff were responsible for patients from admission through discharge, community placement, and aftercare. Shortly thereafter, a day hospital program and a night hospital service were developed to provide supportive service for patients already discharged, as well as transitional services for those patients who were ready for release.

These reforms drew attention to Worcester State Hospital once again. The Worcester experience in census reduction influenced the deliberations of the Joint Commission on Mental Illness and Health (1961) and it provided an empirical example in support of the Commission's recommendations for the conversion of state hospitals from custodial to active treatment institutions (Bockoven, 1972:115). The administrative reorganization of the hospital with its expanded emphasis on outpatient and aftercare services was also featured at a 1961 national conference on the decentralization of psychiatric services and continuity of care sponsored by the Milbank Memorial Fund (Milbank, 1962; Hyde, 1962).

For the next several years, events at Worcester were circumscribed by developments in the mental health field at the national and state levels. Following passage of the National Mental Health and Retardation Act in 1963, an elaborate planning process was initiated for the development of Community Mental Health Centers across the country. In 1965, the Massachusetts Mental Health Planning Project (commissioned to prepare the State Plan mandated by the federal legislation) issued its final report (MMHPP, 1965). It recommended legislative and administrative sanctions for community mental health programs and the reorganization of the Departme〕 of Mental Health into a three-tiered system of state-wide, regior and local catchment area programs.

The paucity of local mental health services in Massachusetts was a direct result of the State Care Act of 1904, which gave the state exclusive jurisdiction over the mentally ill. Furthermore, most of the 351 municipal governments (39 cities and 312 towns) were too small to qualify as federal catchment areas (Marden, 1968). Accordingly, the report proposed a dual role for the future use of the state mental hospitals. Each of the 11 hospitals would serve as a "community mental health center" providing the essential services mandated in the federal guidelines (i.e., inpatient, outpatient, emergency, and partial hospitalization) to the catchment area in which it was located while serving as a regional back-up facility for the other areas in its service region.

In many respects, Worcester represented a model of the new state mental hospital envisioned in this report. While its overall service region encompassed most of central Massachusetts, its primary catchment area consisted of the City of Worcester and its contiguous towns with a population base of over 250,000 persons. The Worcester area had always accounted for the largest proportion of admissions to the hospital, and most of the patients discharged in the 1950s and early 1960s resided in close proximity to the hospital. With the development of outpatient, partial hospitalization, and aftercare programs, its outward appearance had been transformed into a community-oriented hospital. However, all of these service programs were institutionally based and institutionally controlled and, in most respects, the Worcester hospital still functioned as a centralized hospital.

The professional organization of the Worcester hospital in the mid-1960s was the residue of the strong, discipline-based departments that Bryan had created in the 1930s. Bryan's administrative genius rested in his ability to articulate overarching goals for the hospital and in his skill at delegating authority while coordinating departmental programs toward these goals. Over the years, each of the major professional departments (psychiatry, psychology, social work, nursing) had developed a tradition of strong leadership and autonomy. Bryan's management style fostered broad departmental participation in policy formulation and decision-making but maintained ultimate authority for the affairs of the hospital. In contrast, Flower had developed a *laissez faire* approach to hospital management. He was very supportive of his department heads but, when conflicts arose, he refused to mediate the disputes or make unilateral decisions as to their resolution. Department heads were expected to "fight their own battles" and, by remaining aloof from their disputes, Flower avoided charges of favoritism and partiality. This climate reinforced the autonomy and independence of the department heads who knew that they had the implicit support of the superintendent while being unchallengeable by other staff. Indeed, much of the program expansion in the early 1960s resulted from the aggressive pursuit of department-based programs rather than the unfolding of a consensually developed and centrally directed program of reorganization. Department heads controlled staff assignments in the hospital and developed patient-related programs to support the training, research, or clinical interests of their members. In most respects, they presided over miniature fiefdoms.

Flower had adopted a similar nonactivist position toward the communities served by the hospital. Over a period of several decades, community officials and social agencies had expected the hospital to provide total care for the indigent mentally ill. As prevailing definitions of these needs changed, the hospital made internal adaptations to meet these needs. Thus, when Flower initiated his census reduction program in the early 1950s by opening the "back doors" of the hospital, he proceeded to develop a number of support services for patient aftercare and community adjustment. Throughout his superintendency, however, the "front doors" of the hospital remained open and the hospital continued to accept patients who were a social burden to their families and to local hospitals regardless of their need for full-time psychiatric hospitalization. In the late 1960s, for example, the hospital developed an inpatient service to provide detoxification and rehabilitation for chronic alcoholics who were unwanted by other agencies. Community expectations regarding the role of Worcester State Hospital also accounted for the development of institution-based outpatient and aftercare programs and it contributed to the relative lack of alternative services in the Worcester area. The hospital had assumed responsibility for the residual welfare and psychiatric needs of the community. As a consequence, admissions continued to rise during the late 1960s. The result was that Worcester, in a number of respects, was an old institution struggling to survive in a new social context:

In 1966, the Massachusetts legislature passed the Comprehensive Mental Health and Retardation Act which incorporated the essential recommendations of the Mental Health Planning Project. However, the legislature failed to appropriate monies to implement the area programs and the Department of Mental Health proceeded to develop its regional administrative structure that would oversee the state hospitals and promote the development of community-based and community-controlled services.

In early 1969, Bardwell Flower announced his retirement after serving as superintendent for 18 years. During his tenure, the Worcester hospital had been transformed from a long-term custodial institution to an active-treatment, community-oriented hospital. The course of state and national policy would soon disrupt this accommodation and the Worcester hospital would be propelled toward an administratively decentralized as well as a functionally decentralized organizational structure.

## NOTES

1.  Dorothea Dix, who was raised in a town outside Worcester, was largely responsible for the construction or expansion of more than 30 state mental hospitals in the United States. Her "memorial" (petition) before the Massachusetts legislature in 1844 was a major influence leading to the expansion of the Worcester hospital. For a new edition of her memorials on behalf of the insane poor, see Dix (1975).

2.  In recent years, there has been a marked tendency to equate the concept of social control with social repression, especially with regard to the segregation of the mentally ill and other social deviants by powerful elites in society (e.g., Scull, 1977). However, in its classical sociological meaning, the term refers to the capacity of a social group to regulate itself through informal and formal mechanisms (Janowitz, 1975). It is in this sense that the term is used throughout this book. As Grob (1975, 1978) has argued elsewhere, the history of mental hospitalization in America indicates that most admissions were precipitated by families who could not tolerate or support their disabled kin, rather than by community elites who wanted to regulate the poor.

3.  This chapter relies extensively on Grob (1966, 1973) for a reconstruction of Worcester State Hospital's institutional history betwen 1856 and 1920. Information for the period 1921–1968 was derived from the references cited in the text as well as from interviews with several persons who worked at Worcester State Hospital during this period.

4.  The historical record is unclear on the exact time period encompassed by this study. Bockoven (1956, 1972), who rediscovered Park's data in the WSH Annual Reports, has inferred that the patients included in the study were discharged prior to 1847 since the total number followed (1,173) is within 15 of the total number of patients reported discharged as recovered by Woodward during the years 1833–1846 (1,188). However, Grob (1966:254) notes that there is no conclusive evidence to substantiate this claim. In Grob's view, Park's references to the study in the WSH Annual Report for 1881 suggest that patients discharged as recovered after Woodward's tenure were included in the study as well. This interpretation rests on Park's statement that the first 211 questionnaires had been sent out on patients discharged prior to 1840, but "as the cases become more recent, a much greater percent of replies is expected" (Grob, 1966:254).

Nonetheless, consistent with Bockoven's interpretation, if the study was motivated in part by Pliny Earle's interest in disproving Woodward's recovery claims then it would have been essential to restrict the study to patients discharged between 1833–1847. Moreover, Park's reference to "more recent cases" can be interpreted as referring to those discharged between 1840 and 1847 versus those discharged between 1833 and 1839. In any case, Park's study stands as one of the longest follow-up studies in the annals of American psychiatry.

5. The final tabulation of Park's data (completed in 1893) indicated that no information was obtained on 189 of the 1,173 discharged (Bockoven, 1972:60–61; Grob, 1966:254). Of the remaining 984 patients, 568 (57.7 percent) had either died without having a relapse or were still living and had never had a relapse. An additional 67 (6.8 percent) relapsed and were rehospitalized, but were again discharged. Only 143 (14.5 percent) relapsed who were rehospitalized (or sent to almshouses) and not again discharged. Another 142 (14.4 percent) had relapsed and were either still at home or had died while living at home. All told, then, only 210 (67 + 143 or 21.3 percent) of the 984 patients again became a burden to the Commonwealth of Massachusetts.

6. Of the 29 assistants who served under Meyer during his 6-year tenure at Worcester, three (Albert M. Barrett, George M. Kline, and George H. Kirby) later became presidents of the American Psychiatric Association. Others attained fame in different arenas. Isodar Coriat became one of the earliest supporters of Freud in the United States, founded the Boston Psychoanalytic Society, and helped to popularize psychoanalysis. Charles B. Dunlap and Henry A. Cotton went on to distinguished careers in psychiatric research. Overall, the group of psychiatrists who trained at Worcester under Meyer produced a disproportionate share of individuals with national reputations (see Grob, 1966:297).

7. In a national survey of Child Guidance clinics in 1932, the Rockefeller Foundation rated the Worcester Child Guidance Clinic 13 points higher than the next clinic on the national list in terms of service to the community (WSH Annual Trustees Report, 1932:21; Shakow, 1972:83).

8. Although Boisen left Worcester in 1932 to accept a position at Elgin (Illinois) State Hospital and the Chicago Theological Seminary, his students continued the program at WSH. Between 1925 and 1937, a total of 275 trainees from 42 theological schools and 22 different communions had participated in the Worcester program and the graduates went on to establish similar programs at state hospitals and divinity schools throughout the country (WSH Annual Report, 1937).

9. Beginning in the late 1930s, the growing involvement in therapeutic research began to be complemented with a parallel interest in the socioenvironmental aspects of schizophrenia. Géza Róheim, the distinguished analyst–anthropologist, joined the WSH staff in 1938 after fleeing Nazi Germany (Shakow, n.d.). His teaching, didactic analyses, and writings made important contributions to the hospital's educational and staff development programs (see Róheim, 1940a; 1940b; 1943). Howard Rowland (then a doctoral student in sociology at Columbia University) conducted one of the earliest studies of patient social interaction in an American mental hospital at Worcester (Rowland, 1938, 1939). His seminal work identified many of the features of "total institutions" and "patient society" that were to become prominent themes in sociological studies of mental hospitals in the 1950s and 1960s. Also, George Devereux joined the Research Service in 1939 as a staff sociologist and conducted studies of social

therapeutic processes (Devereux, 1939a, 1939b, 1944). The work of Rowland and Devereux made important early contributions to the theory and practice of milieu therapy (see Perrow, 1965:930–934).

10. Among the more prominent members of the WSH Research Service during this period were, in physiology and biochemistry: Hudson Hoagland, Roy G. Hoskins, Joseph M. Looney, and Gregory Pincus; in internal medicine: Harry Freeman, J.S. Gottlieb, and Francis H. Sleeper; in psychiatry: Angus Angyal, D. Ewen Cameron, Hugh T. Carmichael, L.H. Cohen, E. Van Domarus, M.E. Erickson, O. Kant, J.R. Linton, William Malamud, and J.C. Rheingold; in biometry: J.W. Fertig, E. Morton Jellinek, and Forrest E. Linder; in psychology: Tamara Dembo, E. Haufmann, Paul E. Huston, M. Rickers-Ovsiankina, Elliot H. Rodnick, Ann Roe, Saul Rosenweig, and David Shakow; in psychoanalysis: Géza Róheim and Earl Zinn; in social work: I.T. Malamud (see Shakow, 1972).

11. In his subsequent career, Barton did follow in his mentor's footsteps. After a brief period of military service in World War II, Barton became superintendent of Boston State Hospital and later served as president of the American Psychiatric Association. His book on *Administration in Psychiatry* (Barton, 1962) was inspired by Bryan's tutelage and earlier work on the same subject.

12. The late 1940s was a period of significant change in the WSH's Research Service as well. In 1946, Roy Hoskins accepted a position at the Boston State Hospital under Walter Barton, who had recently been appointed its new superintendent. Several other staff members (including David Shakow and William Malamud) also accepted positions at Universities and other hospitals that were beginning a period of rapid growth to meet the renewed emphasis on mental health manpower development and research. Over the next few years, the Research Service phased down its operations (Shakow, 1972:94–100) and the focus shifted to psychological research on coping behavior and prognostic factors in psychopathology, first under the direction of Elliot Rodnick, and then under Leslie Phillips (see Phillips, 1968). Also, in the late 1950s, the Worcester Foundation for Experimental Biology was moved to a new location in Shrewsbury, MA under the direction of Hudson Hoagland and Gregory Pincus. Increasingly, the Foundation began to pursue an independent direction that made it an internationally renowned institute for hormone and steroid research. Among the Foundation's many accomplishments was the discovery of the birth control pill.

13. At the time that Flower and Rothschild inaugurated their census reduction program at WSH in the late 1940s and early 1950s there were few documented reports on similar efforts elsewhere. However, although reports did not reach the United States until the mid-1950s, this was also the period in which the British "open hospital" movement got underway. According to Gruenberg and Archer (1979:491), "three pioneer British mental hospital directors (Duncan MacMillan, T.P. Rees, and G. Bell) tried to change the atmosphere in their hospitals by systematically removing locks from doors, removing restraints, and halting involuntary hospitalization. The pattern of hospital use changed. Long-term stays in the community, interrupted by short-term episodes of hospitalization in periods of crisis, replaced long-term hospital stays." An important ingredient of the British model as well as the program developed at WSH and at the Hudson River State Hospital in New York (Milbank Memorial Fund Quarterly, 1962; Gruenberg, 1966; Gruenberg, 1974) was that the same clinical team of psychiatrists, nurses, social workers, and attendants took responsibility for patient care during both community and hospital phases of care.

14. The precise role of psychoactive drugs in the census reductions at American state mental hospitals during the late 1950s continues to be a much-debated issue. The evidence concerning the discovery and diffusion of these medications is presented in Swazey (1974). The belief that these drugs were the principal cause of the census reduction at state mental hospitals in the United States derives in large part from a series of studies conducted in New York (Brill and Patton, 1957, 1959, 1962, 1966). Opposing views, based on the changes in administrative policies and sociotherapeutic techniques that preceeded the widespread use of these medications can be found in Mechanic (1969:61–62), Scull (1977:79–94), and Gruenberg and Archer (1979:488–493). One of the principal difficulties involved in disentangling the effects of drugs and other factors is that both were occuring at roughly the same time period (Klerman, 1977). Nonetheless, most authorities believe that the psychoactive drugs contributed to the acceleration of census decline through the renewed optimism they generated among the staff of these institutions and/or their effects on symptom control of hospitalized patients.

David J. Myerson

# 4
# Deinstitutionalization and
# Decentralization: 1969–1977

In September, 1969, I was appointed the tenth Medical Superintendent of the Worcester State Hospital (WSH). The following month I was also appointed the first Director for the Greater Worcester Mental Health Area (GWA). That same fall, the 200-acre farm of the WSH was closed and, on this site, construction began for the first state-run medical school in the Commonwealth of Massachusetts. When I resigned from the superintendency and area directorship in October 1977, I was appointed to the full-time faculty in the Department of Psychiatry at the new University of Massachusetts Medical Center (UMMC). The position of Medical Superintendent at WSH was abolished. In its place, the position of Hospital Administrator was created, and it is now occupied by the former Steward of WSH. Similarly, a highly skilled, nonmedical human services manager was recruited as my successor in the Area Director position.

Thus, my tenure of just eight years at WSH spanned the transition from a relatively simple, but highly centralized, institution-based system of care for the mentally ill to one based on a vastly more complex, decentralized network of community services. The old system evolved in response to the reform movement of the mid-19th century, which phased hospitals in, and the new system is emerging out of a series of reform movements during the mid-20th century aimed at the deinstitutionalization and phase-out of state mental hospitals. In this chapter, I intend to describe this transformation—which did not come about easily or smoothly—as I experienced it in the ambiguous, and indeed conflicting, positions of both Superintendent of the old institutional system and Area Director of the new community system.

When I assumed the superintendency, WSH functioned both as the major acute care hospital and the custodial institution for the indigent mentally ill and socially incapacitated individuals in Central Massachusetts. Even though the inpatient population of the hospital had dropped from about 3,000 to 1,000 prior to my tenure, the staffing patterns and the administrative organization still reflected the old system developed during the 19th century when WSH was mandated to provide total medical and custodial care for its inmates. Admission to WSH was easy and discharge was difficult, not necessarily for medical or psychiatric reasons but because the Superintendent was expected to assume total and permanent care of the individuals committed to the hospital. Furthermore, there were no community facilities for their care after discharge. The admission procedures evolved over the past century by a series of legislative acts allowed an efficient mechanism to shunt the indigent mentally ill or incapacitated people from the courts, police stations, certain social service agencies, and the emergency rooms of general hospitals to WSH.

While the potential for violence and self-destruction was emphasized as the key factors for admission of these persons, these traits were really exaggerated and served as a rationale for the easy admission procedures. All the demographic and psychiatric characteristics of admitted patients revealed that indigence, social helplessness, and isolation related to their illness determined admission to, and permanent residence at, WSH. With few exceptions, the affluent mentally ill from supportive families went elsewhere for their psychiatric care. Accordingly, the community agents, police, sheriffs, social workers, and physicians in private practice relied upon easy state hospital admission procedures to relieve the considerable pressure on their respective agencies for the care and disposition of indigent clients. The quality of care rendered to these patients was rarely of concern to these agents, who complained only when WSH staff challenged or delayed the admission of their client.

I soon became aware that I had entered a system in which the Superintendent—the chief administrative and medical officer of WSH—had little or no control over its admission rate. Nonhospital agents made the decision as to who and how many persons were to be admitted, and these agents had no knowledge of (or concern about) the budgetary, staffing, and space limitations of WSH. As I immersed myself in the rich historical records on file at the hospital, the highlights of which have been presented in prior chapters, I came to realize that the one-way flow of admissions from the community to the hospital had haunted each of my predecessors at WSH and that it had led to WSH's greatest problems: overcrowding and an inability to provide high-quality treatment, either for the acutely ill or for the chronically disabled. In effect, the lack of what my sociological colleagues refer to as admissions "boundary control" had served to compromise the organizational integrity of WSH from its founding nearly 150 years ago.

My appointment as Area Director for the GWA entailed other problems that my predecessors at WSH did not have to confront, and for which the historical records offered no perspective or resolution. This position symbolized the revolt against the old system of institutional care and the harbinger of the new system of community care. I was thoroughly aware of the background that led to this reform. In a prior position at the Boston State Hospital, I was involved with some of these problems as that institution began its phase-down in 1967. I had also served on several task forces which influenced the Massachusetts Department of Mental Health (DMH) to decentralize its administration and follow other guidelines of the federal community mental health legislation.

Consistent with these recommendations, Massachusetts was divided into seven administrative regions for the delivery of mental health and mental retardation services. A Regional Director, accountable to the Commissioner of Mental Health and Retardation, was appointed to oversee each regional program. The regions were subdivided into clearly demarcated "areas" of 75,000–200,000 population (with only a few exceptions). These areas were administered by Area Directors who were accountable to a Regional Director. Area programs were to be developed in the community rather than the state hospitals. Ultimately, Area Directors were also scheduled to assume responsibility for the geographic unit at the state hospital that served as the inpatient backup for their specified areas. In addition, the Area Directors related to Area Boards composed of citizens who reviewed programs and budget allotments, but only in an advisory capacity.

When I assumed the positions of Superintendent and Area Director in 1969, the WSH budget passed by the legislature followed the traditional line-method of allotting monies for rigidly defined positions, supplies, maintenance, and the like. Legally, the budget was still under the direct control of the Superintendent. The Regional Offices were allotted only a relatively small amount of funds; the Area Offices, none. Area Directors, however, were mandated by the Commissioner to pry funds from the state hospital budget to develop their community programs which eventually would be budgeted separately and assigned directly to the Area Offices.

The ambiguities of my dual positions under this administrative structure are clear. Throughout my tenure, I was torn between my responsibilities as Superintendent and as Area Director in decisions involving the GWA, and I was in direct conflict with other Area Directors in many matters concerning their inpatient units at WSH. As Superintendent, I was mandated to operate four geographical inpatient units serving different areas while providing space and staff at WSH for a number of region-wide programs. As Area Director, I was responsible for the development and support of community services only in the GWA. Repeatedly, I was confronted with difficult choices, as for example, whether I should assign a nurse to a community clinic in Worcester or to an inpatient ward of the WSH unit serving the GWA. Initially, I rationalized away the weight of these decisions, thinking that if circumstances dictated I could reverse these staff assignments at a later date. My naïveté in this regard became evident on several occasions when I attempted to pull back ward staff assigned to community clinics in the GWA, only to encounter the outrage of community groups protective of "their staff." In contrast, my conflicts over staff allotments with the Area Directors associated with the other WSH geographic units were far more serious from the outset. Here there was no question that, once reassigned, staff positions could never be called back to meet mounting demands on the admissions wards of WSH.

But these role conflicts were only a part of the challenge and paradox of change at WSH. In this chapter I will describe these changes, and the problems that arose in process, as I perceived them from my front-line position. Subsequent chapters in this volume will deal in more detail with the resolution or persistence of these and related problems. Throughout my tenure, I kept a diary of these events and experiences. In addition to this personal record, my observations in this chapter will be based on memoranda and other reports in my files as well as my earlier papers on the phasedown of WSH (Myerson, 1972; Myerson et al., 1974; Myerson, 1975).

This chapter will be organized into several sections that touch upon key aspects of these changes: the social organization of Worcester State Hospital under the old system, with its traditional mandate to provide total care to those people referred by the courts, general hospitals, social service agencies, and private physicians; the response of these agencies when the hospital staff attempted to redefine these boundaries and impose limits on this traditional mandate; the unitization of the hospital and the establishment of community-based clinics as alternatives to hospitalization; the new hospital-based functions and services that began to be offered to the community; and the events that precipitated my resignation from the superintendency of the hospital.

## THE OLD INSTITUTIONAL SYSTEM

The original building at WSH, erected in 1832, was located on a small campus in the center of Worcester. In 1870, with the press of an ever-increasing caseload, a new site was created on a several-hundred-acre tract of land on the northeastern perimeter of the city. In 1956, another eight-story building was erected on this site.

The first building was torn down after 136 years of continuous use. The architectural styles of all the buildings reflect the salient institutional functions of WSH: to provide security for the treatment of acute admissions and basic survival care for long-term institutionalized patients. It is of interest that although facades and floor plans of the two remaining buildings differ considerably, they both provided spacious admission rooms where 80–100 patients were processed per month, large locked wards, each of which housed 30–50 patients, relatively small enclosed nursing stations, and centrally located administrative offices. Each building had its own cafeteria, chapel, beauty and barber shops, and bathing facilities. While the newer building had some space designed for occupational therapy, neither had a gymnasium or space designed for occupational training programs.

Until 1969, the management of the farm, the cafeteria, and the greenhouse relied, to some extent, on patient labor; in other words, the major occupational programs in which patients participated met the needs of the hospital, not the needs of the patient. It was a 19th-century attitude that farming was good for the patients. In reality, the farm was once effective in reducing the cost of patient care. When the farm lost its economic value in the 1960s, it was phased out.

The staffing patterns, too, reflected the acute care and custodial functions of the hospital. Staff were organized along disciplinary lines into the nursing service, the maintenance service, the medical and psychiatric service, the psychology service, and the social service.

Numerically, the nursing service was the largest and consisted of almost 600 persons, including registered nurses, licensed practical nurses, nonprofessional mental health assistants, and a few custodial care positions, such as barbers and beauticians. This service was directed by a registered nurse with a graduate degree. All the supervisors were registered nurses, most of whom had earned advanced degrees during their careers. During the day shift, a registered nurse headed almost every ward. But in the later shifts, there were only enough registered nurses to provide coverage for large sections of the hospital.

Most of the ward care staff were nonprofessional mental health assistants. Their positions were not prestigious, they were relatively poorly paid, and their chances for promotion were almost nil. Yet they had the greatest contact with the patients and were responsible for their custodial management. The better educated and more ambitious mental health assistants stayed only a short time, leaving for higher paying and more prestigious positions. In the old state hospital system, therefore, the sickest patients received most of their care from the nonprofessional staff.

The admission wards that received the acutely ill patients, however, usually had the greatest number of professional staff. But it was a rare ward that had enough staff to provide the patients with a therapeutic milieu even during the day shift. Two registered nurses, one licensed practical nurse, and three or four mental health assistants were considered a good staffing pattern for the day shift on an admission ward. If the ward census remained at 20 patients, the staff was able to consider the therapeutic problems of the individual patients. Frequently, the census reached 30 or more. The concern of the staff then changed from therapy to control. When the professionals and nonprofessionals expressed fear that the violence and self-destructiveness of their patients could get out of control, they requested high dosages of medication and the use of physical restraints for their patients.

The recent legal restrictions on the use of these controls was viewed with concern by the staff, especially when the census on their ward was over 25 or when the staff was depleted by illness, resignations, or job "freezes" (the prohibition of hiring for new, or filling vacant, state positions). In one extreme instance, when the

Governor "froze" all positions, there was an increase in absentee-ism as well as a rise in the inpatient census. The few remaining nursing staff in one ward locked themselves in the nursing station to seek help and protest their dangerous working conditions and their inability to provide even minimal care for their patients. To reduce this extreme tension, the ward psychiatrist discharged about 10 patients, a desperate way to "cure" a problem that clearly arises from the lack of logic of the old system. Clearly, the state govern-ment has a right to economize by holding back funds. But without proportionate decreases in the volume of patients state hospitals have to accept at the will of outsiders, the human costs of these simple economies will indeed be high.

Besides the nurses, professional services in the old system were provided by psychiatrists, physicians, psychologists, and so-cial workers. The psychiatrists consisted of two groups: the staff psychiatrists and the physicians in training or residents. The staff psychiatrists directed professional activities on the wards. They wrote the orders for medication, prescribed all modalities of treat-ment, authorized day passes, and approved discharges. They were also responsible for preparing commitment proceedings. Under this old institutional system, all their treatment activities took place in the hospital. The psychiatrists never left the grounds of WSH for professional purposes. Those patients that were discharged had to return to the hospital for their aftercare treatment. WSH did pro-vide outpatient services, but they were located on the grounds of the hospital.

The main psychiatric activity occurred in the admission unit and the wards that accepted the newly admitted patients. Both res-idents and staff psychiatrists utilized and developed their skills, primarily in the treatment of the new and acutely ill patients. Along with the other professionals, they were interested in pre-scribing up-to-date modalities of treatment, following their patients closely, and discharging them if they could. For the most part, the psychiatrists rarely involved the families of the patients in treat-ment, unless the families were assertive and insisted upon this in-volvement. The psychiatrists usually tried to avoid family contacts, and frequently blamed the patient's problems on their families if they were very assertive.

The long-term patients—those who remained despite all treat-ment intervention or because they suffered from irreversible brain damage or severe developmental disabilities—received only per-functory psychiatric care. A brief monthly visit, a "progress" note, and a medication review were all the psychiatric attention they received. For the most part, the care of chronically institutionalized patients fell under the aegis of the nurses and, if these patients became physically ill, of physicians.

Psychiatric care was the responsibility of the Clinical Director. He was very important, for his professional orientation determined the preferred modalities for treating acutely ill patients. Today, WSH is a veritable museum of institutional psychiatry in America. Scattered throughout its buildings are areas designed for particular modes of treatment when they were in vogue: special baths, facilities for insulin-coma treatment, electric shock treatment, and even group treatment rooms with one-way screens. Each was extensively used for a period of time and then given up. At present, the pharmacy is well stocked with a variety of psychotropic medications, reflecting the current reliance on chemotherapy as the major therapeutic intervention. The choice and abandonment of these diverse techniques reflect the orientation of the different Clinical Directors and the treatment method that was popular during their tenure.

The resident psychiatrists provided 24-hour coverage for the admission room and the hospital. It was difficult to recruit residents from American medical schools because these physicians preferred the prestigious university-based institutions. Consequently many of the residents were foreign medical graduates. The WSH, however, maintained a good reputation as a training institution, and through the high quality of its staff, good salaries, and the provision of housing, it did attract the better-qualified foreign medical graduates as well as a number of American graduates. The WSH has long been used for clinical experience for Clark University, Tufts Medical School, Assumption College, and has come to be used by the University of Massachusetts Medical School.

It is important to note that under this old system, the hospital was responsible for the total medical and surgical care of its patients. Accordingly, WSH had established a surgical service with operating teams as well as an obstetrical service and a nursery. All of these services were being phased out when I arrived at WSH in 1969.

The WSH was unique among state hospitals in that it was able to develop and hold a strong, well-staffed psychological service with an international reputation in research on the problems of schizophrenia and depression. This service also operated one of the best hospital-based psychology training programs in the United States through a grant from the National Institute of Mental Health.

Far more typical of the old state hospital staffing patterns was the social service department. An institution that is geared towards custodial care does not require a strong social service. Social work, as a profession, is community-based and family-oriented. Consequently, as long as the hospital maintained its custodial orientation, it was difficult to recruit qualified social workers even for the few positions that were available in this service.

An important aspect of this institutional system was its maintenance department. The hospital, its subsidiary buildings, and grounds constituted a large plant that required the expertise of engineers, electricians, painters, and the like. All these employees were responsible to the Steward. His functions also included the management of the budget, payroll, and purchasing. Since the Superintendents were all medically trained, the tendency was to assign these important fiscal responsibilities to the Steward. He prepared the budget, kept a running account to prevent deficiencies, and presented the accounting to the state auditors.

Maintenance of two large buildings is expensive. Consequently, perhaps as much as 20 percent of the budget had to be used for purchasing supplies just to maintain the building and grounds. As costs have risen, one of the major arguments for the phase-out of any state hospital is the amount of dollars that have to be used for nonpatient care. For example, should the Steward request $50,000 from the legislature to repair a leaking roof, or for more social workers, or for funds to purchase a community-based residence? As long as patients reside in the hospital, the leaking roof must be repaired. Given the severely limited budget, as well as the inflation, it was difficult to pry money from the WSH budget to establish community programs. The care of the building locked even progressive administrators into perpetuating this old institutional system.

In the typical centralized state hospital, the Nursing Director, the Steward, the Clinical Director, the Medical Director, and the Social Service Director were all responsible to the Superintendent and the Assistant Superintendent. In 1969, both the WSH Superintendent and Assistant Superintendent had to be board-certified or board-qualified psychiatrists. The Superintendent was responsible and accountable for all patient care admissions, discharges, and commitment procedures. It was in his name that each employee was hired, promoted, disciplined, or fired. He was, indeed, the governing body responsible only to a weak, advisory Board of Trustees, the Regional Administrator, and Commissioner. In the past, he lived on the grounds of the hospital, responded to every emergency such as serious assault, suicides, or fires. He had to be ready to intervene in case of controversial or illegal admissions. Up to 1969 the Superintendent of WSH was appointed by the Commissioner who was responsible directly to the Governor. Historically, while the position of the superintendent was rarely a political appointment, the close relationship to the Governor and the legislators placed the Superintendent in a politically sensitive position. In the 1950s, at the height of the state hospital usage, the WSH Superintendent hired 1,000 state employees and cared for 3,000 Massachusetts citizens, each one committed, not to the hospital, but to the Superintendent who therefore was responsible in varying ways for 4,000 people. The Superintendent was answerable for all grievances filed by the employees, the patients, or their families. It was not uncommon for a political opponent of the Governor or Commissioner to attack them through "exposés" of the state hospital. Yet the office of the Superintendent unlike that of the Commissioner was a permanent civil service one, and removal from this office, while possible, was difficult. Suffice it to say that I was the tenth WSH Superintendent since 1833, and the average tenure had lasted about 15 years.

Outside his own constituency, the Superintendent tended to be isolated from the rest of the medical community. He rarely served on the staff of any private hospital. He tended to come up through the ranks in the Department of Mental Health. Usually he was chosen from one of the Assistant Superintendents who, in turn, were chosen from among the staff psychiatrists in any one of the eleven (in 1969) Massachusetts State Hospitals. Until 1969, the Superintendents were a group of psychiatrists with considerable expertise in dealing with administrative and clinical problems of any of the Massachusetts State Hospitals, but with very little experience concerning community problems or the private sector. The Superintendents that preceded me at WSH were all truly public-sector administrative psychiatrists, none of whom to my knowledge had ever done anything else professionally except state hospital work. Unlike my predecessors, I chose not to live on the grounds of WSH. Further, while I had considerable experience in state hospitals, I did not rise up the ranks of this system. I had worked in a number of general hospitals and carried on a private practice. Prior to my appointment as Superintendent, I had directed the first treatment center for drug-dependent people. The center was funded by the state and located at the Boston State Hospital (Myerson, 1953; Myerson, 1956; Myerson, 1966).

Given his authority, any real change in the state hospital system was going to be dependent on the Superintendent. As a rule, Superintendents were conservative, loyal to the old system, and resistant in varying degrees to change. Exceptions like Milton Greenblatt of the Boston State Hospital showed me that an active, progressive, community-minded Superintendent could upset the staleness of the state hospital system (see Greenblatt et al., 1971). It was Dr. Greenblatt who, as Commissioner of the Department of Mental Health, appointed me to the superintendency of WSH.

## FUNCTIONS OF THE OLD INSTITUTIONAL SYSTEM

The claim so often heard that the old state hospital was a static, isolated system not responsive to the needs of the community is simply not true. I soon learned that, as Superintendent, I was expected to follow the tradition of all my predecessors, namely to accept any mentally ill or even socially incapacitated person whose admission was requested by any community agency. An old man, for example, might break his hip and be hospitalized for his surgical procedures in one of the local general hospitals. Following the surgical procedure, he would need a long convalescence; but local nursing home beds were unavailable. If he exhibited confusion or disturbing behavior patterns during his postoperative care, the administrator of the local general hospital could charge him with a minor violation (like disturbing the peace). Two psychiatrists, not connected with WSH, could then recommend to the district court judge that the patient be sent to WSH on a 30-day commitment. As a rule, the judge followed this recommendation and ordered the old patient transferred to WSH. Since this procedure only happened to older men and women without families and money, this 30-day observation was, in effect, a permanent commitment to the state hospital, for at that time there was no other place to send them. I once complained to the district court judge, who condoned this transfer on the basis that it costs four times as much to hold the old person in a general hospital than it did in the state hospital.

It was not unusual for physicians from general hospitals to refer patients even from the Intensive Care Units if they were obstreperous or assaultive. The fact that the state hospital had limited medical facilities was never raised as an issue. In one instance, a physician tried to admit a diabetic woman into WSH because she refused to take her insulin.

The district courts, too, believed that the state hospital was mandated to accept whomever the judge decided to send. Consequently, WSH received arsonists, exhibitionists, alcoholics, and drug users, as well as psychotic people who were detained by the police.

In 1971, the admission and commitment procedures were revised under Chapter 888 of the Massachusetts General Laws. The intent of this chapter was to protect the civil liberties and rights of the patients. The revised statutes encouraged voluntary admission and prohibited involuntary admission to the hospital except when the patients were proven to be physically dangerous to themselves or to others. Only a qualified physician was allowed to determine this degree of dangerousness and mandate an admission to the hospital. One of the crucial features of this law was that it gave the Superintendent the authority to determine who would be accepted as a qualified physician and to withdraw this privilege if the community physician made inappropriate referrals. For the first time, the Superintendent had some authority to control admissions. The law even made psychiatric screening necessary before a judge could mandate the admission of a patient from his court.

This law helped the state hospital administration. At least the general hospitals and other community agencies could no longer commit at will the nuisances, the harmless senile people, or the obstreperous alcoholics. In practice, however, it did not take long before the courts devised another system whereby the judge could order people, more or less at his will, to the hospital (see Chapter 6).

It is of crucial importance in understanding the function of the traditional state hospital to realize that even this moderate degree of control by the Superintendent over the admission rate and one-way flow created considerable friction between the hospital and the agencies that over the years had become dependent on the easy admission policies at WSH.

## REDEFINING THE BOUNDARIES OF
## WORCESTER STATE HOSPITAL

My first confrontation with community agencies involved a new policy concerning the admission of alcoholics to the WSH. In 1967, the previous Superintendent had reversed the policy of no admission of alcoholics. Within a short time, the WSH had to admit as many as 60 alcoholic patients per month. These patients required detoxification, careful medical examination, psychiatric evaluation, and work rehabilitation programs. The courts, family agencies, police, and families inundated WSH with alcoholic patients with the expectation that the hospital would be responsible for their total long-term care. WSH staff struggled valiantly to provide a full range of services until the sheer weight of the patient load overwhelmed the budgetary, administrative, and physical resources. The hospital administration requested additional funds from the legislature. These were refused on the grounds that in Massachusetts alcoholism was a responsibility of the Department of Public Health, not the Department of Mental Health. Accordingly, in 1970, after a few months in office, I unilaterally limited the admission of alcoholics to those whose psychotic features could be clearly defined. The detoxification and the rehabilitation wards were phased-out.

The response of the community to this change in policy was one of fury. At one Area Board meeting, I was accused of being responsible for the deaths of several alcoholics who died after this policy change. Several agencies even tried to force admission through the use of political pressure, but to no avail.

In retrospect, I was correct in changing the admission policy, but erred seriously in the decision to phase out this greatly needed service so abruptly and unilaterally. Had I consulted the Area Board and the other involved agencies, the fury of the community agencies as well as the harmful effects of the disruption of treatment on the alcoholic patients could have been attenuated.

I had to live through this painful experience to learn that the hospital did not exist as an autonomous entity and to understand how dependent the community was upon WSH for the disposition of its social problems. Yet, to change this system, community agencies, too, had to recognize that they could not transfer at will large numbers of maladaptive people to WSH and expect it to provide for their total care.

I did make my point. Like any other agency, the WSH had a finite budget, staff, and space. To function properly, it had to live within these constraints. Moreover, community agencies had ongoing responsibilities for treating alcoholic persons and their families. Such responsibilities couldn't be discharged by transfer to another agency. The question then to be faced was how all of the agencies involved in the care of the alcoholics—Public Welfare, Family Service Agencies, Catholic Charities, Salvation Army Center, Vocational Rehabilitation, state and general hospitals, and the courts—could pool and coordinate their wide array of resources. The result of many meetings, these various community agencies found it possible to coordinate their resources to provide a broad network of alcoholism services. For example, WSH donated a full-time social worker and a nurse to work with these various agencies within the city of Worcester. When needed, a WSH psychiatrist was available to provide evaluation for psychiatric treatment. WSH was also prepared to accept a patient who demonstrated specific psychotic features or severely self-destructive traits that required 24-hour psychiatric nursing and medical care. Several general hospitals provided staff and space for detoxification and outpatient programs. Catholic Charities and Salvation Army offered community residences and family counseling. The Massachusetts Rehabilitation Commission sponsored long-range vocational training programs.

The use of WSH facilities for the drug-dependent and addicted people also became a focus of conflict between the courts and WSH staff. Unlike the policy concerning alcohol programs, the legislature had adopted the policy of funding the Department of Mental Health to develop a variety of drug treatment programs and WSH was assigned some of these funds. Furthermore, as part of Chapter 888, passed in 1970, the legislature mandated psychiatric evaluation and a plan of treatment for every drug offender appearing before the courts on a drug-related charge. We hoped to develop a treatment program with a strong emphasis on a therapeutic milieu which required a high staff–patient ratio. The number of admissions had to be controlled. The pressure from the courts, however, threatened to disrupt the program with unlimited numbers of admissions; this could only lead to institutionalized and security-minded care. We protested the courts' request for unlimited admissions. The protestation led to a confrontation between the judges and the drug treatment staff. In this meeting, the judges claimed that as far as they were concerned, the WSH program was ineffective because it was not designed to meet their needs. I replied that the WSH was mandated to participate in the development of a network of programs and, at that moment in time, no agency could meet the courts' needs without being destroyed as a treatment facility. Gradually, a coalition of agencies (including a crisis center, outpatient clinics, outreach programs, detoxification centers, and self-help groups) did provide a spectrum of services for the drug abusers. Initially, WSH provided the major portion of services in the hospital itself. As the community developed more and more of these programs under the auspices of this coalition, WSH was able to phase down its service and provide only a secure inpatient program for detoxifying severely addicted individuals. Furthermore, there soon were enough community-based personnel trained to meet the requirements of the courts so that every drug-related offender could be evaluated and offered the least restrictive treatment plan commensurate with his or her needs.

The restriction of alcohol and drug admissions to WSH set an important precedent that ultimately included other serious abuses. Among these problems were the unlimited admissions of senile people, and even dying patients. I have mentioned that it was common practice of general hospitals to shunt these severely disabled individuals into WSH, where they occupied the time of large numbers of nursing and medical personnel. It is true that dying patients will die. They clearly need help to die. This may be the responsibility of the family, the general hospital, or a hospice, but not of WSH. People will grow senile, become helpless, and need community support. But WSH could not be the sole provider of care for the indigent senile. The logic is the same as with the drug and alcohol problem. WSH was willing to, and did, provide facilities and staff both in and out of the hospital for such persons, but only in alliance with other agencies which provided preventive and community-based care. With the rise of the nursing home industry and Medicare and Medicaid, some of the pressure on WSH was relieved through the development of alternative facilities.

These experiences taught me an invaluable lesson. I learned that the WSH served a vital function for other community agencies like the courts and the general hospitals. If we were going to interrupt the operations of these important institutions by curtailing their right to send certain patients for care, then these agencies were going to be angry and patients were going to get hurt. Consequently, it was our responsibility to help set up alternative programs, which required, however, cooperation from the same community agencies. The pooling of resources from WSH and the other community agencies was to be the key to its successful phasedown.

## UNITIZATION AND HOSPITAL
## REORGANIZATION

Under the old custodial system, perhaps one of the most significant factors leading to the one-way admission and subsequent institutionalization of patients was the almost random assignment of geographical areas to WSH. The hospital had to receive patients not only from Worcester but from communities as far as 100 miles away. Studies have shown that the greater the distance of the patient from his home, the less likely his family was able or willing to maintain interest, and the more likely this patient was destined for an indefinite stay at the hospital. Further, no matter where a patient came from, he or she was assigned to the ward WSH staff found convenient. Consequently, the mixing of patients from different communities tended to decrease their sense of community identity and to enhance their dependency on the hospital.

To undo this historical fault, the Commissioner mandated the unitization of all state hospitals in Massachusetts. This mandate was the first major step in implementation of the federal and state community mental health legislation. At first, WSH was assigned four distinct areas, but one (Lowell) was still 50 miles away and located in a different region. Later, this assignment was changed, and with the closure of a nearby state hospital (Grafton), WSH provided services to four relatively contiguous areas, all from the same region.

Unitization meant that WSH was to provide contiguous and well-defined ward space for each geographic area so that its Area Director could assume increasing responsibility for the care of patients. Certain programs, like the large Geriatric Service, the Retarded Service, the Medical Service, and the small but highly specialized adolescent and drug programs had to be excluded from geographical reassignment. These services were all included under the fifth unit, known as the Regional Service Unit.

The challenge of unitization was to change the space and staff assignments of an institution designed architecturally to be centralized, and encrusted by a century-old tradition of functioning as a closed, inward-looking organization. That is, as far as the staff was concerned, the residence of a patient at WSH was the primary basis of his social identity, and any relationship to his community or family was of secondary or little concern. Now WSH had to be divided into four distinct units, plus the disparate fifth regional unit.

Every patient, old and new, was supposed to be assigned to a unit representing his geographical area.

The problems were complex. About 80 percent of the admissions came from the GWA, but this unit had proportionately fewer chronic or long-stay patients than the more remote areas. Although these latter units had more chronic patients, they still had to provide some space for the few but significant number of newly admitted patients. There were many chronic patients whose original residence was outside the WSH region. The Department of Mental Health administrators decided that such patients would not be "repatriated" by transfer to other state hospitals now serving these areas. From the point of view of unit staff at WSH, there was no fair way of dividing these out-of-region chronic patients among the GWA unit (with its high admission rate) and the more remote units (that were already overburdened with chronically institutionalized patients).

Further complicating matters, the Regional Service Unit was really a potpourri of disparate entities, each specialized and requiring considerable space and staff. The Medical Service, for example, provided basic medical care for all the units, and in this sense it was a contradiction to the principles of unitization which called for self-contained treatment units.

Beyond the division of space and patient relocation, the problem of dividing and reassigning the staff was even more complex. For the most part, WSH staff had a negative attitude toward unitization. Furthermore, there was not enough professional staff to be divided equally among the five units throughout the three shifts, or even in proportion to their varying caseload demands for acute psychiatric care, chronic care, or medical-geriatric and nursing needs.

My positions as Area Director for the GWA and Superintendent for the whole hospital placed me in unavoidable conflict of interest. As Superintendent, during the early years of my tenure, I had had the final say. I tried to be fair, but there is no doubt that I favored the GWA on the basis of its disproportionately high admission rate.

The assignments of the psychiatrists, high-ranking nurses, and social workers were relatively easy and were decided by their respective department heads. In contrast, the assignment of nursing personnel, particularly the nonprofessionals, was extremely complex and conflict-prone. Among the lower echelons, by agreements with the union, assignments to one of the three shifts, as well as days off, had to be posted and chosen on the basis of seniority. The shifting around of about 600 people could not be done to everyone's satisfaction. In a few instances, we had to break the agreement with the union. We did set up a complicated bidding system, but it took several months to work out the large number of grievances. Finally, after nine months of planning, May 15, 1970 was chosen as the day to move about 900 patients, beds, and about 600 staff to their respective geographically based wards. The day was an eventful one. The patients were moved by a rather excited and loyal staff but at the same time a picket line, albeit a peaceful one, was thrown up for a few hours to protest the unresolved grievances of those who could not get their desired assignments.

Despite these grievances and the grumbling from the other Area Directors, the unitization procedure did accomplish its task. Most of the staff became aware that WSH no longer operated as an independent agency but had some relation to the communities from which the patients came. Unitization tended to decentralize, at least to some extent, the different disciplines. It introduced, in a very practical way, the role of the Area Board (at least for the GWA unit), the members of which gave considerable time and effort to the planning and phasing in of this reorganization. Yet, unitization did not fundamentally change the old structure of the hospital. The budget system was not changed. The directors of each disciplinary group, in the final analysis, still served as "department heads." Psychiatrists were assigned as Unit Chiefs of each geographical area. My position as Superintendent still allowed for centralized decision-making and policy formulation. I consulted only with the Area Board of the GWA. The other Area Directors were barely in place and had no legal authority or experience in coping with such a complex institution. Furthermore, due to insufficient staff, WSH was only really unitized during the day shift. Because of staff shortages, the other two shifts had to combine their resources just to cover the nursing demands of the hospital. In short, despite unitization, WSH still functioned for the most part as a centralized institution.

## THE DEVELOPMENT OF COMMUNITY
## PROGRAMS

The irony of the mandate to unitize and deinstitutionalize was that WSH was not given any additional funds. The Commissioner and the Regional Director told me to pry out of the WSH budget enough staff to provide aftercare programs in the community. But how and where should I attempt to pool the resources of WSH with other community agencies to provide these direct services? Here the Area Board was invaluable. Data from several demographic studies of GWA admissions showed that most patients came from the inner city, contiguous with the section known as the Model Cities Area. Various members of the Area Board opened the doors of several community agencies that provided both space and personnel to work with us to establish necessary community-based programs.

Fortuitously, in 1970, at the time of unitization, the Model Cities Area received federal funds for the development of a mental health component in its neighborhood health center. What better way of pooling resources could there be? The plan that developed called for the GWA Unit to provide a pool of professional staff; the Model Cities Program, in turn, would provide space in that area of its city, indigenous neighborhood workers, professional staff, and an administrator. At first, the federal supervisor of the Model Cities Program objected to the use of WSH staff, but the logic of using state-salaried physicians and nurses, psychologists, and social workers made eminent sense to this community. These professionals, who were already known in the area, received such strong support from citizen groups and from local officials that the federal objections were minimized.

Based in an old remodeled store, WSH and Model Cities personnel were able to provide a wide array of support and aftercare services. Initially, the mental health services provided consisted chiefly of aftercare for those patients who were discharged from the hospital. Then, within a short period, the mental health team came to treat many patients who never had been hospitalized. Furthermore, as already indicated, the staff was able to provide consultation, training, and back-up services for the alcohol and drug programs that agencies such as Catholic Charities, Salvation Army, Crisis Center, and the Worcester Drug Coalition were developing. Vocational counseling services, sponsored by the Massachusetts Rehabilitation Commission, were also added as a vital component to this total array of services.

Organizationally, there were many problems, particularly those pertaining to line responsibility. As the Model Cities funds dried up, this neighborhood health center incorporated, and received funds from other sources. It established a board, 51 percent of whom had to be from the Model Cities area. A Director was chosen who was responsible to the board and for the development of total health care. Mental health care was, of course, only one component. One of the organizational issues was the question of whether WSH employees were responsible to the Center Director or to the Superintendent/Area Director at the hospital which paid their salaries. The solution we reached was that all WSH employees assigned to this neighborhood center would be clinically responsible to the Director, and hence to the citizen board. The Director could ask any or all WSH state employees to leave the center if their work was unsatisfactory. But he could not fire them, and I was responsible for reassignment if any employee were asked to leave. Interestingly enough, this situation occurred only a few times.

That the same clinical team of WSH physicians, nurses, and social workers treated their patients both in the community and in the hospital proved to be one of the rewarding features of this arrangement. As the length of hospitalization shortened to an average of about three weeks for newly admitted patients, most of the care was provided to these patients while they retained their ties with family members, who often became involved in treatment. Thus, another serious cause of institutionalization—the isolation of the staff and patients from families and communities—was modified.

In October 1970, when the Model Cities clinic first opened, the mental health team served 212 patients. By November 1974, the number had grown to 907. These figures underestimate the number of people actually served since these teams did not always have the time or opportunity to record their activities.

A sociological study conducted by Hajib C. Al-Khazraji influenced placement of other personnel during unitization (Al-Khazraji et al., 1970). He defined the sociodemographic composition of the Great Brook Valley Housing Project, located on the outskirts of the City of Worcester. This public housing project was rebuilt with federal funds following a devastating tornado in 1953 that destroyed many dwellings. One of the largest public housing projects in Massachusetts, it offered apartments at low rent to about 3,400 people in 1970. The study revealed that 80 percent of the families were on welfare, that a large number of these families were fatherless, and that there was a considerable elderly population. Although predominantly white in 1970, the area has since had a mass influx of Hispanics. Further, the project was built in an area of the city which is remote from both medical and shopping facilities and has poor public transportation.

In short, the housing project met the criteria of a "high-risk" area with nonexistent health facilities. WSH staff followed procedures that many community-based mental health clinics have outlined. These staff members met with the residents and listened to them talk about their needs. As a result, I assigned a community worker to help the residents organize so that they eventually could seek and receive funds for a neighborhood health center. Also, at the request of the citizens, I was able to assign a geriatrician to help establish preventive medical programs for the older population. In addition, the fledgling mental health team worked with professional staff from other agencies such as a nearby general hospital, the Visiting Nurses Association, Public Health and Welfare Departments, and from the Worcester Housing Authority. Thus, from the outset, the program was multidisciplinary and multi-auspiced.

At first, WSH had to provide funds to purchase office space and equipment for the mental health program since these were not available as they had been in the better-funded Model Cities Center. Gradually, the program succeeded. Like the earlier center, the mental health component first provided aftercare services to about 80 former patients. In time, residents of the project who had not been hospitalized used it for a wide range of mental health problems. Starting in 1974, the clinic began to serve about 300 people, only 100 of whom were WSH aftercare patients. Moreover, by then the residents had organized a board which incorporated and was able to receive federal and local funds for a total health care center. This center now offers medical, social, and both adult and child psychiatric services.

The development of these two clinics has been reported in detail not because they differ from many others that have been developed in recent years, but because in the context of this chapter they illustrate clearly the progress made in redefining the role of the WSH. During the decade of my superintendency a complex network of institutional and community-based services developed around WSH. Additional community clinics were established in storefronts, local churches, a neighborhood settlement house, and in the outpatient department of Memorial Hospital, a private, nonprofit general hospital in Worcester. All of these clinics were staffed by WSH personnel. Special services were created for emotionally disturbed, aggressive, acting-out students from the Worcester Schools (Woodward Day School), retarded youngsters (Quimby School), and for disturbed adolescents (Adolescent Treatment Complex). A forensic psychiatric team served the court and jails; a consultation–liaison program served several local general hospitals.

Additional relationships were established with local social service agencies, the police, regional universities, the Worcester Youth Guidance Center, the Welfare Department, Massachusetts Rehabilitation Commission, and several Worcester area hospitals, including Memorial Hospital which opened a new inpatient psychiatric unit with the assistance of WSH. Many of these programs are discussed in greater detail in subsequent chapters.

These programs demonstrate that the WSH changed from an isolated, centralized institution which provided custodial care to about 3000 people in 1950 to the center of a mental health service system which, by 1975, provided acute and custodial care to about 450 patients and participated energetically and conjointly with many other agencies in the care of about 4000 people who remained closer to their families and communities.

## PROBLEMS IN TRANSITION

The shift of patient care from the centralized hospital to units and to a series of relatively decentralized community facilities presented problems for the psychiatrists and nursing personnel of WSH. Assignments to these community clinics were in conflict with their training and experience, which until recently had been completely hospital-centered with well-defined job descriptions and easily identified lines of authority. In the hospital personnel were in daily contact with their supervisors. When working conflicts or problems arose, they knew to whom they could turn for help. Their job security was protected by the strength of the unions, their professional associations, and civil service. Generally, the rank and file of staff did not understand the reorganization of the hospital with its ultimate accountability to distinct areas and area boards. When they came to perceive this change more clearly, they viewed it with apprehension.

Those personnel who accepted community assignments were faced with new clinical conditions. They worked in nonmedical settings, such as storefronts, apartments, or the basement of a church. They had to cooperate with professionals and nonprofessional workers who not only were non-hospital trained, but often vocally anti-hospital, and who tried to direct the activities of WSH staff. To further complicate matters, the lines of authority were confusing and unpopular. The informal agreement making WSH personnel accountable to clinic directors instead of the Superintendent was repeatedly questioned. In one publicized instance, these staff members were shocked that even my orders were successfully challenged by the director and the citizen's council of one particular neighborhood center where WSH personnel were assigned. In general, the greater the geographical distance between the community clinic and the hospital the greater the administrative conflicts that arose between WSH personnel and the staff in the community facilities. The Model Cities and the Great Brook Valley programs were relatively successfully administered, whereas the programs in the more remote areas controlled by other Area Directors were fraught with many administrative problems.

With the partial shift of staff responsibility to these community centers, their personnel insisted that the WSH staff not only provide aftercare for the discharged patients but primary care service for people who were never hospitalized but who presented a wide spectrum of situational as well as psychiatric difficulties. Accordingly the local staff asked the WSH staff to treat children from disorganized families, unhappy women trying unsuccessfully to cope with fatherless families, isolated, malnourished elderly recluses, aggressive and destructive adolescents, persons involved in marital disputes, and numerous other socio-psychiatric conditions which did not require hospitalization but were a source of concern to the community. Both the nurses and the psychiatrists tended to retain their medical orientation. For example, they tended to label the poverty-stricken woman, abandoned by her husband, as suffering from a "depression" and to rely on the use of psychotropic medication. Only the exceptional nurse and psychiatrists perceived the struggles of their patients as related primarily to social conditions.

In 1973, a questionnaire sent to all WSH personnel assigned to community programs revealed that the vast majority retained their hospital identity. It was a rare nurse or psychiatrist who believed that he or she should be involved in social reform. Nevertheless, it was a challenging experience for WSH staff to "treat" their "patients" as they existed in their crushing social environment rather than in the protection and isolation of the hospital milieu.

Considering the discomfort, the change in line authority, and the broadened responsibilities, it is not surprising that community work was not popular among the rank-and-file nurses and physicians. This created a problem in filling community assignments, which were mushrooming not only in Model Cities and Great Brook Valley but throughout Worcester and the surrounding areas. Because of their training and interest, the social workers and psychologists generally found this community work more acceptable than did the medically trained personnel.

To encourage more active participation, especially among nurses and psychiatrists, we utilized three recruitment techniques. First, we relied on those who actually bid for these community positions. Fortunately, there was a small group of gifted personnel from the different disciplines who willingly accepted the challenge of community work, and preferred to work in the informal community settings rather than in the closely supervised hospital wards. The second technique to aid in recruitment was the establishment of educational programs. The American Federation of State, County, and Municipal Employees (AFSCME) sponsored the first training program. Fifty mental health assistants were selected on a seniority basis for an eight-week course in community psychiatry. Subsequently, AFSCME contracted with several local colleges which provided the instructors and materials for courses that focused on the delivery of mental health services to the community. Once completed, the assistants received a minor salary upgrading, a change in their title to Mental Health Technician, and certification for work in community facilities.

This academic program, with its explicit recognition of community psychiatry, improved the willingness of the nursing service to participate in the community programs. As a result, WSH instituted three similar programs supported out of the hospital budget for the registered nurses. Although they could not receive salary upgrading, they did earn academic credits.

Yet, despite these well-received and popular academic courses, the nursing personnel generally preferred traditional hospital services. Only 8 of the 50 mental health technicians became actively engaged in community programs. When the experimental, community-oriented adolescent program at WSH needed five nurses, only one nurse voluntarily bid for the position. It was necessary to recruit nurses from different hospitals and backgrounds to fill these positions.

To help solve this problem, we developed a third technique to meet the staffing needs of the community programs and clinics. Unfilled nursing service positions were assigned to community programs or facilities whose administrators were authorized to hire the personnel. The only responsibility of WSH was to pay for the salary of the mental health worker, whose training was then the responsibility of the community facility. More recently, after legislative approval, monies were taken out of the WSH budget, assigned to Regional and Area Offices, and used to contract for services through private, nonprofit agencies.

## THE MANDATE TO AREATIZE

By 1976, the community-based programs in Worcester were well in place. The Area Directors of the three other areas were now established and had developed a broad network of services from the funds obtained by the closedown of Grafton and Gardner State Hospitals, two sister institutions that were located in WSH's service region. These Area Directors were now in a position to demand better care and fairer distribution of WSH staff for the wards assigned to them through unitization. The conflicts of being both Superintendent and an Area Director now reached intolerable proportions. It was clear from the mandates of the last three commissioners that the medical superintendency was about to be phased out at all of the state hospitals. The plan was to upgrade the position of the Steward who would oversee the administrative functions of the hospitals. Area Directors would then assume the clinical management of their respective units, which were to be integrated completely into their community programs. The reward for phasing down the inpatient units of the state hospitals was permission to transfer staff positions, or their dollar equivalents, from the hospital budget to their community programs. The Regional Administrator supervised this process and had the final authority to develop further community programs and prevent the state hospital from being completely depleted of staff.

To decentralize administratively, the Area Directors now had to apportion the budget of WSH so that they had fiscal control of their units under the authority of the Regional Director. The Area Directors could then appoint Unit Directors, who then would be responsible for all the clinical services on their units. Psychiatrists were to function not as Unit Directors but part of the clinical team of nurses, social workers, and psychologists. The positions of Director of Nursing, Social Work, and Clinical Psychiatry were also phased out.

It took two years of weekly meetings with the Regional Administrator, her staff, and all of the Area Directors before the budget could be allotted to everyone's satisfaction, or at least to a point where the Regional Administrator made the final decision as to how the budget conflicts were to be resolved. I was given a choice. I could have remained as a kind of watered-down Clinical Director but with no line authority to oversee the clinical management of the patients. Or, I could stay as the Area Director of the GWA. But it was clear that the Area Director was to be a manager. The Department of Mental Health was contracting more and more of its services with other agencies. The Department was allowed to shift its allotted monies from one account to another to pay for professional services, residential care programs, and the like under the auspices of private agencies. One of the responsibilities of the Area Director was to establish and oversee these contracted services. This role required considerable management skill. Since I thought of myself as primarily a clinician, I chose not to seek this position.

Since 1970, the University of Massachusetts Medical Center (UMMC) had developed from a hole in the ground in the former farm of the WSH to a huge medical school and hospital complex. From the beginning of my tenure I had been involved in a variety of training programs for the different mental health disciplines. In 1974 the Commissioner requested that the WSH use its training resources in psychiatry, psychology, and pastoral counseling to develop a consortium with other mental health disciplines and institutions, such as the University of Massachusetts (Amherst), Smith College, and the UMMC. In order to divest the consortium of a state hospital connection, we organized the consortium into a nonprofit, private corporation called the Western Massachusetts Training Consortium (WMTC). We chose a full-time project director, and I became the Chairman of its Steering Committee. The first Chancellor/Dean of the UMMC appointed me Professor of Psychiatry (nonfaculty), and in 1975 the second Chancellor assigned office space at the UMMC for the WMTC. The WMTC set high priorities to develop in-service training programs for state hospital personnel, who were assigned to community clinics after the phase-down and phase-out of the state hospitals in the western part of the state. In addition, we became increasingly aware that it was not feasible for the residency training program to be based at WSH, but rather it had to be transferred to the UMMC.

As a result of my increasing preoccupation with training in the public sector and the Commissioner's mandate to phase out Medical Superintendents, I resigned in October 1977 as the tenth and last Medical Superintendent of the WSH. The Chairman of the Department of Psychiatry at the UMMC invited me to continue my work as a full-time faculty member. In this position I now am the Director of the Residency Training Program, supervisor of the psychiatrists assigned to the GWA at the WSH, and Vice Chairman of the Department of Psychiatry.

# PART II

# Changing Organizational Boundaries

Howard H. Goldman

# 5

# Changing Organizational Boundaries: A Socio-Ecological Perspective

... The Union is on my back about suspending an attendant and the Nurses' Association is angry because I don't back them up with more disciplinary action. The newspaper wants to know what else I'm going to do about these allegations of patient abuse, and the Regional Office wants my job.

The wards are overcrowded and the staff are shorthanded because we've deployed almost everyone available to the clinics. The nursing homes are sending back the patients we placed out during the strike. The psychiatric units at Memorial and St. Vincent and the jail all sent us patients who need emergency commitment.

The Psychology Department wants to maintain its autonomy from Psychiatry and the junior staff continues to complain about the privileges of the senior staff. The legislature has budgeted us for 350 patients and we have nearly 500 . . .

So don't tell me that the residents want more money and less night call . . .

As the above anecdote[1] dramatically illustrates, conflict pervades the contemporary state mental hospital. Within its walls there is tension between patients and staff, professionals and nonprofessionals, physicians and nonphysicians, clinicians and administrators, unions and management. Across its boundaries the state mental hospital is caught up in the tensions between institutional and community-based care systems and between the public and the private service sectors.

The professional and popular literature offer many explanations for conflict in the mental hospital. Most works concentrate on tensions between staff and patients (Stanton and Schwartz, 1954; Belknap, 1956; Goffman, 1961). The sources of this conflict have been linked to role and status differences within "total institutions." Some works have directed attention to tension within the hierarchy and "negotiated order" of the mental hospital (Strauss et. al., 1964). However, few of these studies have viewed the psychiatric hospital as a part of a larger social system.[2]

In this chapter, based on my experiences as a psychiatric resident at Worcester State Hospital during the period 1974–1978, I will attempt to analyze conflicts in and around state mental hospitals within a broader conceptual framework.[3] Earlier studies have viewed the state mental hospital as an isolated, "closed" institution. In contrast, the present chapter relies on a socio-ecological perspective that views the state mental hospital as an open system interacting with a varied social environment. Much of what occurs within such hospitals can be fully understood only with reference to this larger societal context.

## A SOCIO-ECOLOGICAL PERSPECTIVE

A basic premise of ecological theory, known as "The Principle of Competitive Exclusion," has important implications for studies of social relations and social organization (Morowitz, 1975). As formulated in 1934 by the Russian biologist Gause, this principle holds that "Populations of two species cannot persist together for a very long time in the same community when both compete for, and are limited by, a common resource." Ecologists use the term "niche" to describe such a competitive community. A social analogy of this principle suggests that competition between social groups ("species") may be resolved in three ways: (1) extinction or displacement of one group, (2) cooperation between groups, or (3) partition of the niche into territories (Morowitz, 1975).

In the first instance, one of the competing groups is eliminated in the struggle for survival. This may occur actively, when one group overcomes the other or drives it from the niche. Or it may occur passively, when one group competes more successfully for limited resources or adapts to conditions of scarcity, while the other group becomes extinct or is displaced from the community. Genocide, exile, and mass migration are all social examples of extinction or displacement.

In the second instance, the competing groups learn to cooperate and share the limiting resources. This process, which Morowitz (1975) calls "cultural despeciation," decreases competition by changing group values and behavior. Cooperation offers the potential for new solutions to the problem of scarcity. Cultural despeciation fundamentally alters the relationship between social groups, transforming bitter enemies into allies in the struggle for survival.

In the third instance, the niche is divided into territories occupied by separate groups whose relationships are characterized by conflict, competition, and coexistence. Such competitive coexistence partitions nations in times of civil strife, segments society, and divides communities and their institutions. From a socioecological perspective, the boundaries of the niche may be drawn at various levels of social organization. Within each territorial boundary, conflict, competition, and division reflect adaptation to external conditions of resource scarcity.

The contemporary state mental hospital may be analyzed fruitfully from this perspective, as a niche populated by two related "species": the patients and the staff. Further, the state mental hospital system in a particular geographic area may be viewed as part of a larger niche, composed of competing institutional and community-based service units. Ultimately, the mental health and human services system can be described as a complex "ecosystem," roughly divided into public and private sectors.

Mutual dependence on a pool of scarce resources is the common fate of all "species" within these overlapping ecological niches. It is the thesis of this chapter that this mutual dependence promotes competitive coexistence between patients and staff, administrators and employees, community and institution, and public and private sector. Furthermore, resource scarcity and the resultant competition and conflict transcend the boundaries of the mental health system, with ramifications throughout the human services system as a whole.

Examples of these conflicts will be presented against the backdrop of the policies of deinstitutionalization and fiscal austerity at Worcester State Hospital. The analysis will explore the conditions of mutual dependence and competition, both within Worcester State Hospital as a social institution, and more broadly, at several levels within the larger ecological niche in the Worcester area.

## MUTUAL DEPENDENCE ON SCARCE
## RESOURCES

When viewed as an open system interacting with its social environment, Worcester State Hospital (WSH) appears to serve the health and welfare needs of its community, its patients, and its staff. While providing for the care and treatment of its indigent citizens who are mentally ill, WSH also serves as a mechanism of social control for the community. It also provides work for about 1,000 employees and thus is a significant element in the Worcester economy. The health and welfare needs of its patients are met through the provision of basic custodial services; the same basic functions for the staff are realized through its civil service system. Thus, at WSH (as well as other state hospitals) both keeper and kept depend on the institution for survival; both must share its allocation of resources. So, too, the various employee groups, the network of community services, and the institution must share the same limited state mental health budget. In the 1970s, the problem of mutual dependence on scarce mental health resources intensified, not only in Massachusetts but throughout the United States as a whole, as budgetary limitations threatened the very survival of many human service programs.

At WSH, as in other mental hospitals, both patients and staff must coexist because they are mutually dependent. Functionally, neither group could survive without the other. Just as patients require the care of the staff, so, too, staff require patients or their staff role becomes meaningless.

Historically, "total institutions" like WSH have been almost as "total" for the staff as for the patients. In earlier decades, the attendant, nursing, and resident physician staff lived on the grounds of WSH and were subject to strict regulation of their behavior 24 hours a day (Grob, 1966). Some personnel still live on WSH premises, relying on hospital facilities for their daily needs (food, shelter, laundry). Meals in the cafeteria are subsidized by the Commonwealth. In some instances, personnel receive medical care from staff professionals in the WSH dispensary. However, even when staff members do reside off-campus, many of their health and welfare needs are met by WSH through wages, subsidies, benefits, and insurance plans.

The health and welfare functions of state mental institutions may be almost as significant for the staff and the community as for the patients. These institutions characteristically employ more people than they treat at any one time. During the mid-1970s, for example, WSH had approximately 1,000 full-time employees and 500 inpatients. This 2:1 staff–patient ratio is similar to the staffing pattern at other public institutions (Romano, 1974).

The current policy of deinstitutionalization has heightened staff and patient awareness of their dependence on the mental hospital for health and welfare needs. In the 1970s, when Grafton State Hospital and Gardner State Hospital were closed and consolidated with WSH, patients cried "Where is my home?" (NIMH, 1974), and institutional employees complained bitterly that their livelihood was being destroyed (AFSCME, 1975). Local politicians pointed in anger to the economic effect on their communities. The institution had been the only home for hundreds of patients and the largest single employer in many towns. Thus, when state hospitals close, the health and welfare of both patients and employees are threatened.

Federal and state welfare programs came to the aid of many of these deinstitutionalized mental patients, while the employees were rescued by civil service and their unions, welfare systems of a different type. Thus, hospital staff continued to be paid even as patients departed for community residences or were transferred to other institutions. When Grafton State Hospital and Gardner State Hospital closed, some staff followed their patients into the community or to WSH, others continued to report to their jobs, and still others were retired, but all permanent employees continued to be paid (Khan and Kaplan, 1974). The payment of salaries to civil servants whose functions had been terminated parallels the payment of welfare benefits to former mental patients who are unemployed. Both patients and staff had been supported by their respective welfare systems within the hospital niche; support continued even after the niche had been administratively dissolved by closure.

During times of relative abundance patients do not suffer directly from staff salary increases, and the staff does not suffer when spending on patient care increases. When real or policy-imposed scarcity produces a fiscal crisis, however, priority setting becomes a more obvious and threatening process. Patients and staff are placed in direct competition for limited resources. Even in an expanding social welfare system, resources are somewhat limited by the budget, and staff and patients must accept some limitations. But in a contracting, zero-sum market economy, the two groups are likely to see their relationship as competitive (Gil, 1976).

These observations are supported by events at WSH. In 1975,

state workers in Massachusetts were refused a legislatively mandated cost-of-living salary increase. At the same time, the Governor froze welfare payments at the 1974 level. A few state workers protested the welfare cutbacks, but the newly organized collective bargaining units of the unions worked actively to negotiate an employee pay increase. Arbitration was slow and unproductive. In frustration, a general strike (called a "job action") was announced in June of 1976. For a week the nonstriking professionals and administrators at WSH staffed the wards, while support staff and paraprofessionals walked the picket line.

During the strike, approximately 140 of 470 resident patients at WSH were sent home or were discharged to emergency placements in foster homes and intermediate care facilities. On the picket line this strategy was met with a variety of responses. Many workers felt: "It was about time they sent them home where they belonged!" or "Ed didn't need to be on the ward anyway and Joe belongs in jail . . ." Others expressed concern: "Wait 'till they see how tough it is to take care of Doris. Then they'll understand why we're on strike." Most of the attendants were certain that the strike would be successful because "the patients will *really* go crazy if we're not there to manage them." In fact, during the strike there was no more violence on the wards than usual; no one was hurt.

After a few days of around-the-clock duty, the nonstriking staff was exhausted. As the "job action" continued, striking employees became angry and bitter. The atmosphere was extremely tense, especially on the picket line. Longstanding latent conflict between striking nonprofessionals and nonstriking professionals became manifest and even violent. Threats were made and personal and hospital property was destroyed.

During the strike all but the most basic maintenance functions of WSH were halted. There were no admissions, no evaluations, no commitments, and no treatment. There was little danger to the patients, but the staff was tired and the community felt the effect of the slowdown of hospital activity. Pressure began to increase to reopen WSH for emergencies and criminal commitments and to return some of the patients temporarily placed in the community. (Virtually all of the patients discharged prematurely because of the strike eventually returned to the hospital.) WSH and other public facilities were pressured to resume full activity. After one week, the Commonwealth and the collective bargaining units achieved a settlement.

The strike was partially effective: State employees were granted a small wage increase. However, the Governor refused to increase the hospital budgets. The pay hike had to come out of existing allocations that were already strained. There was no money for needed staff positions in the community; ward personnel had to be redeployed to the clinics. Discretionary funds for patients' needs were reallocated to cover the wage increase. The increasing demand on fixed resources made the zero-sum mentality a reality at WSH. As a result, the staff and the patients were brought into more direct competition.

### CONFLICT IN THE HOSPITAL: INTERNALIZING THE LOCUS OF COMPETITION

The job action and the settlement reinforced the staff's ambivalence toward their patients. On the picket line, derogatory comments about patients were mixed with concern for their welfare. Even when not in direct competition for a share of the hospital budget, some staff members perceived many of the patients, especially those unable to successfully hold jobs, as freeloaders on public welfare. Others were angry that some patients were collecting disability and unemployment checks which the staff imagined exceeded their own take-home pay.

The patients in turn complained that staff members refused to help them. Because the staff was protected by Civil Service, patients viewed them as being unsympathetic and lazy. The state hospital provided little reward for initiative, good work, or extra effort. As a result, employees felt justified in not working too hard and in taking days off. Short-staffed, the wards assumed an atmosphere of tension and hostility which resulted in fear and punitive control, rather than understanding and therapeutic limit-setting.

This conflict was most visible in the acute inpatient service at WSH, where both patients and staff were confined in close quarters. On these locked wards, patients were required to ask permission to leave and enter, to smoke, and to get help from the staff. The staff was often short-handed, overburdened with administrative duties, and confined by job descriptions and eight-hour shifts which limited their opportunities to provide direct patient care. They tried to respond to the continuous demands of the disturbed patients and to the dangerous outbursts that occasionally erupted, but the needs of many patients went unmet. The patients, too, were endangered and frightened by the disturbed behavior of their fellow inmates. Patients and staff were surrounded by craziness in a confined, tense environment.

On November 27, 1976 the tension exploded into manifest conflict. Six patients at Worcester State Hospital signed the following statement:

We, the undersigned patients of 4E, are being abused by W.H. on the 2:30–11 shift. We would like the hospital administration to investigate the matter with private interviews of the people signed below and to be kept in confidence. We cannot cope with this situation anymore and are terrified of the situation. We would like immediate action taken for the safety of ourselves and others on the ward.

The next morning, the following incident report was filed by the nursing supervisor.

Patient concerned: Mr. R.M.
Employees: W.H., S.T., M.G.

Mrs. M.G. stated that several patients were upset because of the abusive behavior by the above employees toward Mr. R.M. on the 2:30–11:00 shift, Saturday, 11-27-76. Patients A.P. and C.O. were upset, they were afraid to put it in writing because of what might happen to them for telling. Mr. A.P. finally stated he would write it up. I called Mrs. L.H., LPN who also listened to the report Mrs. M.G. gave me. Later I spoke with Mr. R.M., but he was unable to give me any report as to what happened to him. He appeared fearful, started to cry, but could not express himself, so as to be understood, I later reported the incident to Mr. P.G., R.N., Supervisor.

These allegations of abuse led to investigations by the State Police and by a "Committee to Study Patient Abuse at Worcester State Hospital," composed of hospital staff, Department of Mental Health representatives, and Worcester community leaders. The Report of the Committee (1977) documented 48 incidents of alleged violence or neglect in the hospital during 1976. Twenty one of these incidents record violence by patients or visitors against property, staff, or other individuals. Most of these episodes occurred on the busier admission wards where staff coverage had been reduced by reallocation of personnel to community clinics. The Committee's Report (1977) stated, in part:

With respect to our more general study of patient abuse, we categorized incidents of "patient abuse" as follows:

1) "malicious abuse" in which the abuse derives from specific motivations or intents to do harm to a patient;

2) "reckless abuse" in which abuse occurs from not taking proper and appropriate precautions to protect patients; and

3) "institutional abuse" in which patients are abused or neglected due to the way in which the institution is staffed, financed, or administered.

The individuals with whom we spoke strongly argued that institutional abuse tends to induce tension, anxiety, and irritability in staff members and thereby facilitates the occurrence of both reckless and malicious abuse.

The major patient abuse problems at Worcester State Hospital seem to involve institutional abuse, rather than reckless or malicious abuse. The primary sources of institutional abuse that we have encountered are:

1) Seriously imbalanced staffing pattern across shifts and across wards.

2) A serious imbalance of professional activities and scheduled patient programs across shifts.

3) Insufficient training of ward staff; and

4) Budgeting deficiencies.

The District Attorney for Worcester brought no indictments in the case because blame could not be individualized. However, it was clear that conflict between patients and staff at WSH was a serious problem, rooted in the conditions produced by resource scarcity and societal neglect.[4]

## CONFLICT IN THE COMMUNITY: DISPLACING THE LOCUS OF COMPETITION

As described earlier, the tension within WSH mirrors the resource scarcity and zero-sum market mentality which are fundamental features of the larger society. Therefore, it is not surprising that latent conflict and similar manifestations and responses to this conflict are found in the community-based system of mental health care and human services.

If highly routinized behavior control (along with boredom, nonproductivity, and dependence) are the hallmarks of the total institution, then the deinstitutionalized mental patient may still be a prisoner in "a total institution without walls" (Beck, 1979; GAP, 1978). Reports on the fates of deinstitutionalized patients testify to the poor quality of life they encounter outside hospital boundaries (Arnhoff, 1975; GAO, 1977; GAP, 1978). Although the invisibility of the walls may enhance the patient's feeling of freedom and independence, other constraints help to maintain a kind of institutionalized social control over the patient—social sanctions, dependence on welfare, medication checks, and other aftercare regimens. For better or for worse, some discharged patients in the community completely escape the formal fetters of the state mental hospital. Others sacrifice *asylum* for freedom, only to fall victim to the "street" or some other institution such as the criminal justice system. However, many others are caught in a new coercive system composed of community mental health institutions.

At WSH, patients discharged prior to the expiration date of their civil commitment (permitted by Massachusetts Law, Chapter 123) may be returned to the hospital involuntarily, at the discretion of a clinician or the police. Similarly, criminally committed individuals may be released into outpatient treatment as a condition of parole. Those patients who are not committed to the hospital may be required by a judge to live in a "less restrictive" alternative, to take medication, and to visit an aftercare clinic in the community. If they do not take their medication regularly, they may receive a "depot" injection of antipsychotic medication which will last for several weeks. In many cases, these measures may benefit both the patient and society, but they are not without an element of coercion.

For the patient receiving welfare and Supplemental Security Income (SSI), deinstitutionalization means dependence on inadequate resources, often resulting in confinement to one room in the poorest section of town or to a nursing facility or a board-and-care home. This new living arrangement has been described by many as "reinstitutionalization" and as a "new custodialism" (Frankfather, 1974)—a move from "back wards to back alleys" (Borus, 1978). Welfare dependency also means compliance with regulations, just as discharge means compliance with aftercare. As noted by Beck (1979), deinstitutionalization has not freed the mentally ill from the control of repressive institutions; the "anarchist sentiment" of the community mental health ideology is an illusion.

Conflict is characteristic of the interaction of the patient with the community and the staff of various health and social welfare agencies. Much of the conflict is similar to the tension described within the hospital. The staff in the community mental health clinics are often less interested in the problems of deinstitutionalized chronic mental patients than in the more acute problems of other residents in their catchment area. As a result staff are unwilling to devote their energies to the persistent problems of deinstitutionalized patients. In Worcester the staff in the community clinics are often the same individuals who worked (or continued to work) on the inpatient wards. As a result the clinic patient falls victim to many of the same prejudices previously experienced on the wards. Clinic staff still complain about "lazy patients" taking advantage of welfare. Attendants and nurses still compare their low salaries with the benefits and life-style of some patients on SSI. Staff still seek to control the behavior of discharged patients while subtly competing with them for public resources. Surely not all of the conflict between patients and staff in the community results from competition for scarce resources. One cannot dismiss this source of tension in the community niche, however.

Beyond the boundaries of the institution, competition for limited resources is not confined to patients and staff or even to patients and other individuals in the community. The community mental health system itself may be in competition with the hospital.

## COMPETITION BETWEEN HOSPITAL AND COMMUNITY

The National Association of State Mental Health Program Directors (1979) has called attention to the competition between hospital and community-based programs for a share of the state mental health budget. The closing of Gardner State Hospital, a sister institution to the north of WSH, was necessitated because the limited state appropriation could not support both an institution and a network of community services (Sills, 1975). Like many other states, Massachusetts has a single legislative appropriation to cover both institutional and community-based mental health programs. In some states mental health appropriations expanded to fund community services; in others, the institutional budgets were trimmed to pay for the community programs. In Worcester, the state hospital and the community satellite clinics shared the same budget, administered by the WSH Superintendant, who was also the acting Director of the Greater Worcester Mental Health Area. The budget remained fixed at approximately $10 million per year between 1974 and 1976, a period of inflation and program expansion. In a sense, WSH was victimized by its own innovation. As an early pioneer in community aftercare, WSH had demonstrated the viability of a hospital-sponsored system of satellite clinics in the community, funded out of a single institutional appropriation (Milbank, 1962). With fiscal retrenchment, however, this service network shifted from complementarity to competition.

A freeze on the hiring of new staff resulted in the need for existing professional staff to divide their time between WSH and the clinics. The wards were already depleted of energetic, well-trained staff who were the first to be offered full-time community clinic placements. The inability of the WSH to replace its ward staff was blamed in part for the incidents of patient abuse described earlier. Ward staff complained that the hospitalized patients were neglected by physicians and social workers who were assigned to the community clinics. The clinics, too, were overcrowded and understaffed. Both systems suffered from the scarcity of resources.

Unlike Gardner State Hospital, which was forced to close as a result of competition for scarce resources, WSH endured in a state of competitive coexistence with its community programs. The two systems were able to achieve a measure of cooperation in the Greater Worcester Area only because the hospital and the community clinic staff were the same or had previously worked together. Nevertheless, competition between the two systems took its toll on the quality of both service systems; it stretched adaptive reserves and divided the loyalties of those staff who moved between the hospital and the community. Hampered by scarce resources, WSH and its institutional and community staff struggled to provide continuity of care for their patients.

Discharged patients were considered "hospital patients." As one of the WSH psychiatrists, then working in a community clinic, is alleged to have said: "They are all Worcester State Hospital patients; we just loan them to the community from time to time." Perhaps the identification of these patients with the institution, held in common by the ward staff and the clinic staff, accounted for the comparatively peaceful coexistence between systems in the Greater Worcester area. Each element of the system was familiar with the operation of the other; everyone knew everyone else. However, the identification with WSH may have also led to the continued "institutionalization" of these patients in the community. Rather than freeing patients from the institution, deinstitutionalization expanded the boundaries of WSH to include the patients and staff, hospital programs, and community programs in a complex socio-ecological niche.

## IMPLICATIONS

Mutual dependence on scarce resources produced division and tension within the WSH ecosystem. External environmental conditions were reflected in the structure of the system and in the relationships among groups within that system. At WSH, staff and patients operated within the boundaries of an institutional system characterized by conflict, competition, and coexistence.

Although this chapter has focused on WSH, there is no reason to assume that these phenomena are unique to this particular setting. Because conditions of scarcity have plagued state mental hospitals for 150 years, it is reasonable to generalize the WSH experience.

Resource scarcity brings to the surface the competitive nature of relationships within the mental hospital. Competition is a pervasive value in our social system, and competition gives rise to conflict. The state heightens the perception of competition when it weighs employee salaries against services for current patients or welfare assistance to former patients. Both staff and patients are deprived, but they blame each other rather than the state, which has imposed the scarcities. Administrators, policymakers, and budget-cutters tend to see state employees and the indigent as marginal groups in society. They are the first to have their incomes "stabilized" and their benefits curtailed when resources are limited.

Most hospital employees are poorly paid servants of the state who must work at the difficult task of caring for indigent mental patients. Attendants and patients, as well as some nurses and social workers, come from the same background; they have been neighbors, friends, and classmates. Nursing and attendant staff often know the history of the individual patients and their families. They share a similar sociocultural heritage and value system. This social and experiential closeness between the nonprofessionl ward staff and the patients is both a potential asset and a problem. While it contributes to the perspective of the more distant medical staff and offers a potential for therapeutic understanding, it is also a source of conflict. In a competitive and hierarchal society, the class struggle is most intense between groups that are close together in the social hierarchy (Davis et al., 1941). The attendants are clinging tenaciously to the social ladder only a rung above many of the patients.

The situation has been made worse and more obvious by recent

fiscal policy in many states. The strike at WSH illustrates how patients and staff have been drawn into direct competition for tax dollars. Tension increases, and mental hospitals are at times like
ethnically mixed neighborhoods during economic, political, and
social upheaval, in which groups close together in the social hierarchy are placed in a competitive environment created by a shared
problem.

Within the hospital, competition for scarce resources is inter-
nalized on the wards as conflict between patients and staff. Mutually dependent, patients and staff are "locked" into the state mental
hospital, actually and figuratively. They are in conflict, competing
not only for financial resources but also for time, security, and liberty. Occasionally the conflict manifests itself as violence, as documented by the allegations of patient abuse at WSH. More
commonly, the conflict is latent, taking the form of competitive coexistence, neglect, and "institutional abuse." Under these conditions, the ward as niche is partitioned. The patients, locked into the
"day room," are separated by unbreakable glass from the staff, seeking "asylum" in the nursing station or staff coffee room. This partition is symbolic of the division and conflict within the mental
hospital, described by Bateson and Goffman (1961) as a "binary institution."

In addition to the binary split between patients and staff, further investigation reveals other divisions within the mental hospital. Focusing on the balance of power between all competing
groups within the mental hospital, Strauss and his colleagues
(1964) described the "negotiated order" of such institutions. Consistent with that perspective, this chapter has also examined tensions between hospital employees and the administration, and
between professionals and nonprofessionals. The strike at Worcester State Hospital was a manifestation of the conflict between employees and administration under conditions of limited resources.
The job action also revealed tensions between striking nonprofessionals and the professionals, who continued to work. Division and
hierarchy characterize the public mental hospital, surviving in a
status of competitive coexistence between patients and staff, professionals and nonprofessionals, employees and the administration.

Nonetheless, as noted previously, competitive coexistence is
not the only possible resolution of the Principle of Competitive Exclusion. Extinction, displacement, and cooperation are all potential
alternatives to competition. Extinction is a difficult solution to en-
vision in this example of competitive exclusion.[5] However, Worces-

ter's "total institution without walls" and the competition between hospital and community programs both illustrate displacement. In addition, the relationship between the hospital and the community also demonstrates the potential for cooperation between groups limited by common resources.

Deinstitutionalization and the dissolution of the niche is a variant of displacement in the context of the mental hospital. Displacement of only one species occurs rarely when there is a high degree of functional interdependence. When patients are released into the community, the staff often follows, taking positions in the community mental health system. Thus, deinstitutionalization may be a form of mutual displacement, in which the locus of interaction and potential conflict is moved into the community. The niche is not destroyed, only displaced.

Cooperation between competing groups within the Worcester niche falls short of "cultural despeciation." Although there was some recognition of interdependence, there was never a fundamental transformation in values and behavior. In spite of initial efforts at cooperation, tension continued to characterize the relationship between patients and staff, between hospital and community. In the absence of "cultural despeciation," social groups within the Worcester ecosystem have adapted to resource uncertainty and to the policy of deinstitutionalization by creating new programs and developing cooperative relationships with various community institutions.

## NOTES

1. This is a reconstruction of a conversation that I had with David J. Myerson, late in 1976, when he was Superintendent of Worcester State Hospital and I was a psychiatric resident.
2. The failure of "negotiated order theory" to address the relationship of the mental hospital to the larger social environment has been noted by Day and Day (1977). One exception to this critique is a case history of a state mental hospital by Fowlkes (1975), which views the institution in its societal context. Another exception is a study of Boston State Hospital by Schulberg, Caplan, and Greenblatt (1968).
3. This chapter is an expansion of an earlier paper (Goldman, 1977) which analyzes conflict between patients and staff at Worcester State Hospital as a social analogy to Gause's Principle of Competitive Exclusion.
4. In a separate study of ethics and psychiatry in the state mental hospital, Murray (1979), a former Worcester State Hospital psychiatrist, independently came to

the same conclusion. In that paper Dr. Murray generalized his experiences in Worcester to other public mental hospitals.

5. Extinction could take the form of the elimination of the mentally ill by the staff, as was attempted in Nazi Germany; or the elimination of the staff by the patients, as in completely patient-operated residential therapeutic community. These solutions fundamentally destroy the concept of the mental hospital. Mutual extinction through the elimination of mental illness would also involve the dissolution of the niche and require the reincorporation of former patients and staff into society.

Eric D. Lister
Jeffrey L. Geller

# 6
# Crossing Organizational Boundaries: Pretrial Commitment for Psychiatric Evaluation

The preceeding chapters have amply documented the fact that the use of the term "hospital" with reference to state mental institutions is only a half-truth. Throughout their history in this country, institutions such as Worcester State Hospital (WSH) have served social control and therapeutic functions: sequestering or segregating deviants as well as treating the mentally ill. While the relative emphasis on each function may have shifted at different points during the past 150 years, the enduring organizational character of these institutions has been conditioned, in large part, by this duality of purpose.

State mental hospitals and their social history were foreign to us, however, when as psychiatric residents from Boston's Beth Israel Hospital we first arrived at WSH for a six-month rotation. Our training and clinical experiences in that small teaching hospital had been in psychoanalytically oriented psychiatry. The second-year rotation at a long-term psychiatric facility was designed to expose Beth Israel's trainees to a patient population and a system of organization different from that encountered on a typical psychiatric unit in a general hospital. We choose WSH because of our inter-

This chapter expands upon our article "The process of criminal commitment for Pretrial examination: An evaluation," Am J Psychiatry 135:53–60, 1978. ©American Journal of Psychiatry, with permission of the editor.

est in learning about public sector psychiatry and because of its reputation as one of the leading state hospitals in Massachusetts.

Much of our time was spent caring for hospitalized patients, many of whom had been sent to WSH by the courts for a determination of their competency to stand trial. Most of these patients had been charged with very minor crimes and several, in fact, had no charges pending against them whatsoever. In addition, few wanted to be at WSH. In carrying out treatment responsibilities for these patients, we functioned in an interface between the mental health and criminal justice systems. Our role remained confused and ambiguous no matter how scrupulously we tried to define it. Were we to serve as "the patient's physician," as set forth in the Hippocratic tradition, or were we to serve as examiners for the court? And, subject to the vicissitudes of a patient's hospitalization, how were we to tell which role to play at what time? As de facto officers of the court, we were involved in a process that was not completely open to outside review.

Out of these feelings of frustration and confusion grew our desire to study the process of criminal commitment and pretrial psychiatric examination at WSH.


## BACKGROUND

In 1971, in an attempt to rectify the misuse of civil and criminal comitment and to safeguard the civil rights of the individuals involved, the legislature of the Commonwealth of Massachusetts passed on an act revising the laws regarding the admission, treatment, and discharge of mentally ill and mentally retarded persons. Prior to these revisions, a person "likely to conduct himself in a manner which clearly violates the established laws, ordinances, conventions or morals of the community" was considered mentally ill (Miller, 1976: 13) and commitable to a Massachusetts state mental institution. Those statutory provisions allowed judges to authorize commitment for irritating, troublesome people in the community without clear, consistent legal or medical guidelines. Furthermore, these commitments were not limited in chronological extent, and the nature of the requested psychiatric intervention was ill-defined.

In contrast, among its multiple provisions, the revised statute encouraged voluntary admission to state mental hospitals, spelled out the civil liberties of the mentally ill during hospitalization, authorized commitments by qualified physicians only on the basis of the person's likelihood of serious harm" to self or others, and ended indefinite commitments by limiting court commitments to specific periods (Bayle, 1971).

We were particularly concerned with Section 15 of the revised law, which dealt with criminal commitment for pretrial psychiatric evaluation. Section 15(a) stated that, at the discretion of the court, alleged offenders might be examined at the jail or courthouse by a forensically qualified psychiatrist. This examination might be requested by the judge, by the prosecuting or defense attorney, or by the accused. At the Worcester Central District Court, the purposes of this examination were posted on the desk where examining psychiatrists wrote their reports:

> Attention Psychiatrists—There is a question of his competency to stand trial and his criminal responsibility at the time of the alleged crimes. (The above must be put in your statement upon examination of patients).

On the basis of this examination, Section 15(b) of the law allowed the judge either to bring the alleged offender to trial or to order commitment to WSH for further examination (unless strict security was required, in which case the offender was sent to Bridgewater State Hospital) for a period not to exceed 20 days, with the possibility of one 20-day extension.

During the commitment period, WSH psychiatrists were required to examine the alleged offender in depth, and to evaluate the following: (1) the presence of mental illness, defined by the law as "a substantial disorder of thought, mood, perception, orientation, or memory, which grossly impairs judgement, behaviors, capacity to recognize reality or ability to meet the ordinary demands of life, but shall not include alcoholism" (MDMH, 1971:59); (2) whether or not the defendant is competent to stand trial; (3) whether or not the defendant is criminally responsible; and (4) recommendations to the court for treatment. These recommendations might include "no further treatment," "outpatient treatment," "voluntary inpatient treatment," or "commitment." These evaluations were recorded on a standard form which was then returned to the court.

The research we undertook at WSH was directed at determining (1) whether the new law had any effect (e.g., an increase or decrease) on the number of patients committed to WSH for pretrial evaluations; (2) the characteristics of the alleged offenders (e.g., social demographics, psychiatric history, and pending charges) and their journey through the legal–psychiatric system (e.g., outcomes

at the points of precommitment examination, commitment evaluation, and disposition upon return to the court); and the extent to
which examining psychiatrists at the court, as well as judges, com-
prehended their tasks and responsibilities in these proceedings. In
so doing we hoped to document and understand the delicate balance between clinical needs of the patients, their legal rights, and
community pressure for social control.

## METHODS

To evaluate the impact of the new law on the number of pretrial commitments to WSH, statistical information was compiled
from hospital records on the number of admissions, the number of
civil commitments, and the number of pretrial commitments to
WSH during the 10-year period 1966–1975. The data from these
years bracketed the effective date of the new law (November 1,
1971) and allowed for a trend analysis of pretrial commitments relative to other admissions.

To determine characteristics and careers of alleged offenders,
all individuals committed to WSH under pretrial status between
January 1 and December 31, 1975 were identified. A retrospective
cohort designation method was chosen to insure the availability of
pertinent information on alleged offenders at each stage of their career, from initial examination through final court disposition. The
resultant study group was composed of 80 persons with a total of
87 commitments (4 persons had been committed twice and 1 person had been committed 4 times). These legal proceedings were initiated by 16 courts: 3 in the city of Worcester and 13 in outlying
towns of the WSH service region. The Worcester courts accounted
for 45 (52 percent) of these commitments and the other courts accounted for the 42 (48 percent) remaining cases. Information on
each commitment was abstracted from the medical records at WSH
which contain data on social background and psychiatric history,
as well as from copies of the report filed by the examining psychiatrist at the court, legal charges, and the results of the WSH commitment evaluation. The final court disposition was obtained
directly from court records.

Finally, to determine the understanding of precommitment
procedures by the examining psychiatrists and judges, questionnaires were mailed to the 24 physicians who had written the 69
precommitment evaluations [Section 15(a)] for our study group. (18
of the 87 commitments had been sent to WSH without such evalu-

ations.) Separate questionnaires were sent to the 24 judges who signed any of the commitment papers on the 80 persons composing the study group. The questionnaire sent to psychiatrists included a checklist of factors influencing their recommendations for commitment under Section 15(b). Similarly, judges were asked which factors influenced their decision to proceed with commitment for pretrial evaluation under Section 15(b).

## TRENDS IN PRETRIAL COMMITMENT

One reason that Massachusetts laws were revised was to define more stringently the criteria for civil and criminal commitments and to "voluntarize" the state hospital admissions process. The data, however, indicate that the new law did not have a uniform or stable long-term impact on total admissions, civil commitments, or pretrial commitments to WSH (Table 1).

Following the implementation of the new law, annual admissions to WSH decreased significantly. For the six years prior to its implementation (1966–1971), annual admissions averaged about 1,138, while in the four years after its enactment (1972–1975), admissions averaged only 813, or 325 (29 percent) fewer. The 10-year trend reveals a cyclical pattern indicating that admissions began their decline prior to the new law and that the decline after its enactment was not sustained.

The total number of admissions reached their peak during 1968 (1,403), declined slightly during 1969 (by 7 percent), and then dropped abruptly during 1970 (by 28 percent). In 1971, however, admissions increased by 113 (12 percent). During 1972—the first full year under the new law—admissions again dropped sharply (by 27 percent). Admissions for the next three years, however, repeat this cyclical pattern: an *increase* in 1973 (by 6 percent), a *decrease* in 1974 (12 percent), and an *increase* in 1975 (by 25 percent).

Overall, these data suggests that the short-run effect of the new law did decrease WSH admissions, but that in the longer run admissions were approaching their prechange levels once again.

During the same 10-year period the number of *civil* commitments to WSH decreased significantly. Although the initial decline in these commitments predated this legislation, the single largest annual decrease (266, 72 percent) occurred between 1971 and 1972, the first full year the new law was in effect. For the six years prior to its implementation (1966–1971), civil commitments averaged

**Table 1**
Admission Statistics for Worcester State Hospital, 1966–1975

| Year | Total Number of Admissions* | Number of Civil Commitments** | Number of Pretrial Commitments*** | Proportions | | |
| --- | --- | --- | --- | --- | --- | --- |
| | | | | Civil Commitments: Total Admissions | Pretrial Commitments: Total Admissions | Pretrial Commitments: Civil Commitments |
| 1966 | 1,012 | 712 | 54 | .703 | .053 | .076 |
| 1967 | 1,094 | 648 | 59 | .592 | .054 | .091 |
| 1968 | 1,403 | 611 | 85 | .435 | .061 | .139 |
| 1969 | 1,309 | 607 | 95 | .464 | .073 | .157 |
| 1970 | 949 | 434 | 89 | .457 | .094 | .205 |
| 1971 | 1,062 | 370 | 92 | .348 | .087 | .249 |
| 1972 | 779 | 104 | 53 | .134 | .068 | .510 |
| 1973 | 827 | 104 | 45 | .126 | .054 | .433 |
| 1974 | 730 | 95 | 62 | .130 | .085 | .653 |
| 1975 | 916 | 106 | 87 | .116 | .095 | .821 |

*The number of admissions per year in 1966–1971 was significantly higher than that in 1972–1975 ($p<.01$ by two-tailed t test).

**The number of civil commitments per year in 1966–1971 was significantly higher than that in 1972–1975 ($p<.001$ by two-tailed t test).

***There was no significant difference between the number of pretrial commitments per year in 1966–1971 and that in 1972–1975.
Adapted from Geller and Lister (1978:57).

about 564 per year, while in the four years following its enactment (1972–1975) these commitments averaged about 102 per year, or 462 (82 percent) fewer. Thus, these data offer impressive evidence of the increased "voluntarization" of the admissions process at WSH subsequent to the effective date of the new law. (Also note Table 1, which shows that the percentage of civil commitments to total admissions declined from 70 percent in 1966 to 13 percent in 1972, and then remained relatively constant at 12–13 percent for 1973–1975).

The trend for *pretrial* commitments however, was nearly the exact opposite of the trend for civil commitments. There was no significant difference between the number of pretrial commitments per year during the period 1966–1971 and the number per year in 1972–1975 (79 vs 62, respectively). Also, the annual proportion of pretrial commitments to total admissions in 1975 (0.095) was virtually identical to that in 1971 (0.087).

Despite the downward trend in civil commitments, the proportion of pretrial commitments sharply increased over the 10-year period. Moreover, the new law led to an acceleration in the ratio of pretrial commitments compared to civil commitments, as indicated by the 100-percent increase between 1971 and 1972 (0.249 vs 0.510, respectively) and by the fact that pretrial commitments accounted for 82 percent of the total commitments to WSH in 1975.

Taken together, these trends suggest that the new law had a differential impact on the legal status of WSH's admissions. While the new law initially led to a sharp decrease in total admissions, by 1975 these figures had crept back nearly to their prechange levels (in cycles). The new law did substantially reduce the number of civil (i.e., nonjudicial) commitments and, in this sense, it was successful in "voluntarizing" the WSH admissions process. However, the initial drop in the use of pretrial (i.e., judicial) commitments following the new law was not sustained, and these procedures accounted for the bulk of WSH's involuntary admissions by 1975.

## CHARACTERISTICS AND CAREERS OF PERSONS COMMITTED ON PRETRIAL STATUS

### Social Demographics

Of the 80 individuals committed to WSH under pretrial status in 1975, 65 (81 percent) were men and 15 (19 percent) were women. The average age of the patients was 30.5 years, with a range of 14–67.

Of the 19 patients 21 years old and younger, 8 were from single-parent families, 3 were from foster homes, 1 was adopted and living with both adoptive parents, 1 was living with both natural parents, and the family status of 6 was unknown. Of the 61 patients over age 21, 27 were single, 14 were divorced, 8 were separated, 7 were married, and the marital status of 5 was unknown.

### Prior Psychiatric Hospitalizations

The mean number of previous psychiatric hospitalizations for the 80 individuals was 2.7. Of the total group 24 (30 percent) had no history of prior psychiatric hospitalizations and 56 (70 percent) had one or more. Of the latter subgroup, 6 (8 percent of the total sample) had 10 or more admissions and 37 had been in WSH at least once.

### Charges

According to the law, an individual can only enter the system by being placed in custody by the police and having charges formally filed. In our sample, 4 minors and 4 adults arrived at WSH with no formal charges filed against them. In other words, in 8 of 87 commitment procedures (9 percent) patients were sent for pretrial commitment with no criminal charges pending. One hundred and seven counts were filed in the 79 remaining commitment procedures. Seventy-four of these counts (69 percent) were for misdemeanors, and 33 (31 percent) were for felonies. In 57 commitments, misdemeanors were the only charges filed; in 14, felonies were the only charges filed; and in 8 commitments, both misdemeanors and felonies were filed. "Disturbing the peace" was the only charge filed in 26 commitments (30 percent of the total number of commitments).

### Precommitment Examination [Section 15(a)]

The law requires that the arrested individual first be evaluated by a forensically qualified psychiatrist, as described above. However, 18 (20 percent) of the 87 commitments involved patients who arrived at WSH with no written report from the court psychiatrist. This occurred when either the court psychiatrist communicated verbally with the judge or a report was to follow (it rarely did).

Although questions of competency and criminal responsibility are specifically posed, 45 of the reports (65 percent) made no mention of competency, and 64 (93 percent) made no mention of criminal responsibility. Although questions regarding dangerousness and the need for treatment are not asked, 38 reports (55 percent) labeled the individual as dangerous, and 16 (23 percent) stated that the individual needed treatment (Graph 1).

## Psychiatric Status and Length of Hospitalization

On admission, 56 of the 87 committed persons (64 percent) were diagnosed as psychotic, and 7 (8 percent) received no diagnosis.

Patients were committed for 20 days, with the possibility of one 20-day extension. A patient, however, might be returned to the court earlier if the facility's report was written and the court was willing to hear the case. For our study group, 16 reports (18 percent) were written within 10 days of the patient's hospitalization, 42 more (48 percent) were written before the 20-day limit, and 21 (34 percent) were written afterwards.

Once hospitalized, individuals might legally remain at WSH beyond the period of commitment if the patient signed himself or herself into the hospital as a voluntary admission; if charges were dropped and a civil commitment was issued by the court; or if the patient was judged either incompetent to stand trial or not guilty by reason of mental illness and subsequently committed.

Although 58 reports (67 percent) were written within the requisite 20 days, only 31 cases (36 percent) were discharged from WSH in that period of time. As of January 31, 1976, the median length of stay for the 56 remaining cases (64 percent) was approximately 38 days, with a range of 21 to over 200 days (Table 2).

Of the 56 patients remaining longer than 20 days, 40 had been psychotic on admission, 14 had been nonpsychotic on admission, and 2 had been undiagnosed at the time of admission. Thus 71 percent of patients who were diagnosed as psychotic on admission and 58 percent of patients who were given a nonpsychotic diagnosis when admitted remained in WSH for more than 20 days.

## Commitment Evaluation [Section 15(b)]

The report to the court written by the WSH psychiatrist in charge of a particular patient's case is meant to address the four questions of mental illness, competency, criminal responsibility, and treatment (Graph 2). WSH psychiatrists evaluated 56 cases (67

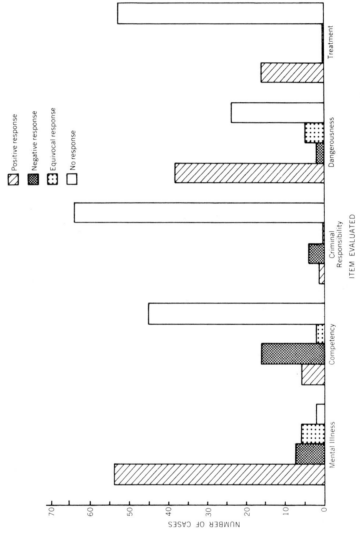

Graph 1. Results of 69 precommitment evaluations of 87 cases of pretrial commitment to Worcester State Hospital.

**Table 2**
Number of Consecutive Days in the Hospital Following
87 Cases of Pretrial Commitment to Worcester State
Hospital as of January 31, 1976

| Number of Days | Number of Cases |
| --- | --- |
| 1–5 | 2 |
| 6–10 | 3 |
| 11–15 | 9 |
| 16–20 | 17 |
| 21–25 | 16 |
| 26–30 | 2 |
| 31–35 | 4 |
| 36–40 | 6 |
| 41–50 | 9 |
| 51–60 | 9 |
| 61–70 | 2 |
| 71–80 | 2 |
| 81–100 | 1 |
| 101–200 | 3 |
| More than 200 | 2 |

percent) as mentally ill, 23 cases (27 percent) as incompetent, 19 cases (23 percent) as criminally responsible, and 52 cases (62 percent) as needing treatment.[1] Of the latter cases, commitment was recommended in 19 reports (37 percent), voluntary inpatient treatment in 20 reports (38 percent), and outpatient treatment in 13 reports (25 percent).

## Court Dispositions

As of November 1, 1976, a record of court dispositions was available for 83 cases (Table 3). When there was more than one count pending in a case, and therefore more than one judicial finding, the disposition for the most severe charge was recorded.

The data indicated that 60 of the 83 cases (72 percent) were dismissed by the court. Of the 23 remaining cases, 14 were found guilty as charged, 2 were found not guilty, 2 were committed, and 5 had their cases filed or continued.

In the 19 cases where WSH psychiatrists requested commitment for involuntary treatment, 11 commitments were granted, 3 were denied, 4 were deferred when patients admitted themselves voluntarily, and one patient escaped. Where voluntary inpatient

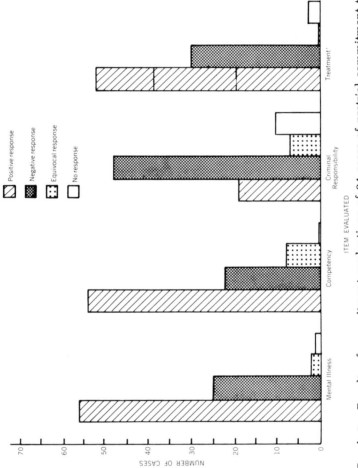

Graph 2. Results of commitment evaluations of 84 cases of pretrial commitment to Worcester State Hospital. (*Commitment was recommended in 19 reports, voluntary inpatient treatment in 20, and outpatient treatment in 13.)

154

**Table 3**
Disposition by the Court of 83 Cases of Pretrial
Commitment

| Disposition | Number of Cases |
| --- | --- |
| Case dismissed | 60 |
| Case continued | 4 |
| Case filed | 1 |
| Found not guilty | 2 |
| Found guilty | |
| Suspended sentence | 2 |
| Probation | 4 |
| Jail sentence | 2 |
| Fine | 1 |
| Monetary restitution | 2 |
| Sentence unknown | 3 |
| Total | 14 |
| Committed to a mental hospital after a finding of "incompetency to stand trial or not guilty by reason of insanity" | 2 |

treatment was suggested (20 cases), 12 patients returned on voluntary admissions. Two of the remaining 8 patients were readmitted within one month under the emergency detention provision of the statute (Section 12).

## DECISION CRITERIA EMPLOYED BY PSYCHIATRISTS AND JUDGES

Responses to questionnaires about decision criteria were received from 16 (67 percent) of the 24 physicians who conducted precommitment evaluations of the patients in the study cohort. These 16 physicians performed 87 percent of the Section 15(a) evaluations. Only 3 of these physicians, accounting for 5 precommitment evaluations, were on the staff of WSH. Respondents, then, accounted for the bulk of the precommitment evaluations and revealed little overlap with the WSH physician population who wrote reports to the court under Section 15(b). Of the 14 judges responding (58 percent), only 10 returned fully completed questionnaires. Responding judges accounted for 62 percent of committed patients, and included judges of the Worcester City and outlying courts.

Two of the 16 physicians indicated they were not psychiatrists and a third, who is a psychiatrist, indicated that a psychologist on his staff actually did the examination on forms carrying the psychiatrist's signature. The responses obtained from the other 13 psychiatrists, who had an average of 19.5 years in psychiatric practice, indicated that many did not understand their designated task under the new commitment law. For example, on the checklist of factors influencing their commitment recommendations, 9 (69 percent) listed need for treatment and 5 (38 percent) listed past history of psychiatric hospitalization as more important than the consideration of criminal responsibility. The recommendation for 15(b) commitment apparently followed from an impressionistic sense of the patient's pathology or a feeling of clinical expediency. The most relevant specifics—competency and responsibility—were often given little or no attention.

Although the evaluation done under Section 15(a) were submitted to the presiding judge, the questions to be answered by this examination were generally not addressed. The judge then had to decide whether to send the accused to WSH under the authority of Section 15(b) for determination of competency/criminal responsibility. From the information supplied by the 14 judges who responded to our inquiry, it became clear that there was significant disagreement as to the criteria for such commitments. For instance, several judges indicated an automatic compliance with the recommendation of the court psychiatrist as expressed in the result of the Section 15(a) examination; others did not. Five judges listed suspicion of dangerousness as a key criteria for Section 15(b) commitment; others did not list it at all. Finally, several judges listed "need for treatment" as a key factor in decision making; others did not rank this factor at all.

### DISCUSSION

The revision of Massachusetts law that took effect in 1971 was designed to encourage voluntary admissions and to control and make explicit the process of judicial commitments to state mental hospitals. According to the WSH data presented in this chapter, these intentions met with only mixed success. The findings clearly indicate that several problems, such as indeterminate confinements and an over-reliance on civil commitment, had been effectively addressed. Moreover, as reported by Morrissey et al. (1979), these legal changes also allowed WSH staff to exercise much more discretion over the appropriateness of voluntary admissions, thereby reducing the number of alcoholic, senile, and medical cases that heretofore would have been routinely admitted to WSH (also see Chapter 4).

Other problems, however, have come more sharply into focus under the provisions of this legislation. In particular, the findings indicate that pretrial commitments for psychiatric evaluation at WSH now account for the bulk of involuntary hospitalizations. In commenting on our original publication of these findings, Stone (1978:62) suggests that these results illustrate the "balloon theory" of incarceration:

> Essentially, the idea is that there is a relatively stable volume of persons who will be confined in any industrial society. If one form of confinement is reduced, another expands. One corollary of this general thesis is that, since civil commitment has been reduced, commitment by the criminal courts will increase.

The individuals in this study who were committed for pretrial evaluation were usually isolated, resourceless, and otherwise disenfranchised. Although these persons were sent to WSH for evaluation of competency and/or criminal responsibility, only 2 of the 87 cases resulted in commitment on these grounds. In the light of this fact, serious attention should be paid to arguments that pretrial commitment—in practice if not in principle—serves to control and sequester deviants.

Procedures for law enforcement in the streets often appear "not determined by legal mandates but are, instead, responses to certain demand conditions" (Bittner, 1967:714). In fact, Stone (1978:62) argues that ". . . the major element in the continuing abuse of competency to stand trial is the discretionary practices of the judiciary." In this study, the judges recognized that many of the individuals who appeared before them with inadequately completed Section 15(a) evaluations could benefit from psychiatric treatment. A significant subpopulation manifested clear symptoms of mental illness. In the face of an overwhelming volume of difficult cases, the judges may order a commitment so that an individual who has been perceived by both the court psychiatrist and the judge as "needing treatment" can be the beneficiary of WSH services.

A marked discrepancy remains between the law as written and its practice. Saran et al. (1978:873) report that, in Vermont as well, pretrial commitment is often ". . . a means for the court to seek more appropriate dispositions . . ." Good intentions and over-crowded conditions, however, should not excuse a tacit social policy with a pretense of following a legally mandated course. The fact that this population is "deviant" as well as mentally ill should not deprive them of the opportunity for treatment. But in responding to expediency, physicians and judges—perhaps unwittingly—abandon their explicit legal mandate. This kind of expediency, regardless of intent, lends itself all too easily to abuse. Numerous other observers (Shah, 1974; Steadman, 1972; Szasz, 1968) have expressed concern about the potential for coercive abuse and implicit control of social deviants through misapplication of pretrial commitment statutes.

This study also suggests that expediency is often compounded with ignorance. For example, in spite of the ostensible forensic qualifications of examining psychiatrists, and in spite of the explicit directions supplied, the majority of the Section 15(a) evaluations on persons included in this study made no mention of competency or criminal responsibility. However, in nearly 44 percent of the cases, examining psychiatrists did address the issue of dangerousness, even though these judgements are not explicitly requested. The validity of these judgements and the willingness of psychiatrists to offer their unsolicited evaluations must be held suspect considering the well-established facts that there is no clear correlation between psychiatric status and legal dangerousness (Brill and Malzberg, 1962; Guze et al., 1974; Zitrin et al., 1976) and that psychiatrists are poor predictors of dangerousness (Rubin, 1972; Shah, 1975; Wenk, 1972).

These data also suggest that judges hold misconceptions of the legal criteria governing pretrial commitments. Many judges point to dangerousness as a reason for commitment, yet this criteria is nowhere to be found in the law itself. Furthermore, on those infrequent occasions when the psychiatric report indicates the defendant is competent and/or criminally responsible, the judge will often respond to a statement of "need for treatment to avoid the likelihood of serious harm" while ignoring the ascertained judgement of competency. It is difficult to determine how much of the judges' tolerance of psychiatrists' inappropriate performance at the court is due to misunderstandings of the law and how much to judicial use of the process as an entry vehicle to the state hospital system.

In an attempt to address these problems, competency screening protocols have been developed by several groups of investigators

(Lipsitt et al., 1971; McGarry et al., 1973; Robey, 1965). One group, working in Massachusetts under National Institute of Mental Health sponsorship, suggested the following among its conclusion: "Serious abuses of due process in the use of competency procedures in the Massachusetts criminal justice system have been found and largely corrected" (McGarry et al., 1973:5). The data presented here suggest that this conclusion is premature. Although the tools for more precise competency evaluations have become available they have not been adequately utilized.

Moreover, technical improvements in the competency evaluation process alone are unlikely to stem the tide of inappropriate uses of state hospitals by the courts. Following completion of this study, for example, WSH established a court clinic staffed by a senior psychiatric resident, a social worker, a nurse, and several outreach workers The new arrangement improved the quality of the precommitment workups, but it could not be sustained when funds dried up under the twin policies of hospital phasedown and fiscal retrenchment. Conditions have since reverted back to their earlier state and the trend toward increased judicial use of pretrial commitments has continued.

Thus, despite efforts at legal and programmatic reform, WSH continues to serve its historic functions of confining social deviants, many of whom are mentally ill, for sequestration and/or treatment under subtle and not-so-subtle coercion. While many of these individuals are in need of treatment and humane care, the process by which they are now shunted from the courts to the hospital makes open debate unlikely and referendum clearly impossible. As long as the interface between the courts and psychiatry remains hidden from public scrutiny, neither civil libertarian nor therapeutic goals will be fully realized.

## NOTES

1.  The data reported in Figure 2 are based on 84 reports. Three patients never had a written report filed during the evaluation period: 1 person was transferred to Bridgewater State Hospital, 1 minor was placed in a foster home, and 1 patient died while hospitalized.

Lorraine V. Klerman, Andrew E. Murray
Clair M. Schmidt, Kevin J. Howley

# 7
# Expanding Organizational Boundaries: The Woodward Day School

The term *deinstitutionalization* is usually associated with the release of the mentally ill from state hospitals. But at this chapter and others suggest, deinstitutionalization may refer to several processes, diverse populations, and many institutions. Not only can the release of the mentally ill be expedited, but their initial or subsequent admissions can be prevented or delayed by community-based services. Similarly, the mentally retarded, the elderly, and the criminal offender have been "deinstitutionalized" or "decarcerated" (Scull, 1977) from state schools, long-term care facilities, and correctional institutions. In those cases when institutional care is necessary, it now is perceived as including rehabilitation and preparation for community life. Ideally, under such a policy, brief periods of institutional care are followed by discharge into a community system providing continued treatment, rehabilitation, and support.

Deinstitutionalization at Worcester State Hospital (WSH) touched several populations. Significant among them were the elderly and the young. Elderly patients on the wards were sent to nursing homes, and new elderly admissions were limited to those who clearly could benefit from psychiatric treatment. Also affected by the deinstitutionalization policy were children with a variety of mental health-related problems: the retarded, the autistic, and the aggressive, predelinquent or the withdrawn, inadequate adolescent.

WSH had a long history of interest in the mental health problems of children. The Worcester Youth Guidance Center (WYGC),

one of the oldest child guidance centers in the country, had its beginnings in the 1920s as the Mental Health Clinic for Children, an
outpatient service of the state hospital. In 1963 it had been provided with land on the hospital grounds to build its headquarters and
main clinical facility. During the middle 1960s, in collaboration
with the previous WSH superintendent, Dr. Bardwell Flower, the
Center had developed programs for mentally retarded and autistic
children whose objective was to prevent their institutionalization.
In 1970, the WYGC in collaboration with the state hospital and the
Worcester Public Schools undertook a program aimed at preventing
the institutionalization of a third youthful group, the emotionally
disturbed adolescent, including those who were aggressive, delinquent, and predelinquent.

Adolescents exhibiting such behaviors were creating problems
in major cities throughout the United States, including Worcester.
They attacked their peers, teachers, and other adults. They vandal-
ized schools and other public and private buildings. They refused
to attend school. When they did attend, they appeared unable to
learn and eager to prevent the learning activities of others. Their
parents were unable to control their behavior and sought help from
the schools and the courts. The schools admitted their inability to
cope and often suspended or expelled such students. The courts
tried a variety of therapeutic and punitive approaches with little
success. The usual children's service agencies such as the WYGC or
the school's Child Study Center had little effect on their behavior.
Massachusetts' training schools received many such youth until
these institutions were closed in the early 1970s (Miller and Ohlin,
1976). The only alternatives for disturbed adolescents appeared to
be adult jails or mental institutions—and in Massachusetts only
one state-operated mental hospital had special facilities for children and youth and these facilities were overtaxed.

In an attempt to prevent the institutionalization of such youth,
in 1968 the Worcester Public Schools (WPS) in collaboration with
Clark University organized an alternative day school. After a year of
operation in a church building the school was in difficulty. Not
only was the building unable to withstand the physical abuse it
was receiving from the students, but the necessary medical and
psychiatric support was not available. State education funds were
depleted, and money was needed to modify the building's construction to meet stringent state and city health and safety regulations. In response to a critical problem, WYGC assumed the
initiative and involved the WSH and the public schools in a series

of planning meetings. In the words of an early WDS report (undated):

> The three respective agencies up to this point had been working individually with this population and each became aware of the limitations of their own agencies in providing comprehensive services. The three agencies were in agreement that a more comprehensive program was desperately needed within the city and pledged their commitment to support such a program.

The result of the collaboration was the opening of the Woodward Day School (WDS), on the grounds of WSH in September 1970. The school was named after WSH's first superintendent, Samuel B. Woodward. The new school's Board of Directors included representatives of the three collaborating institutions. Its initial staff included a director, who was a trained social worker, two teachers provided by WYGC, two additional teachers from WPS, and a psychiatric nurse from WSH. The hospital also donated the physical space for the school, initially one floor in a building formerly occupied by chronic patients, supplied heat, light, maintenance, and other support services, and provided psychiatric backup. WYGC arranged psychiatric and psychological consultation and treatment. WPS gave educational materials, educational consultation, and student transportation.

The school opened with eight students: all referred by the school system, all previously excluded from regular classes, and all too disturbed even for classes for the emotionally disturbed. Initially WDS was limited to Worcester residents and WSH inpatients, regardless of residence, who were between the ages of 13 and 18. WSH desperately needed an educational and activity program for its institutionalized adolescent population, a group which did not fit well into the day-to-day operation of the adult wards.[1] Accordingly, appropriate adolescent inpatients were admitted routinely to WDS. Adolescents referred by other agencies or by families, however, were screened by WDS staff in cooperation with WYGC personnel. The enrollment soon grew to approximately 30 students. A behavior modification program was adopted in an attempt to create a structured environment in which disturbed youth could be reengaged educationally while acquiring socially appropriate behavior.

In its early stages, the WDS provided an outstanding example of a state hospital expanding its institutional boundaries. WSH, in collaboration with WYGC and WPS, had rescued a fragile, community-based program from incipient demise. It had brought the program into a protective institutional environment and provided it with the resources needed to survive. WSH's motives, however, were not entirely community-oriented. The hospital needed WDS to provide services for its adolescent patients who frequently were troublesome during the day.

But WDS did not grow and prosper in a vacuum. By necessity it became involved in the extensive changes in educational and mental health policy which occurred in Massachusetts in the 1970s. In this way its history paralleled that of WSH, simultaneously attempting to meet not only the needs of its client population, but also the demands of society.

### THE WOODWARD DAY SCHOOL IN 1979

Almost ten years after its inception, WDS is still housed in the Woodward Building on the grounds of WSH. The students have found it very difficult to damage or destroy the turn-of-the-century stone structure built for "crazy" patients or to surprise or alarm hospital staff accustomed to the most bizarre forms of behavior. Even more remarkable, the school still is served by its original director and three of the six original staff members. In many other ways, however, the school has undergone significant changes. The total staff now numbers 13 and the physical plant occupies three floors of the Woodward Building. This growth has been in response to changes in the student population, educational program, and scope of operations.

### Student Population

Currently WDS has a census of between 30 and 40. It remains the "school of last resort" for male and female adolescents who are unable to attend public educational programs for various reasons, including hospitalization at WSH. But the student mix has been modified. When the school opened, the overwhelming majority of the students were aggressive, acting-out adolescents. As the staff demonstrated to the public schools that it could provide an educational experience for these youngsters, it began to be challenged by both WSH and WPS to accept adolescents with very different problems, including school phobias, severe social deprivation, and withdrawal. These students also were unable to "make it" in the regular school environment, but seemed to thrive at WDS.

A second change has been in the age span, which has been shifted upward to 15 through 21. This was due partially to the aging of the original population. Admitted at ages 14, 15, and 16, many did not leave at the official "drop-out" age, but stayed on into the later teens. The WPS also developed alternative programs for emotionally disturbed junior high school students, so that they no longer needed to be sent to WDS. Finally, the WDS became involved in two new state-supported programs (Chapter 766 and SHEP, to be discussed subsequently) which mandated services to 21 years.

The geographical distribution of the student body also has changed. An increasing number of students are accepted from adjacent communities. Some are placed in WDS as a result of hospitalization at WSH—and the policy has been maintained of automatically accepting all appropriate WSH adolescent inpatients who can be allowed to leave the wards. A Report by the Task Force on Children's Services at Worcester State Hospital (1978) described the student body in these terms:

> While the clients are primarily day students who live at home, six are currently inpatients at WSH; six more were previously inpatients at WSH; and two were previously inpatients at other state hospitals. Approximately half of the clients, therefore, are, or were, sufficiently disturbed to be inpatients.[2]

But other nonhospitalized, non-Worcester residents are referred by their local educational agency directly to the WDS.

These changes in student population were partially a response to the success of the school in terms of short-range goals. With the exception of WSH inpatients, the adolescents voluntarily come to and remain within a school environment which does not have locked doors. Thus, for at least 50 weeks of the year from 8:30 A.M. to 2:30 P.M., five days a week, they are prevented from hurting themselves, other individuals, or property. Moreover, they do learn, a few in academic fields,[3] but all in the areas needed to survive in the outside world—to read employment ads, to complete driver's license applications, to make change, etc. A follow-up study (Klerman et al., 1979) suggested that the long-range outcomes may be mixed. Of 57 interviewed in 1976–77, between seven months and five years after separation from WDS, 63 percent were either attending school or working, 63 percent had received additional schooling, but only two had been graduated from high or trade school; 88 percent had been employed, but only 41 percent were working currently; and 57 percent admitted to having been in trouble with the law and 39 percent to having spent time in jail or a detention center since leaving WDS.[4]

A governmental social policy also had a strong influence on the selection of students for WDS. A series of court cases in the late 1960s and early 1970s affirmed the right of all children to an appropriate educational placement regardless of physical, mental, or emotional handicap. The response in Massachusetts was the enactment of a law referred to as Chapter 766.[5] Implemented in 1974, it required each local educational agency to provide special educational services for children between 3 and 21 years of age. The presence of WDS enabled WPS to be in compliance with Chapter 766 requirements for the education of severely disturbed adolescents to 21 years. The WDS program was made available to additional categories of emotionally disturbed youngsters unable to cope with traditional or even specialized school programs, and its age range was raised.

Neighboring school systems, in their attempts to be in compliance with Chapter 766, also sought assistance from WDS and WPS. Each system had one or more children who needed a WDS-type educational program, but none had enough to make a separate school economically viable. Home instruction was not educationally sound, and, in fact, was contrary to the "mainstreaming" philosophy of Chapter 766. Early in WDS's history, students from cities and towns outside of Worcester were accepted on an informal basis with the WPS receiving tuition payments. After the passage of the law, many small- and middle-sized communities began to face the problem of finding special education environments for small numbers of students with specialized needs. To meet this dilemma, Special Education Collaboratives were developed through which several communities could jointly sponsor specialized programs. This was the route taken by WPS for WDS.

The Central Massachusetts Special Education Collaborative was formed through the efforts of the city of Worcester and the town of Webster. The WDS continues to be a collaborative program of WPS, WYGC, and the WSH. It accepts only Worcester residents. The Woodward Day School Satellite, basically an extension of the WDS which accepts non-Worcester students, is administered and supported by the Collaborative in cooperation with WYGC and WSH. In the Woodward Day School–Woodward Day School Satellite descriptive brochure (undated), the Collaborative is described as serving "cases of low incidence special needs which can be better met through a collaborative effort providing quality programs in a more cost effective manner. An Educational Collaborative Board determines administrative and program costs which are apportioned among Member Towns and Districts and contracted on a per pupil basis."

Thus, as a result of Chapter 766, the WDS, born in the community but absorbed into the protective atmosphere of WSH as the hospital expanded its institutional boundaries, began to expand its own boundaries and make contacts with new communities. In November 1975, Congress passed Public Law 94-142, "The Education for All Handicapped Children Act," making Massachusetts law into national policy. Communities were placed under even greater pressure to find the most appropriate educational environment for their students and to follow due process in assigning a child to an educational placement. WDS had become a valuable educational resource for central Massachusetts.

The change in student composition, however, did not occur without conflict. One of the earliest problems encountered by WDS as it attempted to establish its organizational boundaries was the determination of the responsibility for admission and discharge procedures. Initially WPS, WYGC, WSH, and personnel from other school systems, human service agencies, and the courts referred prospective students to the WDS on an informal basis for evaluation and possible placement. While WDS personnel might consult with WYGC or WSH staff when it seemed appropriate, the decision generally was left to WDS.

As the school grew in size and influence, and as WPS developed a wider range of alternative programs, school administrators reconsidered these procedures. All prospective Worcester students were to be sent to the WPS's Special Education Department for evaluation and the ultimate decision concerning whether WDS was the best placement. Since the Department presumably had the best knowledge of the capabilities of other school programs, this approach appeared reasonable. However, some students whom the staff felt would have benefited from its program would be sent elsewhere, while it would only be under the most extreme circumstances that WDS would refuse to accept a student referred by the Department. This potentially meant some loss of control by WDS over its student population, although WDS and Department staff conferred and usually reached agreement. Similar arrangements were developed with other cities and towns which referred students. Referrals from the city of Worcester also had to be limited to stay within the guidelines established by the Special Education Collaborative. These stated that 20 students, or approximately half the WDS student body, had to be from outside Worcester.

A similar problem arose in terms of the termination of students. The WDS staff believed that it was in the best position to determine when a student had received the maximum benefit from its program and should be sent to another school or to community life. Under some circumstances, however, students could be forced to leave the WDS before they and/or the staff felt they were ready. Like WSH, WDS had to respond to the courts and other community agencies. For example, most adolescent inpatients at WSH whose behavior was under control and who were academically appropriate were sent to WDS to participate in the educational and other programs. When these adolescents were discharged from the state hospital, they could not remain in WDS unless the communities in which they resided were willing to pay their tuition and were close enough to make transportation practical. Similarly, the Departments of Welfare and of Youth Services in Massachusetts had responsibility for some WDS students while they were in foster care or other alternative living arrangements. If these students were returned to their homes or moved to another home or facility outside of Worcester, they were required to leave WDS unless the new community would assume tuition and transportation expenses. The WDS staff tried to delay the transfer of students whom it felt were benefiting from the program, but it was frequently unsuccessful.[6]

Despite its importance as an educational resource, the WDS did not always have sufficient power to control the admission and discharge of its student population. Its position on the boundary between an institution and the community, while providing it with considerable strength, also created weaknesses. The WDS was forced to mediate the occasionally opposing policies of WSH and WPS. As an element of WSH's institutional system, WDS was responsible for the care of hospitalized and deinstitutionalized adolescents with mental disorders. As an element of a community system, WPS emphasized curriculum, "normalization," and reintegration of WDS students into the public schools. This tension is reflected in the recent history of WDS, both in its changing clientele and in its new programs.

## Educational Program

WDS's initial behavior modification program, which focused on the control of inappropriate and often violent behavior, was essential because many of the early students had a history of being unmanageable within a school setting. WDS staff recall that in the early days of the school it was not unusual for the director, teachers, or the nurse to end the day with torn clothing or minor bruises.

The program had two components: a system of academic points which had been instituted before the school moved to the hospital grounds, and a token economy developed by the WDS staff. Under the point system, for every 15 minutes students engaged in a classroom assignment, they received 10 academic points. Accumulated points could be used to buy sports equipment, clothing, and trips with staff.

The token economy initially provided rewards for the attainment of a very limited goal, containment in the classroom for 15 minutes. During the first year, as the students became able to modify their behavior in exchange for tokens, the behavioral contingencies were made more difficult. Within the same 15-minute span, the student had not only to remain in the area, but also to refrain from disruption and use appropriate language. Tokens could be exchanged for food items such as soda, donuts, and coffee, as well as social rewards, such as a game of pool or an outing with a teacher.

An individual contract was written with some of the more difficult students. These students had to earn a specific number of tokens to remain in school for the full day or to return the following one. Students who formerly had refused to attend school now were willing to behave and work hard for the privilege of being allowed to stay.

As time progressed not only were the students able to comply with more difficult behavioral contingencies, but they also handled the rewards in a more adult manner. Initially the tokens were spent immediately by their recipients. Gradually students began to see benefits in saving tokens for larger rewards in the future, or in sharing tokens. Thus the token economy resulted in several types of positive behavior change.[7]

Over the years, several developments helped alter the noisy, occasionally violent atmosphere, and with it the emphasis on contingency contracting. The first was one of the changes in student characteristics just discussed. After a few years of operation WDS no longer received such a large percentage of the aggressive or violent. As a result, the school's caseload was dominated by withdrawn, school-phobic, and depressed adolescents. Although this mix required an equal if not greater amount of staff attention to ensure that the aggressive did not take advantage of the passive, the diversity of students' problems lowered the overall level of violent behavior.

The success of WDS brought about another change in the referral process which modified behavior. Whereas the original students all had long histories of disrupting classrooms, of which they were somewhat proud and unwilling to relinquish, WPS and other school systems soon began to identify a student needing WDS-type care earlier in his academic career. Some students were referred to WDS before their pattern of aggressive behavior was firmly established.

Changes in student behavior also were due to changes in staff expectations. Originally the staff expected its charges "to raise hell," and they did. Teachers and other staff gradually learned to be less responsive to aggressive behavior. Staff became accustomed to window breaking and were able to convince the hospital steward that it was not too high a price to pay in exchange for removing adolescents from the wards. In addition, the staff became more assured. It stopped worrying about the school's reputation and the need to return students to their referring schools. As staff felt and conveyed less pressure, the students' behavior improved. (Stanton and Schwartz, 1968, report similar changes in their study of a mental hospital.)

In addition, the students began to exercise peer pressure in a positive sense. Many of the adolescents who had spent several months or even years at WDS realized that it provided a haven for them in a hostile world. For some it was a warm and friendly place to escape from an oppressive or abusive home situation. For others it was an alternative to an institution—state hospital, state school, detention center, or jail. Such youth did not want new arrivals to disrupt what they perceived as the benefits of the WDS environment. It was to their advantage to "cool" the new students in collaboration with the staff, or on their own. Finally, the increasing age of the students changed behavior patterns.

For these reasons, the tokens and points of the original behavior modification system no longer dominated the educational environment. The new focus was on an expanded work-oriented curriculum. A small woodworking program was increased in scope so that not only were carpentry and cabinet-making skills taught, but students also learned the arithmetic of measuring and planning for the use of supplies, the economics of merchandising, and the techniques of applying for work. Similarly, a small coffee shop was developed within the Woodward Building. This facility was staffed by WDS students and patronized by WSH personnel, visitors, and patients. As the only place for a coffee break aside from the wards, the coffee shop attracted many of WSH's skilled craftsmen, carpenters, gardeners, and others. They became friendly with some of the WDS students, and, as a result, they were later willing to accept them as assistants in the type of work experiences the students badly needed. Both the coffee shop experience itself and the work situations which developed as a result enabled many WDS students to learn marketable skills.

The WDS staff was pleased with these changes, which they felt realistically responded to the needs and capabilities of the students. WPS felt less positive and curriculum emphasis became another area of conflict between WDS and other agencies. The school officials believed that the major objective of WDS should be reintegration of its students into the public schools. They hoped that after several months or a year at WDS, the students' behavior would be sufficiently appropriate so that they could be admitted to regular classrooms or to less segregated special classes or programs. WDS staff, although originally holding the same hope, soon came to the conclusion that such an objective was unrealistic for the vast majority of its population. Most students who attended WDS were markedly behind in grade level, detested a classroom atmosphere, and had only the most rudimentary skills in reading, writing, and mathematics. It seemed impossible to believe that such students could be brought even close to academic parity with their contemporaries.[8]

Alternatively, the objective which WDS staff set was to teach the students the "survival skills" necessary to participate as independent adults in the community. These included, for example, the ability to read signs, advertisements, and directions, to compute costs and give change, and to complete a variety of application forms. The occasional student capable of reentry was actively encouraged to meet this challenge, as was the student who could pass the General Education Development Test. But for most WDS students, sights were set lower, in terms of adult skills, in order not to repeat past frustrating experiences and in that way further alienate the student.

This conflict between the WDS and the WPS has been almost

totally resolved. Minimum competency testing is accepted in educational circles. The new philosophy is reflected in the Woodward
Day School–Woodward Day School Satellite brochure (undated)
which states

> The ultimate goal of the Woodward Day School and the Woodward
> Day Satellite is to prepare the student first, for possible reentry into the
> mainstream of education of his or her respective school system; second, to
> give the students an opportunity to explore their vocational interest
> through the programs available and to explore the world of work available
> through the Woodward Day programs. Independent decision making and
> adequate social adjustment are also part of the primary goal for each stu-
> dent. The Woodward Day School program provides a broad opportunity for
> these adolescent students to explore and prepare for independent living
> and adequate social adjustment during their stay in the program.

The rhetoric of reentry remains, but for most students the day-to-
day operation is oriented to a terminal placement at WDS and to
survival skill development allowing for transition to community
living.

Thus in several additional respects, WDS's development parallels that of its institutional sponsor, WSH. Both have experienced
difficulty in controlling the admission of a diversity of the most
disturbed clients for whom they represent "the end of the line."
Both are cognizant of their population's limitations, but attempt to
provide services which will enable them to adjust to life in a frequently hostile community.

## Institutional Programs—Attempts to Expand
## the Scope of Operations

Initially, WDS was a small operation which served only adolescents referred to it and whose activities generally were limited to
the Woodward Building. As suggested earlier, the staff's ability to
develop a successful educational program, as well as the passage of
state and national "special needs" legislation caused WDS to expand; to develop a new organizational framework (the Central Massachusetts Special Education Collaborative); and to interact with a
larger group of communities.

WDS was encouraged to expand further its organizational
boundaries when officials of the state Departments of Education,
Welfare, and Mental Health demonstrated a growing interest in the
problems of mentally ill adolescents. Early efforts met with partial
success.

One such venture was begun on the grounds of WSH. In 1977, the state Department of Education made available to each of its regions funds to provide appropriate educational services to youth under the age of 21 who were inpatients in state hospitals. The WDS staff, in collaboration with the Central Massachusetts Special Education Collaborative, applied for and received the State Hospital Education Project (SHEP) funds for WSH. The director of WDS assumed responsibility for the SHEP program as well, and the two programs (WDS and SHEP) also shared a project administrator and a secretary. In addition, SHEP employed an Intake Coordinator and three special education teachers. The shared staffs and commonality of goals made for a mutually beneficial relationship between SHEP and WDS personnel. This had a favorable impact on WSH's adolescent population, which could easily move between the two projects as their mental status changed.[9]

While obtaining the SHEP grant and extending its educational program onto the hospital wards clearly represented a successful expansion effort by WDS, two similar efforts did not. Both involved the state Department of Mental Health (DMH): one was its youth "most in need of services" (MINS) program, and the other its Regional Adolescent Specialized Treatment program.

In 1978 the DPW regional office issued a Request for Proposals for MINS projects. The WDS staff perceived this as an opportunity to make a statement about the unmet needs of emotionally disturbed and mentally ill youth. In its WYGC-sponsored application, WDS proposed a case management program which would be a logical extension of the WDS and SHEP programs. The application (Child Guidance Association of Worcester, Inc., 1979a) stated

> The primary program strategy will be the employment of a team of social workers who will work with existing community-based organizations to improve the capacity of their service delivery systems to meet the needs of this group of adolescents (those enrolled in WDS and SHEP) who are most in need of service. In this regard, the team is expected to identify, develop, expand, and utilize the resources of these organizations to achieve the following goals:
> 1. Increase the rate of deinstitutionalization of adolescents at the State Hospital. Not only will the census be reduced, but length of stay at the hospital is also expected to be shortened.
> 2. Prevent the institutionalization of adolescents who could be more appropriately served in programs outside of the State Hospital.
> 3. Develop an exemplary service model which will result in a more effective and coordinated set of programs for adolescents with severe mental illness.

In the proposed program, two social workers trained as case managers and working under the direction of WDS staff would (1) identify and inventory all adolescent-relevant community resources in the mental health region; (2) develop and expand needed community services when gaps in the system were documented; and (3) increase the level of interagency linkages to develop more coordinated service plans. In addition, the case management team would provide direct services to adolescents in the SHEP and WDS programs. These would include referral to appropriate medical, social, or educational services and the development of individualized service plans with such agencies. The case managers would assess the extent and urgency of needs, counsel the clients, assist them in obtaining services, and periodically follow up on client progress.

Although the proposal was not funded because funds did not become available, it provides an additional example of how the WDS, brought in from the community to the shelter of the state hospital, had matured and was now ready to venture forth and assume a coordination, if not a leadership, role, in relation to emotionally disturbed and mentally ill adolescents in the community. But was the community ready for it to assume such a role?

DMH's attempt to organize a Regional Adolescent Specialized Treatment (RAST) Unit in the Worcester region provided a similar opportunity for WDS to explore its boundaries. The Department proposed a 24-hour, therapeutic, secure residential program for 12 adolescents with severe mental or emotional disorders as an alternative to jails, detention units, or placement on adult mental hospital wards. It was hoped that it could provide intensive treatment for adolescents referred by the state Department of Youth Services, DMH, and other mental health professionals. In 1977, and again in 1978, DMH issued a Request for Proposals to develop such a program. WDS did not respond in the first year. In the second year, through WYGC, it applied for funds to begin an Inpatient Adolescent Facility using a broader definition of need (Child Guidance Association of Worcester, Inc., 1979b). Its proposal was designed to include not only the RAST unit, eligibility for which was commitment to the Departments of Mental Health or Youth Services; but also inpatient adolescent services for seriously disturbed youth with a high probability of becoming RAST-eligible if appropriate services were not available, and adolescents admitted to WSH because of acute psychotic episodes or psychiatric crisis situations. This WDS–WYGC proposal was not approved. The funds went to a Worcester-based community agency which through 1979 was unable to operate an inpatient RAST program because the Determination of Need necessary to institute the program had not been issued by the state Department of Public Health. Meanwhile, the agency provided services to severely disturbed adolescents on an outpatient basis, with the assistance of WDS staff.

Not only were WDS's two attempts to expand its noneducational functions unsuccessful, but its very existence as a collaborative organization on WSH grounds is being questioned. While all three sponsoring agencies (WDS, WSH, and WYGC) and their respective state Departments (Education and Mental Health) agree that the school satisfies an important need and performs in an outstanding manner, financial pressures have caused each to question its sponsorship. The loose coalition, which was adequate to the task of building the program under almost crisis conditions, cannot or does not want to provide the support and direction needed in its expansionist phase. The issue is not whether there is a need for WDS, this has been proven; but where does it belong, who should pay for it, what services should it provide, and to which populations.

The most pressing issue is that of location. The Regional DMH office has seriously questioned the continued location of WDS on hospital grounds. In the era of Chapter 766 and Public Law 94-142, DMH believes that the school should be located in the community and should no longer be supported by DMH directly (through salaries) or indirectly (through space and maintenance). A real possibility exists that WDS will be returned to the community which rejected the alternative school ten years earlier. Although a non-hospital-based facility might have many advantages, such as strengthening ties with community agencies and schools and eliminating the stigma of WSH, it also would have many negative results. The close relationship with WSH would need to be terminated. This would mean a more complicated SHEP program, probably involving busing; no use of WDS by hospitalized adolescents capable of leaving the wards; and a reluctance by WDS to accept or retain the most seriously disturbed adolescents, whom they presently can risk taking because of the immediate availability of WSH personnel and facilities. Nor would the prospective students be the only ones to suffer. WSH pointed proudly to WDS when the hospital accreditation committee came to review its program. Without WDS on its grounds, the hospital's programs for adolescents would appear more limited.

WPS also proudly points to WDS when the state Department of

Education asks how Worcester is meeting its Chapter 766 obligations towards the emotionally disturbed. But it occasionally questions the intrusion of personnel employed by DMH into what it
considers educational matters. It would like to assert more authority over WDS, but is not prepared to manage, in regular or other
specialized programs, the youth it found "unteachable."

Finally, even WYGC has begun to question its fiscal and other
attachments to WDS. Its directors wonder if perhaps the time has
come for WDS to establish itself as another private community
agency, rather than a creature of the public mental health and education sectors. This would be one way to convert the loose administrative structure which characterized the beginning of WDS into
the more stable administrative mechanism which would seem to be
necessary if WDS is to survive and grow.

Although collaborative arrangements clearly have advantages
in terms of combinations of resources and coordination of services,
they also have their drawbacks. They are creatures of convenience.
When it is convenient to claim a program developed under such a
model, this is done. It is equally easy, however, at times of fiscal or
other restraints, to place the responsibility for such a program upon
another organization. The question must arise, but cannot be satis-
factorily answered, "Whose program are you?" This is the situation
currently faced by WDS staff.


## CONCLUSION

The WDS experience to date can be perceived in terms of a
series of trade-offs. In exchange for a protected environment and
considerable financial resources, the original school left the community and located on the grounds of WSH. Its students have been
forced to deal with the stigma of such a location and its staff has
been isolated from the educational bureaucracy.

Multiple sponsorship appeared initially to be a way of
strengthening the fledgling school—three organizations (WSH,
WYGC, and WPS) provided financial input and considerable prestige. In exchange, however, WDS has had to serve several masters,
who did not always agree on policy and programs. Moreover, it is
dependent on each of them in some way and may not chart its
course independently. WDS staff may not always decide which students to accept or when to discharge. They are not in complete control of the school's budget and do not have the secure funding of a

facility funded totally by the Department of Education or the Department of Mental Health.

WDS clearly demonstrates the problems involved when a large institution, such as WSH, attempts to expand its responsibilities. It may also represent what can be expected in terms of social and educational services in the next decade. Few entirely new public programs may be funded. Instead, organizations will increasingly band together to create new semi-autonomous entities. Public agencies will contract with private or semiprivate groups for services rather than enlarge bureaucracies—and from a belief that purchase of services can be used as a more flexible management tool. Responsibilities and authority will be more blurred under these conditions. Many agencies and their staffs will learn to live with the ambiguities and conflicts which characterize the Woodward Day School in its relationships to the community and to Worcester State Hospital.

## NOTES

1. In time even the program provided by WDS was insufficient to meet the needs of the hospital's adolescent population. In 1973 an after-school program was begun which gradually developed into the Adolescent Treatment Complex. Its parallel evolution is the subject of Chapter 6.
2. The WDS staff reports that throughout the school's ten-year history, approximately 50 percent of its students have been present or former inpatients.
3. Currently one-third to one-quarter of the WDS students are in a high school track, studying towards a high school diploma or a General Education Development (GED) Test. In 1979, three WDS students received diplomas from the schools which referred them.
4. The assistance of Linda Farrin and Dennis Poole with the interviewing and data analysis of the follow-up study is gratefully acknowledged.
5. Chapter 766 of the Acts of 1972, the Commonwealth of Massachusetts, an Act Further Regulating Programs for Children Requiring Special Education and Providing Reimbursement Therefor.
6. During the same period, the Robert F. White School, an alternative school for a similar population in Boston, only accepted students if the referring agency agreed to allow them to remain until the school staff believed they were ready to leave.
7. For a more complete description of the WDS program, see Kennedy et al., 1976.
8. WDS and WPS policy, however, is to minimize the gap between WDS and the conventional high school. WDS students must be carried on the rolls of the referring schools, whether in Worcester or a neighboring community. They must receive credit for WDS courses. If they complete their requirements at WDS, they receive their high school's diploma. Some students became very involved in "normalizing" their graduations, including purchasing their class rings and attending the graduation ceremony of their "home" school. Others receive their

diplomas at a luncheon ceremony at WDS in the presence of the director of special education or another representative from the referring school system and invited guests.

9. More complete descriptions of the SHEP program in Worcester, referred to as Project Liaison, can be found in the most recent application (Central Massachusetts Special Education Collaborative, 1979) and a *First-Year Evaluation Report* (Ewald, 1978).

Barry Walsh

# 8
# Transcending Organizational Boundaries: The Adolescent Treatment Complex

This chapter focuses on the evolution of the Adolescent Treatment Complex (ATC), from an institutional program at Worcester State Hospital (WSH) to a network of community-based mental health services. Along with the Woodward Day School (discussed in the previous chapter), the ATC emerged as one of the principal alternative programs developed in the early 1970s as part of the deinstitutionalization and functional realignment of WSH. In contrast to the Woodward program, the ATC not only expanded the functional boundaries of WSH but it has gone on to achieve considerable autonomy from the Hospital. The purpose of this chapter is to examine how the ATC adapted to the policy of deinstitutionalization, under conditions of resource scarcity and the dual pressures of its institutional legacy and community mandate. In so doing, some of the themes presented earlier in this volume—boundary control, organizational conflict, competition, and the development of adaptive interorganizational relationships—will be addressed in the context of human services programming for emotionally disturbed adolescents.

The transformation of the ATC will be presented chronologically within an organizational development framework. The first phase describes the origins of the ATC as an adjunctive activity program for adolescents within the institutional environment of WSH. The second phase focuses on the maturation of the program in the form of a more sophisticated treatment program, the increasing professionalization of its staff, and by the assertion of control over its client intake boundaries. The third phase deals with the differentiation of the program and its early attempts at separation from WSH. During this developmental phase a lack of resources stymied the initial efforts toward independence. Later, while the program continued to rely on WSH for support, the establishment of linkages within community agencies led to stability and the acquisition of a firmer resource base. The fourth phase—still unfolding—concerns the development of organizational autonomy and the problems of a new-found independence as a community-based network of services.

The observations presented in this chapter are based on the author's first-hand experience as Assistant Director, and now as Executive Director of the ATC.

## ORIGINS

Adolescents have always composed a portion of those living in state mental hospitals (Hartman, 1968). As recent studies indicate, the provision of specialized care for adolescents who are psychiatric inpatients is an important variable related to treatment outcome (Gossett, 1977). State hospitals, however, have generally not provided such specialized care. Instead, adolescents have been mixed with adult patients and have been treated as if they were adults. A case in point is WSH in the early 1970s.

During this period there were only two specialized services for adolescents on the grounds of WSH. Both were day schools providing academic and vocational programming. One, the Woodward Day School, described in the preceeding chapter, served a juvenile delinquent and emotionally disturbed population. The other, the Quimby School, served autistic and moderately retarded adolescents. Although both were providing excellent service to their clients, they operated only 5–6 hours per day. Adolescent inpatients, therefore, returned to their wards for significant portions of the day. Like many other state facilities, WSH did not have a specialized inpatient service for these adolescents. The wards to which they returned were populated primarily by acute and chronic adult patients.

This environment was particularly problematic for the adolescents. Such wards were frightening and regressive, frequently exacerbating rather than relieving the behavior problems of the adolescents. Yet, ironically, in the early 1970s the proximity of the day schools to the wards led to a marked increase of adolescent inpatient admissions to WSH.

This increase created tensions at all levels within the facility. The administrators were aware that the adolescents were not receiving adequate care and that they were a highly visible group. The ward staff was concerned with the increased number of management problems which the adolescents presented. In addition, the adult patients were stressed by the volatile and "bizarre" behavior of the adolescents.

Accordingly, the consensus among hospital administrators, ward staff, and even some patients was that a considerable increase of service for these adolescents was needed. This opinion was echoed by the various local child welfare agencies that were aware of WSH service deficiencies. More problematic, however, was determining what *type* of service was needed and how to provide the *resources* to establish it.

The Superintendent of WSH was the key person involved in shaping these decisions. During the early 1970s, as noted in Chapter 3, the superintendent had considerable power. It was, in effect, Dr. Myerson's decision whether to establish a specialized inpatient service for adolescents or to expand day program services with an eye toward community-based care. He chose the latter for a variety of reasons. An attempt at operating an adolescent inpatient ward a decade earlier (in the mid 1960s) had proved disastrous. Ward management problems had been extreme, requiring periodic state police intervention. No one was eager to repeat this experience. In addition, expanding daytime programming was considerably less expensive than establishing a three-shift, 24-hour ward. And, finally, a new day service providing increased community activities for adolescents was more consistent with the goals of deinstitutionalization.

In June of 1973, Dr. Myerson redeployed four psychiatric nursing positions to staff a modest afternoon and evening program for adolescent inpatients. The initial program was located on an old vacant ward and offered primarily recreational services. Its purpose was to remove the adolescents from their wards after the school day ended to provide them with age-appropriate activities. Within several months, the staff was augmented with three attendant positions. In addition, a full-time graduate social worker was hired to direct the program and to provide the basic clinical services of individual, family, and group therapy. By late 1973, between 9 and

12 adolescents regularly participated in the program. These adolescents were drawn from the Woodward Day School and Quimby School populations of severely disturbed and mild-to-moderately retarded clients.

Even this modest program, however, created considerable tension within the hospital community. The Director of Nursing, for example, complained that the redeployed nurses and attendants were needed on the understaffed wards. Ward psychiatrists objected that their case management power was diluted by the new, actively involved, program. Hospital business administrators asserted that establishing a new program was ill-advised given the scarcity of resources. Without the active, often daily, intervention of the Superintendent, the program would surely have been short-lived or at least reduced to a token activity.

Another key source of support during this early period was a newly organized "interdepartmental team" of local child welfare agencies. The members included area representatives from the state Departments of Mental Health, Public Welfare, Youth Services (for delinquents), the Division of Special Education, Office for Children (for child advocacy), and the Massachusetts Rehabilitation Commission (for vocational rehabilitation). This "team" had a multiplicity of other functions, but it was of particular assistance to the new day program. Specifically, the team monitored and screened referrals to the program and prevented the rate and quantity from exceeding a manageable level. Without this "protective" assistance the new program either would have been overloaded or criticized as unresponsive. The team also was able to divert many marginally appropriate adolescents away from admission to WSH, thus avoiding the risks described above. More concretely, one of the team members, the Office for Children, provided the day program with a small grant for supplies and recreational expenses for community activities.

Thus the ADP's early development was characterized by a number of key elements. Those most crucial to its implementation and continuation were the following:

1. The presence of consistent, high-level administrative support within WSH. This support was able to overcome the resistance and opposition from all levels of the existing WSH services.
2. The willingness of program staff to operate with very modest resources. For example, the activity budget for the first year was $1,200, with staff using their own vehicles for client transportation.

3. A philosophy of community-based care. Although the program was located on the WSH grounds, Superintendent Myerson and the day program staff emphasized "normalizing," community-oriented activities from the start.
4. The existence of external supports from child welfare agencies. The administrators of these community-based agencies recognized that support of the new day program was in their own best interest. This cooperative attitude lessened competition between agencies and reduced the fragmentation of services for adolescents.

## MATURATION

By 1975, the staff of the adolescent program had become increasingly professionalized. Another graduate social worker and a part-time psychiatric resident had been added. A "volunteer" senior Ph.D. psychologist from the WSH Psychology Department was now responsible for the majority of staff training and case supervision. Under his influence the activity program became increasingly sophisticated. The recreational focus gave way to a more skillful counseling and behavioral contingency management orientation.

Other Psychology Department staff also provided family therapy and "grantsmanship" consultation and the service of a part-time clinician. This assistance was significant in that Psychology was the first WSH department to actively support the ADP. There were several reasons for this support. Because of limitations in clinical resources at WSH, this department was under mounting pressure to become oriented more toward direct services and less toward research. The psychologists involved with the ADP staff were attracted by the energy and enthusiasm of the new program. These psychologists were aware that the ADP was "green" and unsophisticated and that its staff could benefit from the clinical expertise of their Department. In time, as this affiliation developed, Superintendent Myerson was able to lessen his direct involvement somewhat, without threatening the continuation of the program.

There were other important changes during 1975. The admissions criteria for the ADP were narrowed to include only psychiatrically disturbed adolescents. The small number of retarded clients who had previously been referred from the Quimby School were excluded. The rationale for this decision was that the previous mixture had been too heterogeneous to permit adequate peer group socialization. ADP staff had discovered that their most difficult clients were often the retarded who were the slowest to improve. Increased control over entry into the ADP reduced staff frustration and organizational stress. Interestingly, this redefinition of ADP boundaries was easily accepted both inside and outside the organization. Other community agencies were amenable to the exclusion because alternative community-based programs for retarded youngsters were simultaneously being developed under other auspices. These new day and residential programs had been created by court order, and at that time, they were considerably more comprehensive than the ADP. Thus it was felt that Quimby School clients and other retarded children would benefit more from these new programs.

An additional change in the ADP's boundary definition was the acceptance of community referrals from the Departments of Education, Public Welfare, and Office for Children. These were emotionally disturbed adolescents who lived with their natural families or in foster care, but who nonetheless were in need of extensive day-care services. Following the community orientation of the ADP's original activities, the acceptance of outpatient referrals was the second step in the transformation of the ADP from an institutional to a community-based program.

However, accepting referrals from the community was not without its problems. One source of resistance came from several of the adolescents themselves, who balked at attending a program located at WSH. The hospital setting carried the stigma of deviance and mental illness which some clients understandably wished to avoid. Fortunately, as clients became involved in the recreational and social activities offered by the ADP, their resistance tended to diminish.

Another form of resistance came from the Director of Nursing and the WSH Business Manager. They argued that scarce resources were now being used for patients who were not even a responsibility of WSH. Arguments based on the principles of prevention and community mental health could not convince these opponents. It was ultimately Dr. Myerson's intervention which again permitted change to occur.

By 1975 the staff of the ADP had an emerging sense of the population it could best serve. One group, primarily inpatient, consisted of acutely ill schizophrenics or impulse disordered clients exhibiting violent aggression, sexual deviance, or fire-setting. The other group, primarily outpatient, consisted of more "stabilized," process schizophrenics or unsocialized depressives. Both groups were generally from impoverished, highly disorganized families with multigenerational histories of mental illness and deviance.

As the target population gradually became better defined, a distinctive model of treatment also emerged. Given the severity of the problems that engulfed these adolescents and their families, the ADP staff recognized that a "multiple intervention treatment model" was necessary. By 1975 the services which the ADP was able to provide were individual, group, and family therapy, psychopharmacology, and daily activity programming. In addition the WDS provided comprehensive, specialized schooling and WSH maintained the "back-up" inpatient service.

## DIFFERENTIATION

### Transition to the Community

In early 1975, after the ADP had been in operation for nearly two years, a number of its inpatient clients were ready for discharge. These clients were candidates for placement in several types of existing community residential settings. Two were placed, for example, in halfway houses, serving delinquents. The settings proved unsuccessful because socially sophisticated psychopathic residents easily victimized the ADP's emotionally disturbed adolescents. In addition, the staff of these programs was uncomfortable with the "bizarre" behavior of the ADP clients. Placing older adolescents in their own apartments with the ADP supplying support services was also attempted. Without live-in supervision, however, these clients quickly regressed and returned to the hospital.

As a result, the Program Director and Dr. Myerson decided that a community residence specifically designed for the ADP population was needed. To establish such a residence a number of steps had to be taken:

1. Establishing (or preferably affiliating with an existing) private, nonprofit corporation to serve as host agency for the residence;
2. Locating an appropriate site conducive to a surrogate family environment;
3. Obtaining the resources to support the program;
4. Gaining community acceptance for such a residence; and
5. Designing a highly structured treatment program specific to the needs of ADP clients.

Dr. Myerson's "linkages" within the Greater Worcester Area social service community helped to identify a sponsor and a suitable site. He became aware of a local agency, Greendale People's Church, which was active in providing residential care for the elderly and had considerable experience with third-party funding. In addition, the church was interested in "expanding its ministry" to include adolescents, and it owned a soon-to-be-vacant nursing home which might serve as a site. With Dr. Myerson's support, initial funding was also obtained. The Department of Mental Health was willing to fund the new residence for its first year of existence. Although the funding level was only $32,000, considerable in-kind services were supplied by the ADP and People's Church.

Establishing the residence was much easier than obtaining adequate maintenance resources and gaining community acceptance. The Department of Public Welfare (DPW) was approached about being the primary sponsoring and funding agency for the residence. DPW was receptive in that it had responsibility for many adolescents who were severely disturbed, while there were few residential programs which would accept them. Despite this initial interest, however, it proved onerous to complete the myriad of bureaucratic tasks necessary to obtain DPW support. The process of securing DPW funding took over two years. During the interim, the residence was forced to operate on a subsistence level.

Community opposition was also a formidable problem. When neighbors of the vacant nursing home were approached about the proposed new use of the facility, they panicked, citing the dangers of Sirhan Sirhan and psychopathic killers. And, perhaps most significantly, they called City Hall and fought the residence with all the power they could muster.

The resulting court litigation took two years to resolve and it cost the already under-funded residence $3,000 in legal fees. Briefly, the legal process included a defeat for the new program at the local Board of Appeals, but subsequent victories at the District, Superior, Appellate, and State Supreme Judicial Court levels. The legal argument which was used successfully consisted of defining the residence as an educational facility which offered a structured daily curriculum regarding basic living skills and socialization. As an educational facility licensed by the Office for Children and supported by a public agency (DMH) the program was not, therefore, subject to local zoning restrictions (Massachusetts Supreme Court, No. STC-1114). Without the advocacy of both the Office for Children and DMH during this period, it is doubtful whether the residence would have survived.

With the various administrative, financial, and legal issues at least partially resolved, the staff of the new residence was finally able to provide some service. The residence was named CLEAT, an acronym for Community Living Education Aiding Teens. Its treatment program was designed with considerable input (again) from the WSH Psychology Department.

These clinical components have been discussed in detail elsewhere (Walsh and Rosen, 1979; Rosen et al., 1980). Briefly, CLEAT may be described as a family-style, behavior modification community residence. A basic aspect of the program is its high degree of structure. There is a rather strict regimen, for example, in the form of a point and level system which rewards prosocial and adaptive living skills. This system assists the residents by compensating for their characteristic cognitive disorganization and behavioral impulsivity. In turn, the structure also minimizes the staff–client conflict and management problems which contribute so much to residential staff "burnout" and turnover.

The client population of CLEAT is essentially identical to that of the ADP (although actively psychotic or dangerously impulsive clients are not accepted). The program is co-ed with a capacity of eight. The residents are 14–18 years old and are required to have a full-time job or school program. Most residents also attend the ADP part-time or at least receive their individual therapy, family therapy, and medication through the day service. The length of stay for residents is usually protracted, ranging from six months to two years. Upon graduation, they may return home, live independently or move to the Cooperative Apartment program to be described later.

The staff for the CLEAT program consists of two sets of houseparent couples, one full-time, the other weekend relief. There are also clinical and administrative directors and a community liaison worker. Significantly, the clinical director of CLEAT is also the clinical director of the ADP. This results in especially close coordination between the programs.

## Continued Institutional Support

An important aspect of any community residential treatment program is the availability of "back-up" support for those residents who require suspension or dismissal. Occasionally, the problematic behavior of a resident will necessitate his or her removal from the program. Antecedents of a client's regression can involve many factors including an inability to handle internal or external stress, acting-out behavior, deliberate manipulation, and (unfortunately) staff inconsistency. Regardless of the form of the regression, a client's removal can be a pressing necessity in order to avoid a contagion effect on other residents.

For a program like CLEAT, an adequate back-up service must include three elements. It must be quickly available; otherwise, the prolonged presence of an out-of-control resident can wreak havoc on the program and alarm the neighborhood. It must also provide secure, humane, and therapeutic treatment. Regressed adolescents typically require supportive, but restrictive, care. And, it should operate in close coordination with the referring residential program. This permits the client to return to the community-based program as soon as possible.

It was clear from the early planning stages of CLEAT that WSH would be its backup. But WSH, as noted earlier, could not provide specialized care for adolescents. This problem was diminished through yet another affiliation with the WSH Psychology Department.

Psychology had operated a co-ed "open-door" ward since 1967. This ward was generally acknowledged to be the superior inpatient service at the hospital, due largely to the close supervision of the Chief of Service (a Ph.D. psychologist), and the involvement of students from the Psychology Department's predoctoral internship program. Each year five or six psychology interns were assigned to the ward and were responsible for five or six patients. This resulted in a higher staff–patient ratio and closer case management than the other wards could provide.

Because of the previous affiliations with Psychology, CLEAT and the ADP were able to arrange for the open-door ward to provide the majority of its backup. Most adolescents initially required a locked, inpatient setting. As soon as they were stabilized, however, a transfer to the Psychology Ward was usually possible. From there, the client gradually returned to CLEAT whenever possible.

A case example from CLEAT's second year of operation (1977) is illustrative of the type of coordination which developed.

A 17-year-old girl had lived in CLEAT for eight months. She had been attending the WDS and the ADP daily. Due to increased use of street drugs and conflict with her disorganized natural family, she became increasingly psychotic. Continued family therapy, a change in medication, and other interventions failed to produce improvement. Within a month, the girl's behavior at CLEAT had reached unmanageable proportions. Even the other CLEAT residents complained about her bizarreness.

Accordingly, CLEAT staff decided to suspend the girl and within hours she was admitted directly to the Psychology Ward at WSH. She responded well to the less demanding ward atmosphere and recompensated quickly. Within eight days she began her reentry to CLEAT and within two weeks she had returned there full time. During the entire period, she continued to attend WDS and the ADP.

Predictably, this new arrangement between CLEAT and Psychology was not without its detractors. Staff from other wards which also referred patients to the open ward complained that adolescents were given preferential status regarding admission. Several nursing administrators complained that catchment area requirements were being violated in that some CLEAT residents were not originally from Worcester. Still, by this time the opposition was considerably less than in the past. By 1977, the ward staffs seemed to acknowledge the value of the "new" adolescent services. And, in turn, staff from the ADP and CLEAT were becoming more aware of the need to cooperate with the "old" institutional services—if for no other reason than to provide adequate back-up care for their clients.

## EMERGENT INDEPENDENCE

### Inadequate Resources

By 1976, the experience of operating the ADP and CLEAT programs led to identifying an additional service need of the severely disturbed adolescents. It became clear that a significant percentage of clients would require care well into adulthood. Some clients, for example, completed the CLEAT program successfully (in the process acquiring many of the necessary social and living skills), yet they were still not ready for totally independent living. There were also older ADP clients (ages 17–19) who needed community residential care, but for whom the younger population at CLEAT and the family model were not appropriate. Instead, these two types of clients seemed to need a facility specifically designed for psychiatrically disturbed *adults*. One model which was familiar to the program staff was the "Cooperative Apartment" first utilized by Chien in the late 1960s (Cole, 1978). For the original "Co-op," Boston State Hospital staff obtained apartments near the hospital for soon-to-be discharged patients. Hospital staff provided support services such as medication and informal counseling on a weekly home visit basis. In turn, the discharged patients were responsible for all areas of their daily lives, including paying rent and other living expenses and providing their own day programming. With this program model, receptive owner-landlords were sought who were willing to provide living skill training to their tenants; thus landlords also provided a component of support services. This experimental program proved to be an effective deinstitutionalization technique and was widely copied in Massachusetts and elsewhere. The staff of CLEAT and the ADP drew heavily on the original Co-op model, but made adjustments to address the specific needs of the adolescents.

The model which the ADP and CLEAT staff envisioned as necessary would (unlike the original Co-op) utilize live-in supervisors. These were seen as necessary in that the older adolescent clients were thought to be more volatile than the middle-aged adults of the Boston program. Also, the living-skill deficits of these adolescents were seen as requiring more attention and direct supervision than a nonprofessional landlord could provide. An additional factor was a sensitivity to criticism about the trend of "dumping" mental patients in the community with less-than-adequate follow-up care.

The need for a Co-op program had been discussed for several months prior to learning of a potential funding source. In this case, the source was DMH Mental Retardation funds designated to reduce the census of retarded people living in state hospitals and state schools. Since a number of the ADP clients were both inpatients of WSH and borderline retarded, the ADP via its nonprofit affiliation with the People's Church was seen as eligible for such funding. As a result, People's Church submitted an application for funds to establish a single Co-op apartment and received $12,365 for the first year—a level of funding which had become a familiar problem.

To a considerable extent, the amount of funds obtained dictated the type of service which could be provided. The contracted funds were used entirely to hire two live-in supervisors. Each supervisor worked three or four days per week and then was relieved by the other. The setting for the new Co-op was a three-bedroom, relatively low-rent apartment in a large, low-income housing project. Initially, four male clients resided in the program. The client residents were responsible for the rent and phone expenses as well as their food, transportation, supplies, and living costs. Since there was no "start-up" money provided, furniture, kitchen equipment, and other items were either "scrounged" from local merchants or donated by People's Church.

The population residing in the Co-op was an older component of the ADP and CLEAT client groups, requiring many of the same services: individual and family therapy, psychopharmacology, structured recreational activities, continued living skill and socialization training, etc. Obviously the Co-op budget did not permit provision of these services within the Co-op program itself. Instead they were supplied on an in-kind basis by the ADP as they also were for CLEAT. Thus, the ADP functioned as the "hub" or core clinical service component for the two residential programs. In addition, the ADP was actively involved with those clients receiving short-term, back-up, inpatient care on the Psychology Ward at WSH. Accordingly, the administration and staff of ADP, CLEAT, and the Co-op began to conceptualize these programs as an interrelated "Complex" of services. The three programs, therefore, became known as the Adolescent Treatment Complex (ATC).

It is important to emphasize that within the constraints of limited resources the network of the ATC was developed directly in response to the needs of the ADP client population as described above. These were adolescents with multiple "handicaps." Given the multiplicity of their problems, the "multiple intervention model" evolved in response to these needs. Thus, by 1977, the treatment philosophy of the ATC was to provide long-term, continuous care ranging from brief, "restrictive," inpatient treatment to relatively independent, adult co-op living. As a result, some clients might progress from the inpatient service to the ADP to CLEAT (while still maintaining the ADP) to the Co-op. Others might utilize only one or two of these components as their specific needs require.

## Adequate Resources

Program changes which have occurred since 1977 have been consistent with the multiple intervention model. The most recent programatic change in the ATC has been the expansion of the Co-op program. By early 1978, the top priority for DMH was the continued reduction of the inpatient census of state hospitals. This effort required a reciprocal expansion of community-based programs, particularly community residences. As a result, the Greater Worcester Area Office of DMH issued a "request for proposal" for a 10-bed, co-ed residence based on the cooperative apartment model. People's Church responded to this request and was awarded the contract. Because of the amount of the contract ($27,000 for start-up costs, $62,000 for the first year) the ATC was for the first time able to begin a new program with relatively adequate resources. Perhaps adequate funds were provided because deinstitutionalization had become an actual *political* priority and not merely a preferred treatment philosophy.

The contract enabled the staff to develop an improved, co-ed version of the original Co-op. Four adjacent, two-bedroom units were rented in a pleasant garden apartment complex. Those adolescents living in the original Co-op were phased into the new facility. Staff was expanded to include full-time male and female live-in managers and three weekend relief managers. In addition, a full-time M.A. psychologist was hired as clinical director to do intake, records, case management, and staff supervision for the program. A half-time M.A. psychologist was hired as a clinician to provide individual and family therapy and community liaison work, and a psychiatric consultation was also employed for medication monitoring.

Establishing both the original and expanded Co-op programs in the community was considerably less difficult than starting CLEAT. Renting the first unit in 1975, for example, produced no community opposition. The ATC approached the Worcester Housing Authority for approval to locate a residence of the Co-op model in the Plumley Village Housing Project. The Housing Authority was most receptive to the proposal. Perhaps this cooperation was in part due to the moderately high percentage of vacant units in the housing project at the time. An additional factor may have been the presence of a small DMH-sponsored satellite clinic in the Plumley Village project. Because the mental health clinic had been in place for several years and was seen as an important resource for the project, the Housing Authority may have been receptive to another DMH-sponsored program.

There was also no opposition from the neighborhood. The absence of neighborhood resistance seemed to be attributable to two factors. First, renting an apartment requires none of the formal civic and legal approval involved in establishing a free-standing residence. Not having to complete such formal and public procedures greatly reduces the advance visibility of a new program. As a result the Co-op staff and residents simply moved in and began operation. Second, the neighborhood already had a relatively high tolerance for "deviance." The crime rate in the area was rather high and alcohol and drug abuse among adolescents was prevalent. If anything, then, the inclusion of the more withdrawn, passive, Co-op clients went relatively unnoticed.

When the Co-op expanded and relocated in 1978, there was also little community resistance. The private owner of the apartment complex initially was concerned that the presence of a Co-op might cause other tenants to leave. After receiving a positive recommendation from the Housing Authority and suitable credit references, however, the owner became receptive. In fact, within several months, he offered to rent additional units, which the program could not afford.

Perhaps ironically, the only major source of resistance came from the staff of one inpatient ward at WSH. This ward was supposed to be an important source of referrals for the Co-op. Nonetheless, the staff of the ward was unified in its belief that discharging patients to a Co-op setting was "wrong." The staff explained its opposition by stating: (1) "WSH is the home of these patients. To throw people out of their only home is cruel." (2) "Co-op apartment programs are in it for the money. Why should a patient leave a place where he lives for free and go someplace where he has to pay rent?" And (3) "Moving these people out is deluding them; they'll never make it. They'll come back to us like they always have."

An additional, albeit unspoken, reason for opposition was a fear of losing jobs. Most of them had already been reassigned once or twice as wards at WSH had been closed or consolidated. By now they were intuiting correctly that the long-term plan was to close their ward as well, although no formal decision had been announced. It is understandable, therefore, that the anxiety level of the staff would be high regarding this most recent effort at census reduction. In fact, the anxiety was so high, and the opposition so strong, that the Co-op eventually gave up recruiting candidates from that ward and concentrated on other sources. Ultimately the ward was closed and patients and staff transferred to other wards. This process involved a loss of status and power for the redeployed workers.

## AUTONOMY: A COMMUNITY BASED
## NETWORK OF SERVICES

The final step toward autonomy to be discussed is the development of the ATC as a nonprofit, community-based, corporate entity and the effects of this development on the provision of service. By mid-1977, all three ATC programs had private nonprofit status through affiliations with People's Church. The funding sources and cooperating agencies had already been reviewed for CLEAT and the Co-op. An additional key development was the affiliation of the WSH-based ADP with People's Church. By attaining nonprofit status, the ADP was able to secure a new source of third-party funding, Special Education money. These funds are mandated for special-needs children by Massachusetts Law, Chapter 766, the state counterpart to P.L. 92-142. The ADP qualified for these tuition funds because the service it renders is deemed necessary in assisting special-needs adolescents to remain in school. It is an especially important source of funds for two reasons. First, it provides the ADP with an operating budget (of about $30,000 per year) to complement the in-kind DMH-WSH staff positions. Thus, for the first time, the ADP has a relatively stable source of income for community recreational expenses, client rewards for behavioral contracts, supplies, food, transportation, staff training, and other basic costs. Second, these funds will allow the ADP to move off the WSH grounds in the near future, joining CLEAT and the Co-op as truly community-based programs.

The emergence of the ATC as an autonomous, private, nonprofit corporation has also generated considerable internal tension. One area of stress has been related to the task of developing adequate administrative and financial expertise. When the ADP first started, the administrative and financial components were supplied by the larger institution, WSH. But as the program developed and CLEAT and Co-op were added, the ATC needed its own administrative organization. In part this has been supplied by the parent corporation, People's Church. However, its expertise was limited; the ATC's third-party contracts were with divisions of public agencies with which the Church had no experience. Over time, some staff, originally hired as clinicians, assumed greater administrative and financial responsibilities. Since these clinicians were without management training, financial planning and policy-making proceeded on a trial and error basis. Only recently have adequate bookkeeping, accounting, and management practices been implemented.

This management "skill deficit" had programmatic ramifications. The administrators were not always able to assess accurately the financial resources of the programs. A financial conservatism resulted, which restricted the adequacy of client service. For example, an initial distrust of DPW's reliability in reimbursing the CLEAT program caused the director to provide a very constricted budget for the program. This led to a less than optimum atmosphere for clients: Recreation was restricted and home improvements were delayed. It is a simplistic but important point that the adequacy of administrative organization in many ways determines the adequacy of direct service.

Another source of tension has been the "unit of service" mentality basic to community-based mental health care as it is being implemented in Massachusetts. "Unit of service" refers to the actual number of days a client participates in a program per month. Typically third-party contracts have rigid requirements about frequency of client participation. Thus if a residence falls below 80-percent occupancy, the program is threatened with a reduced level of reimbursement or eventual cancellation of its contract. Although this may at first seem to be only a reasonable attempt at accountability by the public agencies, the "unit of service" requirements have significant negative effects.

Disturbed adolescents are by nature a volatile, crisis-ridden group. They require periodic changes in programming such as brief rehospitalizations, suspensions, or periods of intense work followed by therapeutic "vacations." This kind of flexibility is basic to the multiple intervention model. "Unit of service" requirements often work against the responsible utilization of this model. Clinical decision-making is compromised by "irrevelant" concerns about levels of participation and census quotas. In turn, conflict develops between the more purist direct-service clinicians and the administrators worried about reimbursement and future fundability. This remains an ongoing dialectic for the ATC and it appears to be insoluble as long as "unit of service" requirements remain inflexible.

## RETROSPECT AND PROSPECT

The ATC has been transformed from an institutional program of WSH into a largely independent community-based network of services. This transformation has occurred by adapting to internal demands and external pressures. Adaptation to environmental conditions produced a variety of organizational responses at each phase in the developmental history of the ATC. A review of these adaptive responses reveals the central theme of this chapter and provides an important perspective for understanding the deinstitutionalization of WSH.

The impetus towards developing the ATC arose from a complex interorganizational "consensus." Internally, Superintendent Myerson's commitment to a philosophy of "normalizing," community-based services for adolescents was the primary determinant. Externally, the policy of deinstitutionalization of the larger mental health system (DMH) and the advocacy of local child welfare agencies also contributed. This "consensus" led to the establishment of the original modest service component, the ADP.

This first step generated considerable resistance within all sectors of WSH. Only the consistent high-level administrative support was able to overcome this resistance to organizational change. Although the opposition was not successful in preventing the establishment of the ADP, it was not without effect. The primary result was that the opposition considerably restricted the resources which the Superintendent could provide to the new program.

In response to this resource deficiency the ADP adapted in a variety of ways. Internally, the staff of the ADP maximized its use of what support was available from the Psychology Department and Dr. Myerson. And externally, the ADP affiliated with a supportive nonprofit corporation and obtained additional funding. With internal support at key places within WSH and external support from diverse sources within the community, the program matured. In the process the ADP was able to increase its professionalism, boundary control, and resources. As resources increased more community activities were possible, but the program continued to rely on WSH for resources and administrative support.

Programmatically the next phase was to establish a community residence. This was supported by DMH and the child welfare agencies, but vehemently opposed by citizens and local government. Again the support of high-level administrators was crucial. In this case, the local and state courts upheld the legality of the program's philosophy.

The theme of resource scarcity continued during the early phases of the CLEAT program. In this case, the deficiency was not due to an interorganizational "compromise," but was due to bureaucratic inertia. The skills of coping with scarcity learned during the origins of the ADP continued to be utilized during this phase of expansion and organizational differentiation.

Only with the establishment of the larger Co-op program were adequate resources provided. In addition, community opposition was minimal. Still, the capacity for institutional resistance remained as "old guard" WSH staff fought the program as they perceived a threat to their job security.

Other significant obstacles remain before the ATC can achieve viability as a young organization in the community of local mental health and social welfare agencies. Management skills must continue to improve. The conflict generated by "unit of service" requirements must be addressed both within the ATC and in relationship to its contracting agencies. More broadly, the absence of stable, long-term funding remains as a major source of uncertainty for the fledgling ATC. The fragile resource base of the program has been pieced together in an ad hoc and opportunistic fashion with the assistance of agencies such as the Department of Mental Health, Public Welfare, Education, the Office of Children, and the People's Church. Whether these arrangements will survive the current fervor in Massachusetts for tax caps and roll-backs in human service budgets remains to be seen. Predictably, when the budgets of state agencies are cut, their administrators react reflexively in protecting well-entrenched programs that have vocal constituencies among the electorate. As a result, the motivation to share resources and effect cooperative, multiagency ventures such as the ATC is quickly eroded.

Perhaps the most significant problem yet to be resolved is the tension between the institutional legacy of the ATC and its community mandate. The programs of the ATC were created to serve *severely disturbed* adolescents *in the community.* Originally designed to supplement the treatment of adolescents hospitalized at WSH, the ATC now provides a wide array of community services for a selected clientele. This transition from an institutional program into a non-profit, community-based network of services has largely been accomplished. Most adolescents can now avoid hospitalization through participation in the WDS, ADP, CLEAT, or Co-op. Nonetheless, a few retarded and seriously dangerous adolescents (perhaps five or six at any one time) continue to be admitted and remain long-term in WSH because they present risks which prevent community placement. Ironically, they resemble a portion of the population whom ADP originally was created to serve. Accordingly, some segments of the social service community feel that the ATC has abandoned its original mandate. The ATC continues to rely on some WSH resources and consequently there is pressure to serve the institutionalized population. On the other hand, some argue that the ATC has been consistent with its community mandate and should not attempt to treat clients incapable of community-based care. This attitude is reinforced both by the prevailing DMH deinstitutionalization philosophy and by the policy of contracting for service, which promotes the "creaming" or selective intake of clients who are more likely to remain in placement and have successful treatment outcomes. Thus, while the ATC has expanded and improved services to disturbed adolescents in the Worcester Area, its community-based network has not fully supplanted the reliance on institutional confinement at WSH. To do so will require much more community acceptance, additional resources, and new forms of innovative programming. These remain as major unfinished tasks in the deinstitutionalization of WSH adolescents.

Howard H. Goldman

# 9
# Linking the Public and Private Sectors: Psychiatry in the General Hospital

The theoretical perspective which guides this volume suggests that the development of organizational boundaries and interorganizational relationships represent adaptive responses of a social system to environmental pressures. Earlier chapters have explored the realignment of organizational boundaries at Worcester State Hospital (WSH) under conditions of resource scarcity and changing social policies. They have described the divisions within the hospital system and analyzed relations between the hospital and other community institutions. This chapter extends that analysis, examining the relationship between WSH and The Memorial Hospital (TMH), a voluntary, nonprofit general hospital in Worcester.

The creation of a linkage between the public and the private mental health services sectors in Worcester deserves careful analysis for practical and theoretical reasons. The President's Commission on Mental Health (1978:12) encouraged such relationships as a mechanism for improving services, and a consideration of such linkages provides an opportunity to expand our knowledge of "organizations in action" (Thompson, 1967). The focus of this chapter is a newly established inpatient psychiatric unit at TMH and its relationship to WSH.[1]

The significance of this relationship can only be appreciated in a historical context. The division of the mental health care system in the 19th century into a public and a private sector was due to the reluctance of community general hospitals and private asylums to provide treatment for the indigent mentally ill. Thus, public resources were allocated for the establishment of separate asylums, since private resources were almost exclusively used to build and finance facilities for paying patients. As the system evolved, the public sector institutions tended to specialize in long-term, custodial care for poor, disturbed, involuntary patients, and the private sector offered treatment to wealthier, acute, quiet, voluntary patients.[2]

Over the past century, the differentiation of the mental health care delivery system has resulted in a pluralism of institutions, methods, theories, and ideologies. The hospitals in each sector were partially isolated and partially interdependent. The divisions between them were characterized by latent conflict, inherent in the societal conditions that gave rise to their original differentiation. Until recently, the hospitals have had little formal contact with each other, except for the occasional transfer of patients. However, recent changes in mental health policy have encouraged relationships between public- and private-sector institutions. Viewed in this historical context, this chapter considers whether linkages between WSH and TMH signal a change in the fundamental conditions which split public and private psychiatry or represent only a temporary organizational adaptation to local environmental conditions in Worcester.

## PSYCHIATRY IN WORCESTER

For more than 100 years WSH dominated psychiatry in Worcester. The hospital was engaged in service, research, and manpower development. A psychiatric residency program at WSH trained physicians in the techniques of hospital practice and the psychodynamic approach to outpatient therapy. Some graduates of the program remained on the staff at WSH; others went into private practice. Some did both. Staff psychiatrists at WSH frequently supplemented their salaries by treating private patients. Occasionally a psychiatrist at WSH would establish such a large private practice that he or she would leave the WSH staff. However, prior to the early 1950s there was no other inpatient facility in Worcester specifically designed for psychiatric care.

In 1954 St. Vincent Hospital (SVH), a community general hospital under the direction of the Roman Catholic Diocese of Worcester, opened a 36-bed inpatient psychiatric unit. The unit was expanded to 50 beds in 1965 and was affiliated with the University of Massachusetts Medical School in 1971. The psychiatrists at SVH had a predominantly "directive–organic" orientation, although some of the staff had been trained in dynamic psychiatry at WSH. In fact, in 1976 at least half of the private psychiatric staff at SVH had some prior professional affiliation with WSH. Not one member of the WSH staff, however, admitted private patients to SVH.

There was little contact between WSH and SVH. Relations between them were strained by tensions derived from different practice styles and attitudes. The two institutions served distinct populations. However, occasionally a patient required transfer from SVH to WSH—either because the patient required involuntary commitment or the patient's insurance or financial resources were exhausted. Usually the patient would be admitted to WSH, but at times, transfers from SVH were refused. These transfers increased the tension between the hospitals. WSH resented being "dumped on"; SVH resented being refused.

Limited contact between WSH and SVH reduced active conflict between the public and private sector in Worcester, but it also deprived WSH psychiatrists of a private practice site in the community. However, in 1971 a former WSH psychiatrist helped to open an 8–10 bed "special care unit" in Holden Hospital, a private suburban hospital. Several WSH psychiatrists were invited to join the staff and admitted private patients to the "special care unit." Most of the psychiatrists found the unit small, improperly staffed, and adequate at best—but they had no alternatives. Other general hospitals in Worcester admitted patients with psychiatric diagnoses to their medical and surgical services, but none had a separate unit. Frequently patients hospitalized for somatic complaints or patients being evaluated in the outpatient clinics required psychiatric consultation. To meet this need general hospitals in Worcester employed part-time psychiatric consultants. Only SVH and Holden Hospital had specialized units.

## PSYCHIATRY AT THE MEMORIAL HOSPITAL

Prior to the 1960s, psychiatric services at TMH had been limited to consultation for emotionally disturbed patients who presented management problems to the medical and nursing staffs. For a short time in the 1920s the newly established Worcester Youth Guidance Center was housed at TMH. However, when the Youth

Guidance Center moved to its own quarters in the 1930s, it no longer needed the affiliation with TMH and it developed autonomously.
During the 1960s, however, several part-time members of the Department of Psychiatry began to care for mentally disturbed children and adults in TMH's ambulatory "Nerve Clinic." Primarily
private practitioners who admitted their psychiatric inpatients at
SVH, the psychiatrists of the "Nerve Clinic" saw poor patients in
the ambulatory department without a fee. A small group therapy
program for children was established, but most of the care consisted of supplying medication to patients. The "Nerve Clinic" served
a limited, charitable function and suffered from marginal status at
TMH.

   Although the development of an inpatient psychiatric unit had
been discussed earlier by the Board of Trustees and the Medical
Staff at TMH, other programs and hospital expansion had taken priority. In 1969 during TMH's third phase of development, a study
was undertaken to assess the need for and the potential role of such
a unit. Ultimately, a 20-bed unit was included in the plans for the
new South Wing building, scheduled to be completed in the early
1970s.

   At about this time the Chief of Psychiatry at TMH died and was
succeeded by a psychiatrist from SVH who had been trained in the
public sector and understood the value of many modes of treatment. In an attempt to revitalize the moribund "Nerve Clinic" he
developed an informal relationship with Dr. Myerson, Superintendant at WSH. Dr. Myerson needed both a community agency to
house a WSH satellite aftercare clinic and a general hospital affiliation to broaden the scope of WSH's psychiatric residency training
program. TMH agreed to provide space for the aftercare clinic;
WSH would provide the professional and paraprofessional staff.
The older psychiatrists who had staffed the "Nerve Clinic" left, returned to SVH, and thus maintained their separation from the public sector. The Chief Psychiatrist of the WSH unit serving the
Worcester catchment area surrounding TMH was appointed Clinic
Director.

   Although expert opinion had been sought concerning the architectural design of the new unit, very little attention had been devoted initially to operational issues. The hospital administration
and representatives of the nursing department, however, had expressed dissatisfaction with the directive–organic orientation of the
Department of Psychiatry. Some felt that medication and electroconvulsive therapy were used excessively at SVH, where the TMH

psychiatrists admitted their patients. An ad hoc planning group for the new psychiatric unit at TMH preferred a therapeutic community approach to inpatient care. The group, composed of hospital administrators, physicians, and nurses, visited other psychiatric units in community hospitals in the area and concluded that a private practice model with a full-time unit director located at TMH would be ideal.

When TMH applied to the State Department of Public Health for a Certificate of Need, it was referred to the Central Office of the Department of Mental Health, which suggested that TMH consult with Dr. Myerson at WSH and with the Department's director in the Worcester region. Doctor Myerson and the Regional Director helped TMH to obtain a Certificate of Need. Already committed to a community mental health approach, they supported the concept of an inpatient psychiatric unit in a Worcester general hospital, particularly if it established a relationship with WSH and the public sector. TMH was an ideal site because it already housed the WSH aftercare clinic which had replaced the old "Nerve Clinic."

TMH had felt no concern about staffing the new unit. The administration anticipated that the new unit would attract some of the established psychiatrists in Worcester, as well as encourage new psychiatrists to move to the community. The presence of the new medical school was considered an added inducement for new physicians to relocate in Worcester. An infusion of psychiatrists was needed in the area. Some of the older practitioners were nearing retirement and there were waiting lists at both SVH and Holden Hospital.

Nor was there concern about the supply of patients. Private practitioners would bring their own patients and the WSH aftercare clinic also would be a source of referrals. However, the financial viability of the inpatient unit *was* a cause of concern. Would aftercare clinic patients have insurance coverage? Could the unit afford to admit Medicaid or nonpaying patients?

These questions offered Dr. Myerson an opportunity to develop his plan for expanding WSH's affiliation with TMH. He vigorously opposed another predominantly private "elite" inpatient unit such as that at SVH. He felt that the public sector psychiatrists, including WSH psychiatric residents, and their disadvantaged patients should have access to the inpatient unit at TMH. He reminded TMH of its obligation to provide care to the indigent as a consequence of the use of Hill-Burton funds in its building program. Doctor Myerson also suspected that WSH staff psychiatrists would move their private practices from Holden Hospital to TMH if given the opportunity. He also recognized the necessity of a closer affiliation between WSH and TMH if WSH's residency training program was to continue to be accredited.

## MEMORIAL HOSPITAL AND THE PUBLIC
## SECTOR: PARTIAL HYBRIDIZATION

Doctor Myerson found TMH staff "surprisingly receptive" to his egalitarian ideology and his plans for affiliation. Apparently there was a substantial area of agreement between TMH and the public sector. They shared elements of a commitment to provide equal access to mental health services and a belief in the merits of a psychodynamic approach to treatment complemented by judicious use of medication and electroconvulsive therapy. They had cooperated at policy-making/administrative levels and WSH staff were already working comfortably in the aftercare clinic at TMH. Psychiatrists at WSH sought a new private inpatient unit for their private practices and TMH needed a psychiatric staff.

Although it was clearly in the private sector, the inpatient unit would admit public-sector patients within a private-practice model. This combination represented a form of "partial hybridization" in organizational terms. Interdependency and commonality of goals, resources, and technology were inadequate for the actual merger that would yield total hybridization. The degree of interdependency and sharing of goals and ideologies was sufficient, however, to permit a close affiliation which would partially affect the development and character of this new unit.

Having seen the direction the new inpatient unit was taking and pressed by other commitments at the University of Massachusetts Medical School, the Chief of Psychiatry at TMH decided to resign and accept the post as Chief of Psychiatry at SVH. He wanted to continue his position at the medical school and he anticipated that the job at TMH would be very time consuming. The unit at SVH was well-established, larger, and its practice style was more congruent with his orientation. He continued, however, to support the different ideological direction of TMH's inpatient unit. He felt certain that the unit was viable and given the presence of a waiting list would not seriously compete with SVH for patients. He also believed that some patients would prefer the approach at TMH to the directive–organic orientation at SVH, but that others would be unwilling to participate in the therapeutic community proposed for the unit at TMH.

The former Chief of Psychiatry at TMH agreed to serve on the search committee to select his replacement, who would act as Director of the inpatient service at TMH. Doctor Myerson was offered the position, but declined, preferring his post at WSH, in spite of its difficulties. Myerson, however, joined the search committee which contacted several excellent psychodynamically oriented candidates with experience in therapeutic comunities. With very little conflict or disagreement the search committee chose a new director in the Spring of 1975.

The unit was scheduled to open in the Fall or Winter of 1975 and a great deal of on-site planning and staff recruitment needed to be completed. In spite of the apparent ease of developing the working relationship between WSH and TMH many problems lay ahead. The public and private sectors in Worcester had maintained little contact. The minimal interaction had been marked by tension, ideological differences, and occasional manifest conflict. The fundamental problems which had divided the mental health system into two separate sectors had not altered. The two systems differed in ideology, resource base, target population, technology, and practice style. In the early planning stages of the new unit, TMH administrators scheduled a meeting at a local exclusive club for all the psychiatrists in Worcester. They naively called together two groups of physicians who had rarely spoken to each other. Many had never met, yet they knew each other by name and prejudicial reputation. Some came purely out of curiosity and discovered that they had more in common than they imagined. This recognition of commonality, which became an oft-repeated cliché, was an encouragement to those who wished to see the unit as a vehicle for rapprochement between the public and private sector.

## THE PSYCHIATRIC UNIT AT MEMORIAL
## HOSPITAL

Although both WSH and TMH recognized the possibility of mutual benefit from their initial cooperation, continued negotiation between the public and private sectors was essential. This process was to reflect old tensions and to produce new conflicts.

## The Director: Private Practice, Public Spirit

The new Director of Mental Health Services at TMH had been trained in a strongly psychoanalytically oriented residency in Boston. He also had experience in the public sector as a Public Health Service offices at St. Elizabeth's Hospital in Washington D.C. and as chief resident on an inpatient unit at Boston State Hospital. Prior to his two years in private practice, he was associate director of the inpatient psychiatric service at a large municipal hospital. He indicated, however, that his training should not be confused with indiscriminant eclecticism. He believed in the principles of dynamic psychiatry and would apply them on the new unit.

The unit at TMH would be guided by the psychoanalytically based model of psychopathology which emphasized the use of psychotherapy in the treatment of mental dysfunction. Although all forms of psychotherapy would be employed in conjunction with milieu therapy and somatic therapies (psychotropic medication and electroconvulsive treatment), the emphasis would be on dynamic concepts in crisis intervention and understanding the nature of the recent insult to the patient's psyche. Treatment plans would be individualized. "Patients shouldn't be fit into boxes," the new director noted. "We wouldn't want to turn anyone away."

In order to inform the professional community of the opening of the new unit, the Director sent out a letter of introduction describing the goals of the unit and the means for achieving them:

Dear Colleague:

The Memorial Hospital is pleased to announce the opening of a 20-bed psychiatric in-patient unit on the 6th floor of the new South Wing.

The goal of our unit is to implement the full range of modern, comprehensive psychiatric care. Each patient's treatment will be highly individualized on the basis of a thorough understanding of the individual, his family, and his social network.

The unit will accept patients over the age of 16 on a voluntary basis who can benefit from acute, intensive psychiatric care (a few days to a few months) on an unlocked unit. We cannot accept patients who are committed, who require long-term hospitalization, who need detoxification from heroin, or who are sufficiently ill physically to require treatment on a medical or surgical unit.

Each patient will have a thorough individual evaluation by one of our attending psychiatrists and, where indicated, psychological testing by a consulting psychologist. We have two social workers to ensure that each patient's family is evaluated and assisted to whatever extent is needed. Our nursing staff and occupational therapist will implement an active therapeutic milieu, which will include daily community meetings and a variety of specialized therapeutic activities. Somatic therapies, such as medication, will be used according to the judgement of the attending psychiatrist. Our physical plant facilitiates an active therapeutic milieu by means of a large day room–dining room surrounded by an occupational therapy workshop, a patient's laundry room, an open kitchen, a library–reading room and an outdoor recreation terrace.

To ensure effective collaboration by the various professionals working with each patient, we will have daily staff conferences led by the Chief of Psychiatry who is full-time at The Memorial Hospital. The complete medical resources of The Memorial Hospital are available for those patients who need them. The psychiatric staff is available to consult on the emotional problems of the patients whose physical illnesses require inpatient treatment in other units of the hospital.

Admissions to the Psychiatric Unit may be made through any psychiatrist who has admitting privileges at The Memorial Hospital. Inquiries about admission may also be made directly to the Psychiatric Services, weekdays, from 9:00 A.M. to 5:00 P.M. or at other hours directly to the unit. The referring person or patient will be asked if he or she prefers any particular psychiatrist or wants the Chief of Psychiatry to select an available psychiatrist. A list of staff psychiatrists will be provided on request.

Referring physicians and other health professionals without privileges will be welcomed as consultants while their patients are on the unit. A referring psychotherapist may continue to work with the patient where appropriate although the direct professional responsibility for the patient will belong to the attending psychiatrist.

We look forward to serving you and the public and welcome any inquiries or suggestions.

Sincerely,

Chief of Psychiatry

## The Psychiatric Staff: Private Practice, Public Servants

When the inpatient unit at TMH opened, six psychiatrists from WSH and two from SVH joined with the Director at TMH to form the core staff of physicians admitting private patients. The psychiatrists from SVH were drawn by the availability of additional beds on the new unit at TMH. The WSH psychiatrists were attracted by a new practice site to replace the limited "special care unit" at Holden Hospital, which had served their private practices. In addition, the WSH psychiatrists already had a relationship with TMH based in the aftercare clinic in the outpatient department.

Doctor Myerson, Superintendant at WSH, was among the public-sector psychiatrists who used the unit at TMH. Although he admitted very few patients, he agreed to participate in teaching conferences and to conduct psychiatric consultation rounds on the medical service at TMH. He was accompanied on these rounds by WSH residents in order to expose them to consultation–liaison psychiatry, otherwise missing from the WSH residency curriculum. Largely because of the deficiencies in the residency, Myerson worked hard to maintain ties with TMH.

In addition to Myerson, the Assistant Superintendant at WSH initially became actively involved in the activities on TMH's inpatient unit, but within a few months he discovered that his WSH duties were too demanding. With his characteristic enthusiasm he had admitted not only private patients but also some WSH patients who needed special care. On several occasions he asked WSH psychiatric residents to attend to these patients on the ward at TMH.

Four other WSH psychiatrists joined the psychiatric staff at TMH. Three of them had small private practices and admitted relatively few patients. The fourth was the director of the aftercare clinic at TMH and a unit chief at WSH. In this dual role he saw many patients suitable for the inpatient unit at TMH. It is not surprising, therefore, that he admitted more patients than any other psychiatrist from either WSH or SVH. However, dividing his time between public and private practice became too exhausting and created too much conflict in both sectors. He was unable to fulfill his obligations and responsibilities at both WSH and TMH. In July, 1976 he resigned from WSH and was employed by TMH on a part-time basis as Director of the Psychiatric Outpatient Clinic. In this capacity he continued to oversee the WSH-TMH aftercare clinic and to admit patients to the inpatient unit at TMH.

Other WSH staff left the public sector to work at TMH when the new inpatient service opened. Three young staff nurses, a nursing supervisor, and a nursing instructor from WSH joined the staff at TMH, adding to the drain on WSH resources. Although lured by higher salaries, the selected patient population, and the opportunity to work on a unit in a therapeutic community, these nurses contributed to the public-sector perspective of the partially hybridized unit. They also encouraged the unit to accept patients from the aftercare clinic and from WSH.

## The Patients: Private Practice,
## Public Contact

The dual public–private affiliations of the staff and the developing relationship between TMH and WSH encouraged a higher degree of heterogeneity in the patient population ("case-mix") than is usually found on an inpatient unit in a nonpublic general hospital.[3] The stereotype of the patient on such a general hospital psychiatric unit is a young, insured, employed adult. One would also expect that most patients would have acute, nonpsychotic disorders predominantly and that few patients would have had prior hospitalizations, and almost none in the public sector.

An analysis of the first 12 months of operation of the unit at TMH suggests that partial hybridization had marked effects. Most striking was the number of patients who had prior contact with the public sector. On three successive monthly spot-checks late in 1977, 20 percent of the patients on the unit previously had been inpatients at WSH and 40 percent had prior contact with the WSH aftercare clinics, most frequently at the TMH outpatient department. Another 10 percent had been patients in SVH's psychiatric unit, and a small number had been at Holden Hospital. This clearly was not an "elite" population of first admissions.

The diagnostic categories also revealed some deviation from the norm for general hospital units. TMH's unit cared for a larger percentage of psychotic patients (41 percent) than the average for all general hospital units in Massachusetts (29 percent) or for SVH (31 percent) (see Table 1). This difference probably was due to the unit's greater opportunity for contact with psychotic patients, often admitted through the aftercare clinic. More importantly, however, it reflected a willingness by the director and staff of the unit at TMH to expend the extra effort necessary to care for these difficult patients. This commitment permeated the whole staff, perhaps influenced by the prior experience of many in the public sector. The psychiatrists and nurses from WSH were most outspoken in their support of treating these patients rather than transferring them to WSH.

The ward atmosphere and the degree of patient psychopathology on TMH's unit, however, was considerably less disturbed than that which characterized WSH's locked wards. This was due to the voluntary nature of the admissions to the unit and to the refusal to admit violent or out-of-control patients. The unit at TMH was so much more "normal" than the wards at WSH that a paranoid for-

# Table 1

Characteristics of Admissions to Worcester State Hospital and to Psychiatric Inpatient Units at St. Vincent's Hospital, The Memorial Hospital, and at a Sample of Other General Hospitals in Massachusetts.

| Facility and Admissions Characteristics | Worcester State Hospital — Greater Worcester Unit Admissions Wards | | Private Non-Profit General Hospitals | | | | | |
| --- | --- | --- | --- | --- | --- | --- | --- | --- |
| | | | St. Vincent's | | Memorial | | Statewide Sample of 22 Hospitals | |
| Time Period | May–June 1977 | | June 1976–May 1977 | | October 1976–September 1977 | | Fiscal Year 1974 | |
| Number of psychiatric beds | 60 | | 51 | | 20 | | 599 | |
| Number of admissions | 96 | | 1033 | | 246 | | 7618 | |
| Average stays (days) | 22[a] | | 17 | | 26 | | 20 | |
| Legal Status | N | % | N | % | N | % | N | % |
| Voluntary | 66 | 68.8 | 1033 | 100.0 | 246 | 100.0 | 7547 | 99.1 |
| Involuntary | 30 | 30.2 | 0 | 0.0 | 0 | 0.0 | 71 | 0.9 |
| Total | 96 | 100.0 | 1033 | 100.0 | 246 | 100.0 | 7618 | 100.0 |
| Payment | N | % | N | % | N | % | N | % |
| Insurance | —[b] | — | 1067 | 53.9 | 173 | 70.3 | 3885 | 51.0 |
| Medicare | — | — | 318 | 16.1 | 17 | 6.9 | 1235 | 16.2 |
| Medicaid | — | — | 280 | 14.1 | 42 | 17.1 | 1615 | 21.2 |
| Self | — | — | 189 | 9.5 | 11 | 4.5 | 533 | 7.0 |
| Other | — | — | 127 | 6.4 | 3 | 1.2 | 350 | 4.6 |
| Total | — | — | 1981[c] | 100.0 | 246 | 100.0 | 7618 | 100.0 |

| Diagnoses | N | % | N | % | N | % | N | % |
|---|---|---|---|---|---|---|---|---|
| Subtotal psychotic | (79) | (82.2) | (611) | (30.9) | (100) | (40.7) | (2230) | (29.2) |
| Organic | 5 | 5.2 | 38 | 1.9 | 4 | 1.6 | 69 | 0.8 |
| Schizophrenic | 55 | 57.3 | 235 | 11.9 | 43 | 17.5 | 1376 | 18.1 |
| Other | 19 | 19.8 | 338 | 17.1 | 53 | 21.6 | 785 | 10.3 |
| Subtotal non-psychotic | (13) | (13.6) | (1370) | (69.1) | (146) | (59.3) | (5388) | (70.8) |
| Neurosis | 2 | 2.1 | 668 | 33.7 | 100 | 40.7 | 2952 | 38.8 |
| Personality disorder | 6 | 6.3 | 80 | 4.0 | 19 | 7.7 | 533 | 7.0 |
| Alcoholism | 3 | 3.1 | 435 | 22.0 | 4 | 1.6 | 533 | 7.0 |
| Other | 2 | 2.1 | 187 | 9.4 | 23 | 9.3 | 1370 | 18.0 |
| Unknown | (4) | (4.2) | (0) | 0.0 | (0) | 0.0 | (0) | 0.0 |
| Total | 96 | 100.0 | 1981[c] | 100.0 | 246 | 100.0 | 7618 | 100.0 |

Source: Data for Worcester State Hospital, St. Vincent's Hospital, and The Memorial Hospital were obtained from the medical record office at each hospital. The state-wide sample data were obtained from the Massachusetts Hospital Association, Report of the Task Force on Psychiatric Services, January 1976.

a Based on Data for 1973.

b The cost of care at Worcester State Hospital is paid by the state in most instances. Specific figures on self-payment and third-party reimbursement for the minority of patients whose changes are not covered by state appropriations were unavailable.

c Includes primary and secondary psychiatric diagnoses.

mer WSH patient refused to believe that she was in a psychiatric unit when she was admitted to TMH for treatment. She begged to be transferred back to WSH: "At the state hospital everyone is really sick like me. These people are all spies; they aren't patients at all but disguised staff here to help me."

The former WSH staff shared an element of this patient's perception. They were impressed by the relative health of the patients at TMH and surprised by their social resources. Unlike their counterparts at WSH, the patients at TMH generally had families, jobs, and homes. They also had health insurance—the most direct reflection of a patient's financial resources and a key to admission to the new unit. About half of patients admitted to the unit at TMH had Blue Cross–Blue Shield coverage, and another quarter had either commercial insurance or Medicare—all of which pay the hospital and the psychiatrist adequately for their work. The remainder either had Medicaid or no third-party source of payment. In the latter category were those who were poor but ineligible or who had not applied for Medicaid. Almost no patients were able to pay for their hospitalization "out-of-pocket." None of Worcester's gentry and few professionals were admitted to the unit at TMH. This was also the pattern at other local facilities. Apparently, the wealthier elements in Worcester were hospitalized in nonpublic psychiatric centers elsewhere in New England.


## CONFLICT ON THE INPATIENT UNIT: THE PRICE OF PARTIAL HYBRIDIZATION

The mixture of elements of the public and private sector on the inpatient unit at TMH created tension and conflict. Some conflict was latent, inherent in the essential differences between the public and private sectors. Other conflict was manifest, involving issues of responsibility for admissions of disadvantaged patients, patient transfer, and coverage of psychiatric emergencies. Conflicts surfaced at the boundaries between WSH and TMH.


### Patient Selection: Boundary Control

Control over admissions was one of the more important processes governing the "case mix" on the unit (Morrissey, 1976). This important function of "boundary control" (Thompson, 1962) was managed by the inpatient unit director and his secretary. The Director was employed by TMH on a full-time basis. In addition to managing private patients and serving as the administrator of the ward, he and the director of the aftercare clinic were expected to take referrals from the clinic and outside sources. The clinic director had primary responsibility for the clinic admissions; the unit director received calls from agencies and staff physicians. The hospital did not require, however, that salaried physicians admit every patient who requested admission. As a result the unit director made many referrals to other psychiatrists at TMH and other facilities. He reserved discretionary control over admissions.

The most commonly cited "source of referral" listed on the face sheet of patient records was the name of the admitting psychiatrist. The admission history, however, suggested a more complicated route to TMH. Sometimes a primary care provider would refer a patient to a private psychiatrist or to TMH's aftercare clinic and then, after an initial or extended period of evaluation, the person would be admitted to the unit. Occasionally a consultation to the medical or surgical service would lead to an admission to the unit. TMH's aftercare clinic was also a common source of patients, many of whom had previous experience in the public sector, especially at WSH. This was due to the cooperative nature of the clinic, where WSH staff followed former patients and others with psychological problems who could not afford or would not seek psychiatric care in a private office. Some potential admissions were too disturbed to be admitted directly to TMH; others were sent to WSH or to SVH to wait for a bed to become available at TMH. Some patients were transferred directly from WSH to TMH for specific treatment, such as electroconvulsive therapy, unavailable at the state hospital.

Not all referrals were routed directly through the Director or another TMH psychiatrist. The unit secretary received calls from individuals and families, human services professionals within and outside the hospital, members of TMH's medical staff, and from WSH. Some calls were requests for admission, others were inquiries about outpatient referrals. When the needs were unclear, the secretary would refer the call to a psychiatrist or social worker on the inpatient unit for evaluation—either privately or through the aftercare clinic.

These calls were managed according to an unwritten policy which reflected the constraints of the unit. A patient first needed to be judged appropriate for the unit: Did he/she require inpatient treatment or was outpatient care sufficient? Was he/she able and willing to sign a voluntary commitment paper? Was he/she an alcoholic or drug dependent person requiring detoxification? Did he/she require high security or a locked facility because of unusual violence? Where the decision was difficult, it was made by a unit psychiatrist, occasionally in cooperation with a clinic psychiatrist or other therapist. "Inappropriate" patients were referred elsewhere—to WSH, drug and alcohol treatment centers, and the police.

Once a patient was determined to be appropriate for admission to TMH, the secretary used another formula to assign a psychiatrist. If the patient was relatively well-to-do, or had insurance or Medicare, she generally was able to arrange for a psychiatrist to take responsibility for the case. Some of the psychiatrists, however, rarely accepted referrals, choosing to hospitalize only their own carefully selected private patients—one or two at a time. Most had a limit on the number of patients they would accept on referral; few psychiatrists felt comfortable treating more than four inpatients at any one time. Occasionally they would exceed this number, but only in an emergency, as a special favor, or when providing coverage for another psychiatrist.

If the patient was on Medicaid or had no third-party coverage, it was more difficult to find a psychiatrist willing to admit the patient. Reimbursements from Medicaid were much lower than insurance reimbursement ($12.50–$17.50 versus $30.00–$40.00 per inpatient visit). According to the psychiatrists, Medicaid payments were also slow in arriving and accompanied by excessive "red tape."

The hospital-based psychiatrists, the inpatient unit, and the aftercare clinic directors had a responsibility to take a "fair share" of the patients without "adequate" third-party coverage. The hospital had an informal commitment to take patients referred by its aftercare clinic, a frequent source of disadvantaged patients often with a history of admissions to WSH. The hospital also had an obligation to fill a proportion of its beds with nonpaying patients because of its use of Federal funds in its building program. The inpatient director helped TMH meet this responsibility both by treating these patients himself and by negotiating with other staff psychiatrists to share this responsibility with the unit and the hospital. All psychiatrists were expected to do their share in helping with this commitment to disadvantaged patients. The staff recruited from WSH, predictably, were more willing to do this than those recruited from SVH.

Occasionally, however, a patient could not be matched with a psychiatrist or there was no bed available immediately. In these cases, the patient would be referred elsewhere, or if it was not an emergency, would be placed on a waiting list until a bed and/or a psychiatrist could be found. The most common reason for referral elsewhere, after ruling out "inappropriate" individuals, was the absence of a bed, followed in frequency by the lack of a psychiatrist. The latter was especially true for disadvantaged patients. This was a source of conflict for the unit because of TMH's commitment to the public sector.

There were a number of mechanisms used to reduce this tension and increase the capacity of the unit at TMH to accept disadvantaged patients. If a co-therapist could be found, a TMH psychiatrist might be willing to accept a Medicaid or other disadvantaged patient, knowing that the reduced payments would be defrayed by a reduced commitment of time spent caring for the patient. Co-therapists were found among the patient's counselors or case workers in other agencies, or in a social worker or a nurse therapist from the aftercare clinic.

Occasionally, an inpatient nurse who had established an important therapeutic relationship with a patient during a previous admission might be co-opted into taking a more active and time-consuming role with a disadvantaged patient on a subsequent admission. Sometimes the nurses had difficulty refusing a psychiatrist's request for assistance with patients and accepted more responsibility than they had time for or than they really wanted. Moreover, at times competent nursing staff were given assignments which exceeded their feeling of expertise. Their workloads were further increased when they were unable to locate a psychiatrist for consultation or to obtain authorization for an order. This was a major source of intrastaff conflict for the unit.

The social workers also occasionally acted as co-therapists, especially if patients were admitted primarily for family or couples therapy or for social service problems. For disadvantaged or chronic patients they would assume a major role in the management of the case, allowing the psychiatrist additional time for other aspects of work.

Psychiatric residents, too, helped to care for disadvantaged patients for whom a private psychiatrist could not be found. Even before a formal relationship was developed with the WSH residency program, psychiatric residents from WSH treated patients on the unit at TMH. By the first birthday of the inpatient service, one WSH resident was regularly assigned to TMH's inpatient unit, primarily treating disadvantaged and difficult patients. As the linkage between WSH and TMH developed, the public sector psychiatric residents increasingly were drawn into roles mediating conflict within and between the boundaries of the two institutions (Goldman, 1978).

### Patient Transfer and Emergency Coverage

Patient selection provided a mechanism for reducing tension and fiscal uncertainty for the inpatient unit by controlling the "case mix" prior to admission to TMH. Patient transfer and referral was a method for adjusting the mix after admission. Insured patients whose behavior became unmanageable on the ward were occasionally transferred to a private psychiatric hospital. Poor and very disturbed patients, many with prior WSH experience, created special problems for the unit. When indigent patients became unmanageable they were transferred to WSH, but not without difficulty.

Patients resisted transfer to WSH and the WSH staff resented its role as a backup for TMH. When transfers required involuntary commitment, WSH staff and administration made the process difficult in order to minimize the "dumping" of unwanted patients. The psychiatric residents from WSH were involved most frequently in this transfer process—on both sides of the boundary between WSH and TMH. Occasionally patients regarded as inappropriate for TMH did not meet the criteria of dangerousness necessary for involuntary commitment at WSH. Some of these patients were evaluated at WSH and released. Often this situation led to a series of acrimonious debates which promoted animosity between TMH and WSH. While these problems are typical of relations between private and public institutions, feelings were intensified because of the developing link between the two hospitals. Staff in both institutions felt a sense of disappointment and betrayal—a sense of exploitation and compromise, when confronted with the persistent differences between them.

Animosity and conflict permeated other relations between WSH and TMH, such as the coverage of psychiatric emergencies at the general hospital by WSH staff. An agreement between TMH's psychiatric staff, many of whom were WSH psychiatrists, and Dr. Myerson called for the psychiatric resident on-call at WSH to serve also as "backup" for psychiatric emergencies at TMH's inpatient unit, medical and surgical services, and emergency ward. Although the private psychiatrists at TMH were assigned on rotation to cover psychiatric emergencies, they were occasionally unavailable, especially on weekends or in the middle of the night. Despite the fact that WSH had played this role prior to the expansion of TMH's Department of Psychiatry, the continuation of this policy after the development of the inpatient unit was particularly resented by the WSH residents. They received calls and emergency transfers at any hour of the day or night.

Patients were also transfered from the inpatient unit to the aftercare clinic at TMH. Just as WSH psychiatric residents and nonmedical ward personnel absorbed some of the burden of caring for nonpaying and difficult patients during hospitalization, these same professionals provided aftercare to disadvantaged patients following discharge from the unit at TMH. On several occasions private patients were referred by their psychiatrists to the aftercare clinic when their insurance benefits expired or were exhausted. Troublesome or noncompliant patients were referred to the aftercare clinic as well. Like the inpatient unit, the clinic at TMH, combining elements of the public and private sectors, was partially hybridized— simultaneously a source of tension and a mechanism for reducing conflict at TMH.

## LINKING THE PUBLIC AND PRIVATE SECTOR: WHO BENEFITS?

In spite of differences between public- and private-sector psychiatry in Worcester, the relationship between WSH and TMH developed through the late 1970s. Differences and conflicts arose but mechanisms for reducing tension helped WSH and TMH adapt to their evolving relationship. But does this new link between public and private psychiatry in Worcester signal a change in the fundamental conditions which historically have separated them, or does it represent temporary adaptation to local conditions?

There is no evidence of fundamental change in any of the forces which resulted in the differentiation of the mental health care delivery system into public and private sectors. The institutions in each sector remain partially competitive and partially interdependent. The relationship between WSH and TMH developed because of mutual benefits as both expanded their mental health services: TMH needed to staff an outpatient clinic; WSH wanted a new community clinic. WSH psychiatrists desired a private practice site; TMH needed a psychiatric staff. TMH had to meet a commitment to its disadvantaged community; WSH had disadvantaged patients with special mental health needs. WSH's residency training program sought a general hospital affiliation; TMH desired the status as a training site and benefitted from the additional manpower provided by the psychiatric residents. The linkage between them was characterized by partial hybridization.

As we have seen, hybridization resulted in tension and conflict related to the basic differences between WSH and TMH at the same time that it satisfied mutual needs. The linkage between public and private sectors in Worcester exaggerated the difference between them. This seeming paradox can be explained by looking closely at the "creaming process" (McKinlay, 1975) as it occurred in Worcester.

The creation of the psychiatric unit at TMH began by skimming off the energies of Dr. Myerson and other Department of Mental Health administrators, and then further diverted the attention of the psychiatrists at WSH away from the wards. Already involved in private practice, the WSH psychiatrists found the new unit to be an excellent and congenial practice site. Further, some of the younger and more energetic nurses left the WSH wards to work at TMH. Finally, some of the more desirable and manageable patients from the public sector were "creamed" for treatment at TMH. Some were transferred from the wards; some were admitted from the aftercare clinic at TMH; and others were referred from the emergency service at WSH. Typically, these patients were "appropriate" for TMH: voluntary, nonviolent, and amenable to treatment. Often, they were less chronic, more motivated, and better insured than the average WSH patient. As a result, these "more desirable" patients, who had been treated at WSH prior to the era of general hospital psychiatry, were admitted to TMH.

The "cream" of the public sector was skimmed off by the private sector. What resulted was an enlarging gulf between WSH and TMH, spanned by a bridge traveled by patients and staff. In the short run, the bridge helped WSH to adapt to scarcity and changing mental health policies. The link benefited the private practices of WSH psychiatrists; it benefited the psychiatric residency at WSH; and it benefited the few WSH patients fortunate enough to be admitted to TMH. However, WSH's resources were depleted and its patient population was reduced to a residual of the poorest and the most difficult. In contrast, TMH was able to deliver high-quality psychiatric care to carefully preselected patients. This was possible because it controlled sufficient resources to attract high-calibre staff, because it had the autonomy to govern its own admission's policy, and because it could rely on WSH to shoulder the responsibility for the tasks and patients unwanted by the private sector. In the long run, in the absence of fresh resources and a change in its historical mandate, WSH continues to be responsible for the disadvantaged, the involuntary, and the most chronic and disturbed. In this capacity WSH fulfills a public duty and maintains the privilege of private practice.

## POSTSCRIPT

With the demise of WSH's medical superintendency and the subsequent transfer of its Residency Training Program to the University of Massachusetts Medical Center (see Chapters 4 and 11), the inpatient unit at TMH began to move more fully into the mainstream of private psychiatry in Worcester. Public-sector psychiatric residents no longer worked on the unit and the organizational linkages described in this chapter came undone. However, TMH continued to operate its aftercare clinic in conjunction with the Greater Worcester Area Unit at WSH and a few of the senior psychiatrists who left WSH for full-time private practice maintained their affiliations with TMH. In addition, TMH continued to care for a mix of patients drawn from the public and private sectors. Thus, in spite of the termination of innovative linkages for the staffing of a hybrid public–private sector inpatient unit, a residue of public sector involvement could still be found at TMH.

Whether this involvement will provide a base for future collaboration with public sector psychiatry remains to be seen. The historical record of TMH and WSH does provide a precedent for the on-again, off-again convergence of their mutual organizational interests. In the 1920s, during the heyday of the mental hygiene movement, TMH provided the first site for the Youth Guidance Center organized under the auspices of WSH. After a hiatus of nearly 50 years, the fates of these two hospials were reconnected by the programs described in this chapter. Opportunities for their reemergence in the immediate future will be conditioned by ongoing policy debates concerning the role of the general hospital inpatient unit. In 1980, a coalition of interests was exerting strong pressures on local general hospitals to assume major responsibility for involuntary treatment (Leeman, 1980; Leeman and Berger, 1980) as a step toward closing the remaining state hospitals in Massachusetts. As in past eras, the outcomes of these extra-local policy debates will shape the enduring roles of TMH and WSH as part of the functional ecology of mental health services in Worcester.


**NOTES**

1. This chapter is based on over two years of direct observation of the creation and maturation of a new inpatient psychiatric unit at The Memorial Hospital (TMH) in Worcester, Massachusetts. The details of the methods and findings of this investigation are presented in the author's doctoral dissertation (Goldman, 1978). As a participant observer, the author participated in negotiations concerning the functioning of the new unit, served as a psychiatric resident in the aftercare clinic for almost two years, and worked on the inpatient unit for 25–30 hours per week during a six month period.
2. This brief historical review is derived from the author's monograph (Goldman, 1977) based on multiple secondary sources (including Grob, 1966; Grob, 1973; Rothman, 1971).
3. The characteristics attributed to patients in nonpublic general hospitals are derived from the unpublished chartbook of data collected in the sample survey of general hospital psychiatric units conducted in 1975 by the American Hospital Association and the Division of Biometry and Epidemiology, National Institute of Mental Health.

E. Milling Kinard

# 10
# Beyond Institutional Walls: Discharged Patients in the Community

In this chapter, the emphasis shifts from the organizational process-es of deinstitutionalization in the Worcester area to a consideration of the posthospital fates of patients in the community. Focusing on patient outcomes provides a means of assessing the extent to which community programs spawned under the twin policies of deinstitu-tionalization and "communitization" of mental health care have ac-tually met the aftercare needs of former mental hospital patients. Reactions to the state hospital deinstitutionalization movement have culminated in a "backlash," heightened by numerous reports in the professional and popular literature documenting wide-spread abuse and neglect of chronic mental patients in the commu-nity. Knowledge about patient outcomes is, therefore, politically and programmatically crucial to the ongoing debates about the success-es and failures of deinstitutionalization and the future role of state mental hospitals.

The research presented in this chapter focuses on the posthos-pital experiences of a cohort of patients released from Worcester

The study reported in this chapter was conducted as a collaborative project between the Brandeis-Worcester Training Program in Social Research and Psychiatry and the Division of Research and Evaluation of the Massachusetts Department of Mental Health. The Brandeis-Worcester Training Program in Social Research and Psychiatry was a joint program sponsored by Brandeis University, Worcester State Hospital, and the Worcester Youth Guidance Center, and was supported by a grant from the National Institute of Mental Health (MH-13154).

State Hospital (WSH) and two other nearby state hospitals to communities in central and eastern Massachusetts during 1974. At the time this study was in the planning stage, WSH had already discharged the majority of its chronic, long-stay patients no longer requiring continuous hospitalization (Myerson et al., 1974). The Massachusetts Department of Mental Health (DMH) was interested in further census reduction, but was concerned about the extent to which such a policy might be contraindicated by the outcomes of patients then being discharged from the state hospitals. DMH was especially interested in patients released to noninstitutional placements in the community in order to assess whether the shift from hospital to community living represented an improvement in the patients' environment and whether aftercare services were fulfilling their intended objectives.

The choice of the other two hospitals for this study was also determined by DMH policy interests. Central Massachusetts was served by three state hospitals located within 25 miles of each other in Gardner, Westboro, and Worcester. As part of the DMH regionalization and area planning process, the closure of the hospitals in Gardner and Westboro and the reassignment of their service regions to Worcester was under active consideration.[1] In terms of both physical proximity and future utilization, then, a study involving these three hospitals was seen as highly desirable.

## METHODOLOGY

### Subjects

The selection criteria used to designate a patient cohort at each hospital were (1) age 18–70 years at index release; (2) diagnoses of functional psychoses or neuroses at index release; (3) independent living settings at index release, that is, living with families or living alone; and (4) continuous stays in the community since the index release. Excluded from the eligible population were patients with primary diagnoses of organic brain syndrome, mental retardation, or drug or alcohol abuse; those discharged to nursing homes or congregate care facilities; and those rehospitalized between the index release and the follow-up interview.

The original design proposed interviewing a total of 300 patients (100 from each of the three hospitals) from the total eligible population of 583 patients released between January 1 and September 30, 1974. The sample was to be selected from the eligible population at each hospital utilizing random numbers; the selection process was to continue until the desired total of 100 patients from each hospital had been interviewed.

However, due to difficulties in locating patients in the community and refusals from some patients, the entire population of 583 cases was exhausted before reaching the desired sample size. A total of 176 patients were interviewed between May and October, 1975. The time period between the index hospital release and the follow-up interview ranged from 8 to 21 months, with a mean of 12.7 months.

## Procedures

Interviews were conducted with patients in their homes after consent forms were received from each patient in response to a letter from the superintendent of the hospital from which the patient was released describing the study and requesting participation. Questions focused on patients' lifestyles both before and after hospitalization and their use of aftercare services and assessment of the adequacy of these services. Information about the index hospitalization was abstracted from hospital records.

SAMPLE BIAS

Potential bias in the study sample due to attrition, a common problem in follow-up studies of released patients (Bachrach, 1976a, 1976b), was determined by comparing the interviewed with the noninterviewed patients. Contingency table analysis showed no statistically significant differences on socio-demographic characteristics between the 176 interviewed patients and the remainder of the eligible population ($N = 407$). Only one significant difference occurred on hospitalization characteristics: interviewed patients were more likely than noninterviewed patients to have drugs prescribed at discharge. Considering the number of statistical tests performed, this one difference may well have occurred by chance alone. Thus, the interviewed sample seems to be broadly representative of the eligible population.

The three hospitals were also compared with respect to socio-demographic and hospitalization characteristics for both the eligible population and the interviewed sample. Of the total interviewed sample, 68 (38.6 percent) were from Worcester, 76 (43.2 percent) from Westboro, and 32 (18.2 percent) from Gardner State Hospitals. Although contingency table analysis revealed some statistically significant differences among the three hospital subsamples, the differences were minor. Consequently, the groups from the three hospitals were pooled so that a sufficiently large sample size would be available for the analysis of patient outcomes.

## SAMPLE CHARACTERISTICS

The sample as a whole tended to be evenly distributed across the categories of age, marital status, and education (Table 1). Only two significant differences between males and females were noted: males were more likely than females to be young and single. Most of the study sample had diagnoses of functional psychoses, had short-term stays for the index hospitalization, and had one or more drugs prescribed at release. The large proportion of study patients (73.4 percent) who were prescribed drugs at the time of release from the hospital supports the belief that psychotropic medication has been vital to the deinstitutionalization movement. The most common drugs prescribed were antipsychotic medications (68.1 percent).

The majority of the patients had previous psychiatric hospitalizations, either at the same hospital from which they had been released or at other psychiatric institutions. The number of prior admissions to the index hospital ranged from 1 to 6, with a mean of 2.2. Half of the respondents (51.4 percent) had prior admissions to the index hospital; similarly, more than half (58.1 percent) had prior admissions to other psychiatric facilities. The frequency of multiple psychiatric hospitalizations and of short stays for the index hospitalization suggests that the study sample may exemplify the "revolving door" patients who continue to be readmitted to state hospitals across the country despite deinstitutionalization (Goldman, 1979).

## POSTHOSPITAL LIFE STYLES

### Living Arrangements

Living situations were classified into three types: (1) families of procreation; (2) families of origin; and (3) nonfamily settings, that is, living alone or with unrelated individuals. A comparison of prehospital and posthospital living arrangements showed a strong significant relationship (Table 2), indicating that little change occurred from before to after hospitalization. Almost all who did not return to families of procreation or origin shifted to nonfamily

**Table 1**

Socio-Demographic and Hospitalization Characteristics
of Study Sample

| Variables | Male N | Male % | Female N | Female % | Total* N | Total* % |
|---|---|---|---|---|---|---|
| **Socio-Demographic Characteristics** | | | | | | |
| Age at Release from Hospital † | | | | | | |
| 18–24 years | 22 | 28.6 | 18 | 18.9 | 40 | 23.3 |
| 25–34 years | 30 | 39.0 | 22 | 23.2 | 52 | 30.2 |
| 35–44 years | 14 | 18.2 | 26 | 27.4 | 40 | 23.3 |
| 45–65 years | 11 | 14.3 | 29 | 30.5 | 40 | 23.3 |
| Marital Status at Interview ‡ | | | | | | |
| Single | 40 | 50.0 | 22 | 22.9 | 62 | 35.2 |
| Married | 21 | 26.3 | 33 | 34.4 | 54 | 30.7 |
| Separated, divorced, or widowed | 19 | 23.8 | 41 | 42.7 | 60 | 34.1 |
| Education | | | | | | |
| Grade 9 or less | 21 | 26.6 | 27 | 28.1 | 48 | 27.4 |
| Grades 10–11 | 14 | 17.7 | 19 | 19.8 | 33 | 18.9 |
| High school graduate | 22 | 27.8 | 29 | 30.2 | 51 | 29.1 |
| Beyond high school | 22 | 27.8 | 21 | 21.9 | 43 | 24.6 |
| **Hospitalization Characteristics** | | | | | | |
| Diagnosis | | | | | | |
| Functional psychoses | 58 | 72.5 | 63 | 65.6 | 121 | 68.8 |
| Neuroses | 16 | 20.0 | 28 | 29.2 | 44 | 25.0 |
| Other | 6 | 7.5 | 5 | 5.2 | 11 | 6.3 |
| Previous Psychiatric Hospitalizations | | | | | | |
| Yes | 64 | 82.1 | 67 | 69.8 | 131 | 75.3 |
| No | 14 | 17.9 | 29 | 30.2 | 43 | 24.7 |
| Length of Stay | | | | | | |
| Under 1 month | 46 | 59.1 | 58 | 62.4 | 104 | 60.8 |
| 1–3 months | 26 | 33.3 | 19 | 20.4 | 45 | 26.3 |
| Over 3 months | 6 | 7.7 | 16 | 17.2 | 22 | 12.9 |
| Number of Drugs Prescribed at Release | | | | | | |
| None | 23 | 30.7 | 20 | 23.0 | 43 | 26.5 |
| One | 33 | 44.0 | 39 | 44.8 | 72 | 44.4 |
| Two–Four | 19 | 25.3 | 28 | 32.2 | 47 | 29.0 |
| Months Since Release | | | | | | |
| Under 1 year | 34 | 43.6 | 30 | 31.6 | 64 | 37.0 |
| 12–14 months | 28 | 35.9 | 30 | 31.6 | 58 | 33.5 |
| 15 or more months | 16 | 20.5 | 35 | 36.8 | 51 | 29.5 |

*Total may not equal 176 because of missing data.

† $\chi^2 = 11.574$; $p = .010$.

‡ $\chi^2 = 14.625$; $p < .001$.

**Table 2**
Living Arrangements Before and After Hospitalization

| Prehospital Living Arrangements | Posthospital Living Arrangements | | | | | | | |
|---|---|---|---|---|---|---|---|---|
| | Procreation Family | | Origin Family | | Nonfamily | | Total* | |
| | N | % | N | % | N | % | N | % |
| Procreation family | 73 | 94.8 | — | — | 4 | 5.2 | 77 | 100.0 |
| Origin family | 1 | 2.1 | 35 | 74.5 | 11 | 23.4 | 47 | 100.0 |
| Nonfamily | 4 | 7.8 | 9 | 17.6 | 38 | 74.5 | 51 | 100.0 |
| Total | 78 | 44.6 | 44 | 25.1 | 53 | 30.3 | 175 | 100.0 |

\* Total is less than 176 because of missing data.
$\chi^2 = 193.680$, p < .001;
gamma = .889, p < .001.

settings. Those who changed from nonfamily situations tended to return to their families of origin rather than establish their own family units. These findings held for both males and females.

The majority of the study patients (62.0 percent) resided at the same address after release as before admission. All of those who changed address also changed living arrangements. Most former patients lived in single family houses (41.0 percent) or apartments (50.6 percent). Very few (8.4 percent) were living in the kinds of residences—boarding houses, rooming houses, hotels—commonly described as "dumping grounds" for former mental hospital patients (Etzioni, 1975; Lamb and Goertzel, 1971; Reich and Siegel, 1973).

## Employment

Three categories described employment status: (1) employed, (2) not employed, and (3) housewife. For posthospital employment status, the "not employed" category was further subdivided to distinguish between those not employed at the time of interview but employed since hospital release, and those not employed at all since hospital release.

As Table 3 shows, posthospital employment status was significantly related to prehospital employment status, thus revealing little change. For those who did change, nearly half employed before hospitalization were not employed at the time of interview. Sizeable proportions of patients not working prior to hospital admis-

**Table 3**
Employment Status Before and After Hospitalization

| Prehospital Employment Status | Posthospital Employment Status | | | | | | | | | |
|---|---|---|---|---|---|---|---|---|---|---|
| | Employed at interview | | Employed since hosp., but not emp. at interview | | Not employed since hosp. | | House-wife | | Total | |
| | N | % | N | % | N | % | N | % | N | % |
| Employed | 49 | 55.1 | 20 | 22.5 | 16 | 17.9 | 4 | 4.5 | 89 | 100.0 |
| Not employed | 16 | 34.8 | 9 | 19.5 | 20 | 43.5 | 1 | 2.2 | 46 | 100.0 |
| Housewife | 5 | 12.2 | 8 | 19.5 | — | — | 28 | 68.3 | 41 | 100.0 |
| Total | 70 | 39.8 | 37 | 21.0 | 36 | 20.4 | 33 | 18.8 | 176 | 100.0 |

$\chi^2 = 104.167$, $p < .001$;
gamma = .587, $p < .001$.

sion, whether unemployed or housewives, had worked at some time following discharge. These results were not related to sex.

For the 70 patients employed at the time of interview, two-thirds (67.2 percent) worked in blue collar occupations, while the remainder held white collar positions. The majority (71.0 percent) of this group of employed patients worked on a full-time basis; the rest had part-time jobs. Most expressed satisfaction with their jobs (79.7 percent). Of those who had been employed since release from the hospital but were no longer working at the time of the interview (N = 37), most (78.4 percent) had been in blue collar jobs and the remainder in white collar occupations.

Respondents who were not working at the time of the interview were asked whether they were interested in working. The majority (60.0 percent) indicated an interest in working, while the rest reported no interest in employment. The latter group was asked if there were any particular reasons for their lack of interest in working. The most frequently cited reason was the belief that they were not yet well enough to function in a job (64.3 percent). Several (14.3 percent), all females, stated that they could not take a job because they had no day care available for their children.

### Financial Support

Source of support was classified into three types: (1) independent (income only from wages of respondent and/or spouse); (2) partially independent (income from wages of respondent and/or spouse and from benefits, either public or private, and/or relatives); and (3) dependent (income only from benefits and/or relatives). As with the previous lifestyle variables, the before- and after-hospitalization measures of financial support were significantly related (Table 4).

Half the sample reported no change in the source of financial support. When changes occurred, they tended to be more often toward increased dependence than toward increased independence. An inspection of individual cases revealed that most of the change to increased dependence was due to the loss of employment following hospital release. The patterns of change for males and females were similar to that for the sample as a whole.

### Household Role Functioning

Role functioning within the household was reflected in the assignment of responsibility for five household tasks: preparing morning and evening meals; planning the menu for evening meals;

**Table 4**
Source of Financial Support Before and After
Hospitalization

| Prehospital Source of Support | Posthospital Source of Support | | | | | | | |
|---|---|---|---|---|---|---|---|---|
| | Independent | | Partially Independent | | Dependent | | Total* | |
| | N | % | N | % | N | % | N | % |
| Independent | 46 | 54.8 | 17 | 20.2 | 21 | 25.0 | 84 | 100.0 |
| Partially independent | 8 | 22.9 | 9 | 25.7 | 18 | 51.4 | 35 | 100.0 |
| Dependent | 10 | 20.0 | 9 | 18.0 | 31 | 62.0 | 50 | 100.0 |
| Total | 64 | 37.9 | 35 | 20.7 | 70 | 41.4 | 169 | 100.0 |

* Total is less than 176 because of missing data.
$\chi^2 = 24.665$, $p < .001$;
gamma $= .503$, $p < .001$.

grocery shopping; cleaning the house; and household repairs. Responses were classified according to whether responsibility was assumed by the respondent alone, was shared with others, or was held by others only. The sum of scores across the five tasks provided a measure of the overall level of responsibility.

As shown in Table 5, role responsibility following hospital release was significantly related to role responsibility prior to admission. Overall role responsibility did not change for most respondents, whether male or female. When change did occur, it shifted only slightly more frequently toward increased responsibility than toward decreased responsibility.

**Table 5**
Role Responsiblity Before and After Hospitalization

| Prehospital Role Responsibility | Posthospital Role Responsibility | | | | | | | |
|---|---|---|---|---|---|---|---|---|
| | Low | | Moderate | | High | | Total* | |
| | N | % | N | % | N | % | N | % |
| Low | 37 | 62.7 | 15 | 25.4 | 7 | 11.9 | 59 | 100.0 |
| Moderate | 9 | 15.8 | 40 | 70.2 | 8 | 14.0 | 57 | 100.0 |
| High | 4 | 7.3 | 11 | 20.0 | 40 | 72.7 | 55 | 100.0 |
| Total | 50 | 29.2 | 66 | 38.6 | 55 | 32.2 | 171 | 100.0 |

* Total is less than 176 because of missing data.
$\chi^2 = 99.037$, $p < .001$;
gamma $= .749$, $p < .001$.

## Decision Making

Patterns of decision making within the household after hospital release were determined for five areas: choosing where to live; spending personal money; making major household purchases; managing household money; and disciplining the children. As with role functioning, three classifications were used: respondent only; shared with others; and others only.

A summary score reflecting overall responsibility for the first four decisions indicated that two-fifths (39.5 percent) had high levels of responsibility, one-third (34.1 percent) had moderate levels, and the remainder (26.4 percent) had low levels. Disciplining children was applicable in only 70 cases; of these, most either shared decision making (50.0 percent) or made decisions alone (40.0 percent). Only a few (10.0 percent) took no part in this decision.

## Social Participation

A composite measure of posthospital social participation was derived from respondents' reported frequencies of seeing friends or relatives, talking with friends or relatives by telephone, seeing one person to whom the respondent feels close, writing letters, going to meetings, and attending religious services. The sample was approximately evenly distributed among high levels of social participation (34.3 percent), moderate levels (33.1 percent), and low levels (32.5 percent).

The use of leisure time following hospital release was determined by participation in five leisure activities: watching television; listening to the radio or records; working at a hobby; reading books, newspapers, or magazines; and going for walks. More than half the respondents (54.4 percent) took part in four to five of these activities on a regular basis. One-fourth (25.2 percent) engaged in three activities, and the rest (20.5 percent) in at least one or two activities.

### USE OF AFTERCARE SERVICES

The community-based aftercare systems associated with the three study hospitals were well developed and closely tied in to the discharge planning process. For WSH, the main psychiatric aftercare service network consisted of community clinics located in the city of Worcester and several surrounding towns and rural areas

staffed, in part, by WSH personnel. WSH itself served as the primary inpatient facility for these catchment areas without any inter-
posed general hospital psychiatric unit. Strong ties were thus
promoted between the WSH and community programs. At the
Westboro State Hospital, only patients released from the geographic
unit serving the Cambridge-Somerville catchment area were included in the study. The major psychiatric aftercare resources for these
patients were community clinics in Cambridge, Somerville, and
surrounding towns. The Cambridge-Somerville Community Mental Health Center at the Cambridge City Hospital provided local inpatient services with regional back-up facilities at the Westboro
State Hospital, located some 35 miles away. For Gardner State Hospital patients, psychiatric aftercare responsibilities resided with the
Gardner-Athol Mental Health Center and the North Central Mental Health Center located at the Burbank Hospital in Fitchburg. Local inpatient services were provided at the Burbank Hospital with
regional back-up at the Worcester State Hospital following the close
of Gardner State Hospital.

## Referrals

According to hospital records, referrals were made at discharge
for most (83.0 percent) of the sample. As Table 6 shows, the majority of patients were referred to community mental health facilities.
There were some referrals to other medical sources, such as private
clinics or general hospitals, but only a few referrals to nonmedical
sources, such as rehabilitation programs or agencies providing assistance with housing, employment, or finances. Those who were
not referred generally had left the hospital without authorization or
had refused referrals.

COMPLIANCE WITH REFERRALS

To assess continuity of care between the hospital and the community, the extent to which patients complied with discharge referrals and used aftercare was examined. Three levels of compliance
were determined: (1) full compliance, that is, receiving care from
the places to which referrals were made; (2) partial compliance,
that is, receiving more than one referral but complying with only
one of the referrals or receiving a referral and complying with that
referral but also receiving services from another source without a
referral; and (3) noncompliance, that is, receiving aftercare from
sources other than those to which referrals were made or failing to
receive any care. Most (59.9 percent) of those referred complied

**Table 6**
Types of Referrals at Hospital Discharge

| Type of Referral | Referred N | % | Not Referred N | % | Total* N | % |
|---|---|---|---|---|---|---|
| Community mental health clinics/centers | 116 | 67.8 | 55 | 32.2 | 171 | 100.0 |
| Other medical sources | 30 | 17.5 | 141 | 82.5 | 171 | 100.0 |
| Nonmedical sources | 16 | 9.4 | 155 | 90.6 | 171 | 100.0 |

* Totals are less than 176 because of missing information.

fully with these referrals. Partial compliance was noted for about one-fifth (19.7 percent), and noncompliance for the remaining fifth (20.4 percent).

Patterns of association between compliance and socio-demographic, hospitalization, and posthospital lifestyle variables were examined using Pearson product-moment correlation coefficients. For this analysis, composite measures were used to represent chronicity,[2] posthospital lifestyle,[3] and change in lifestyle from before to after hospitalization.[4] Greater compliance was associated with having high chronicity, drugs prescribed at release, no environmental problems (such as unemployment, financial difficulties, marital discord) as reasons for the index admission, and more dependent lifestyles posthospital (Table 7).

These data were further analyzed using a stepwise discriminant function technique (Table 8). The first discriminant function indicated that posthospital lifestyle and chronicity were the most powerful predictors of compliance. Compliance was associated with high levels of chronicity and dependent lifestyles. In the second discriminant function, compliance was associated with low

**Table 7**
Correlations of Independent Variables with Compliance with Referrals

| Independent Variables | Compliance with Referrals r | p | N* |
|---|---|---|---|
| Chronicity | −.256 | .001 | 142 |
| Drugs Prescribed at Release | −.252 | .002 | 134 |
| Environmental Problems | .242 | .002 | 135 |
| Posthospital Lifestyle | .150 | .037 | 142 |

* N for compliance with referrals is based only on cases with referrals.

**Table 8**

Discriminant Function Analysis for Compliance with
Referrals

| Independent Variables | Standardized Discriminant Function Coefficients | |
|---|---|---|
| | *Function 1* | *Function 2* |
| Chronicity | .732 | .125 |
| Environmental reasons for admission | −.270 | .441 |
| Suicidal, withdrawn behavior as a reason for admission | .259 | .329 |
| Posthospital lifestyle | −.851 | −.066 |
| Change in lifestyle | .370 | −.481 |
| Decision making | −.146 | .672 |
| Number of problems | .339 | .069 |
| Eigenvalue | .293 | .152 |
| Canonical correlation | .476 | .363 |
| Wilks' Lambda | .671 | .868 |

This analysis was based on 110 cases; 32 cases were excluded because of missing information on the independent variables. Criteria for the selection of variables was the maximum $F$ ratio for the differences between group centroids. Additional variables included in the analysis but not entered into the equations were sex, age at hospital release, education, acting-out behavior at admission, major psychiatric symptoms at admission, number of drugs prescribed at release, posthospital role functioning, change in role functioning pre-post hospitalization, and social participation.

levels of responsibility in decision making and, to a lesser extent, positive change in lifestyle following hospitalization and no environmental problems as reasons for the index admission. When the discriminant functions were used to classify cases, the proportion of correct classifications (52.9 percent for full compliance, 46.4 percent for partial compliance, 62.1 percent for noncompliance) considerably exceeded the a priori probabilities (33.3 percent), thus underscoring the importance of these functions as predictors of compliance with aftercare referrals.

These findings suggest that the less chronic the illness and the more independent the lifestyle, the less likely the patient is to receive aftercare. The tendency for environmental problems to be associated with decreasing compliance may reflect difficulties patients have in obtaining assistance with these problems at community mental health facilities. As previously noted, few referrals were made to agencies specifically offering such assistance.

## Services Received

Nearly all (91.8 percent) of the released patients received some type of aftercare after leaving the hospital. Examining correlates of receiving care revealed that those who obtained aftercare were more likely to be chronic, to have drugs prescribed at hospital release, and to report more problems after release than those who did not receive aftercare (Table 9).

Respondents were asked about the types of service providers used, the places where they were seen, and the frequency of contacts. More than half the total sample (55.2 percent) reported seeing psychiatrists or psychologists who were most often located at community mental health centers or clinics. It must be noted, however, that respondents were not asked about the nature of the contact. Thus, "seeing" a psychiatrist or psychologist may reflect a variety of styles of interaction, from brief contacts for regulating medication to longer sessions for individual psychotherapy.

Aftercare was obtained from a nurse for more than one-third (36.2 percent) of the total sample of released patients. Some respondents (27.6 percent) received aftercare from social workers located as often at community mental health clinics as at outside agencies or at the state hospital. Other kinds of providers, such as nonpsychiatric physicians or nonpsychiatric groups like Alcoholics Anonymous, were used by a few respondents. Regardless of the type of provider, the last contact was most often during the four weeks preceeding the follow-up interview.

Of all respondents receiving aftercare, half (50.6 percent) used only a community mental health facility, either a clinic (outpatient

**Table 9**

Correlations of Independent Variables with Aftercare Received

| Independent Variables | Aftercare Received | | |
|---|---|---|---|
| | r | p | N* |
| Chronicity | −.222 | .002 | 171 |
| Drugs prescribed at release | −.167 | .018 | 158 |
| Number of problems after release[†] | −.186 | .007 | 170 |

* Totals are less than 176 because of missing data.

† Number of problems is the sum of responses indicating difficulties encountered after hospital release with getting medication, employment, housing, counseling, meeting people, medical care, shopping, or transportation.

services only) or a comprehensive center (both outpatient and inpatient services). Facilities outside the community mental health system, such as private practitioners, hospitals or clinics, or social agencies, were the sole source of care for about one-fifth (18.1 percent) of those receiving care. Some respondents (12.5 percent) used both community mental health facilities and outside agencies. A small number were served by outpatient facilities at the state hospitals or by various combinations of the different kinds of facilities.

### Rating of Aftercare Services

Nearly three-fourths of the total sample (74.6 percent) reported satisfactions with aftercare services, ranging from general comments that the people were nice and kind to more specific references about positive gains in terms of mental health. Very few (9.5 percent) stated that they had no satisfactions with services.

Dissatisfactions were mentioned by 51.8 percent of the respondents. Complaints were most often concerned with treatment programs or medications (40.5 percent), for example, a lack of individual therapy, or insufficient contact with staff. The remaining complaints were mainly about operational characteristics, such as long waits or inconvenient hours.

Despite dissatisfactions with services, less than half the respondents (45.8 percent) had suggestions about changing the system for providing aftercare services. Suggestions for improving or increasing treatment programs or medications were the most frequent (27.7 percent). Improvements in discharge planning, followup, and operating characteristics of aftercare programs were suggested by a number of respondents (21.7 percent). A few (9.0 percent) wanted more assistance with environmental problems, such as employment, financial support, or housing.

### REHOSPITALIZATION

In August, 1979, hospital records for the WSH subsample of interviewed patients were examined to determine the frequency and duration of rehospitalizations at WSH subsequent to the follow-up interview. These data provided a basis for assessing the extent to which these WSH patients were able to remain in the community without rehospitalization for a five-year period.

During the period between the index hospital release in 1974 and July 31, 1979, two-thirds (67.2 percent) of the interviewed patients in the WSH subsample remained out of the hospital, while one-third (32.8 percent) experienced at least one rehospitalization at WSH. Since no information was available about psychiatric admissions to other facilities during this period, these figures may not be completely accurate reflections of recidivism. However, the tendency for the study sample as a whole to exhibit stability in household composition and place of residence after hospital release suggests that the rate of readmissions to WSH is a reasonable approximation of the extent of recidivism for this patient cohort. This finding is lower than statewide figures on readmission rates for patients released from state mental hospitals. However, it must be remembered that the study results do not reflect the total hospital population, but rather a select group of patients considered likely to have successful outcomes following hospital release.

For the one-third rehospitalized, the number of readmissions ranged from one (11.9 percent) to 17 (1.5 percent), with a mean of 4.7. Readmission stays tended to be relatively short: the proportion of the five-year follow-up period spent in the hospital ranged from less than 1 percent to 22 percent, with a mean of 4.5 percent. Thus, at least some of the rehospitalized patients illustrated the "revolving door" concept of patients with multiple short-term hospital stays.

Relationships between rehospitalization and socio-demographic, hospitalization, and lifestyle characteristics were examined using Pearson product-moment correlation coefficients (Table 10). Rehospitalization was more likely to occur for those with high levels of chronicity, major psychiatric symptoms as reasons for the index admission, low levels of posthospital role responsibility, and low scores on the VIRO scale (Kastenbaum and Sherwood, 1972).[5] Although no standard measures of overt symptomatology were used in the study, major psychiatric symptoms at admission, such as bizarre behavior, hallucinations, confusion, or rambling speech, served as an approximation of overt symptomatology. The findings thus suggest that patients with overt symptoms, whether bizarre and erratic behavior as measured by major psychiatric symptoms, or lethargic and depressed behavior as demonstrated by the VIRO scale, were at high risk for rehospitalization.

A stepwise discriminant function analysis of rehospitalization derived one discriminant function with considerable power to distinguish between the rehospitalized and nonrehospitalized groups

**Table 10**
Correlations between Independent Variables and Rehospitalization for
Worcester State Hospital Subsample

| | Rehospitalization | | |
|---|---|---|---|
| Independent Variables | r | p | N* |
| Chronicity | .354 | .01 | 67 |
| Major psychiatric symptoms | | | |
| as reasons for index admission | −.261 | .05 | 67 |
| Posthospital role responsiblity | −.269 | .05 | 67 |
| VIRO scale | −.259 | .05 | 67 |

*N < 68 due to missing data.

(Table 11). According to the chief components of the function, dependent lifestyles, positive change in lifestyle following hospitalization, high chronicity, and major psychiatric symptoms at the
index admission were strong predictors of rehospitalization. The
proportions of each group correctly classified using the discriminant function were greater than the a priori probabilities, giving
further evidence of the function's discriminating power: 68.9 per-

**Table 11**
Discriminant Function Analysis for Rehospitalization

| Independent Variables | Standardized Discriminant Function Coefficients |
|---|---|
| Chronicity | .558 |
| Posthospital lifestyle | −.662 |
| Change in lifestyle | .628 |
| Posthospital role functioning | −.279 |
| VIRO scale | −.235 |
| Age at release from hospital | −.248 |
| Major psychiatric symptoms as reasons | |
| for index admission | −.479 |
| | |
| Eigenvalue | .498 |
| Canonical correlation | .577 |
| Wilks' Lambda | .667 |

This analysis was based on 67 cases. Criteria for the selection of variables was
the maximum F ratio for the differences between group centroids. Additional independent variables included in the analysis but not entered into the equation were
sex; suicide and withdrawn behavior at admission; acting out behavior at admission;
change in role functioning pre-post hospitalization; number of problems encountered after hospital release; and aftercare received.

cent of the nonrehospitalized group and 77.3 percent of the rehospitalized group were correctly identified. Although the tendency for rehospitalized patients to have experienced positive changes in lifestyle seems contrary to expectations, it may be that some patients are not sufficiently improved to handle positive changes, particularly in employment. The fact that change in lifestyle did not enter the equation until after posthospital lifestyle suggests that once the degree of independence in lifestyle is controlled, it is change toward greater independence rather than maintenance of independence that contributes to a greater risk of rehospitalization.

## SUMMARY OF FINDINGS

This chapter has focused on the outcomes of deinstitutionalization for patients released from WSH and two nearby state hospitals to noninstitutional living situations in the community. Outcomes were assessed for three dimensions: lifestyles following hospital release; use of aftercare services; and, for a subgroup of the sample, rehospitalization.

### Posthospital Life Styles

Most of the study patients returned to their prehospital living arrangements following release, but approximately two-fifths experienced changes in employment, half in the source of financial support, and one-third in role functioning. Changes in employment and financial support were more often negative than positive, that is, toward greater dependence than independence. These findings suggest that some patients are not sufficiently rehabilitated by hospitalization to resume the work role and thus may become burdens on the public welfare system following hospital release. It may be that patients are released from the hospital too quickly or that community aftercare systems do not provide sufficient assistance with life situation problems such as employment. The former explanation is supported by the finding that many who were unemployed after hospital release indicated a desire for employment, but stated that they were not well enough to work; the latter by the finding that few aftercare referrals were made to agencies providing assistance with employment.

Changes in role functioning were slightly more often positive than negative, that is, toward increased rather than decreased responsibility. The tendency for role responsibility to increase may be a function of decreased employment: loss of jobs may provide more time for household duties. This result also suggests that household functioning is not impaired to the same extent as functioning outside the household. Although there was no prehospital measure for decision making, the finding that most respondents had sole or shared responsibility for making decisions is in accord with the patterns of role responsibility, thus further supporting the ability of discharged patients to function within the household.

### Use of Aftercare Services

Most of the patients in the study sample were referred for aftercare, indicating that efforts were made to transfer patients to community-based care at the time of release. Absence of referrals was due largely to patients leaving the hospital without authorization or refusing referrals.

Successful transition from institutional to community-based psychiatric care for the mentally ill may depend upon continuity of care between the state hospital and the community aftercare program. Despite the desirability of continuity of care, Kirk and Therrien (1975) have suggested that achievement of this goal is more a myth than a reality. Using compliance with referrals as an indicator of continuity of care, the present study found a considerably higher rate of compliance than a previous investigation addressing that issue (Wolkon, 1970). Since characteristics of the samples were similar, this difference may stem from the nature of the referrals: the previous study examined referrals to only one aftercare program, while the present study looked at all referrals regardless of where the referral was made. Wolkon (1970) found that patients with financial support from public agencies were more likely to comply than those with no public assistance. Similarly, in the present study, greater dependency in lifestyle (which included source of financial support) was related to compliance. On the other hand, Wolkon found no relationship between either previous psychiatric hospitalizations or diagnosis and compliance, but found that shorter stays for the last hospitalization were related to compliance. In the present study, chronicity, an index composed of diagnosis, length of stay, and previous psychiatric hospitalizations, was related to compliance: the greater the chronicity, the greater the likelihood of compliance.

Regardless of whether patients received referrals or complied with them, nearly all patients in the present study received some form of aftercare. Other studies have reported lower proportions of patients receiving aftercare, but most focused on only one aftercare facility or one type of facility, whereas the present study evaluated aftercare regardless of where the care was obtained.

In the present study, patients with higher levels of chronicity were more likely to receive aftercare. Those with more independent lifestyles posthospital tended to be less likely to receive aftercare, while those with a greater number of problems after release were more likely to obtain care. The finding that patients having drugs prescribed at hospital release were more likely than those without drug prescriptions to comply with referrals and to obtain aftercare suggests that aftercare services may focus more on the use and regulation of medication than on the provision of assistance with emotional and environmental problems.

### Rehospitalization

The success of aftercare programs has often been measured in terms of the extent to which patients remain out of the hospital. Studies examining recidivism (Anthony and Buell, 1973; Byers et al., 1978; Kirk, 1976; McCranie and Mizell, 1978; Winston et al., 1977) have shown a remarkable consistency in the proportions of patients experiencing rehospitalization. The readmission rates varied from 24.1 to 40.0 percent, but were comparable to the one-third proportion found in the present study. These readmission rates were similar despite follow-up periods ranging from six months to five years. In contrast, earlier studies noted an increase in recidivism with increasing follow-up time (Anthony et al., 1972). Perhaps rehospitalization rates may have stabilized, with approximately one-third of patients released from mental hospitals requiring rehospitalization in the future.

In the present study, greater chronicity was a strong predictor of rehospitalization. Further indication that rehospitalization may depend on the psychiatric condition was given by the finding that patients with overt psychiatric symptomatology were likely to be rehospitalized. More dependent lifestyles following hospital release were also related to rehospitalization.

## IMPLICATIONS FOR INSTITUTIONAL
## BOUNDARIES

The study findings have several important implications for the deinstitutionalization movement. Increased economic dependence for some patients following release from the hospital without adequate plans or preparations for resuming the work role lends credence to the criticisms concerning rehabilitation leveled by Kirk and Therrien (1975) against the community mental health movement. Although patients with low chronicity and independent lifestyles were at high risk for discontinuity of care, they were not likely to be rehospitalized and thus may be able to function in the community with minimal assistance from mental health facilities. Despite a greater likelihood of continuity of care, the more chronic, dependent patients were the most likely to be rehospitalized, suggesting that some form of inpatient care will continue to be required for patients with enduring psychiatric liabilities.

It may be that the success of deinstitutionalization depends on the organizational structure of aftercare services available for use by released hospital patients. In another assessment of deinstitutionalization at Westboro State Hospital, Feldman et al. (1979) compared two models of aftercare service delivery: (1) *integrated*, characterized by consolidated administrative responsibility over the components of the system, formal linkages among agencies and programs throughout the system, and patient advocates who follow patients through the system and intervene on their behalf; and (2) *nonintegrated*, exemplified by fragmented administrative responsibility, lack of coordination between agencies, and no patient advocates. They found that the catchment area with the integrated model was more successful than one with the nonintegrated model in implementing deinstitutionalization, as indicated by lower admission rates, shorter hospital stays for rehospitalized patients, and longer community stays for released patients. As previous chapters have indicated, WSH has emphasized the integrated approach in the development of the mental health care service system in its region with community clinics staffed, in part, by WSH personnel. This structure may have contributed to the apparent success of many of the present study patients in their transition from hospital to community-based care.

Although integrated aftercare service delivery systems show promise for maximizing the effectiveness of community aftercare programs, the findings of the present research and Feldman's study indicate that even excellent systems cannot entirely supplant mental hospitals. Psychotropic medication and community-based aftercare programs have made possible the release of large numbers of patients from state mental hospitals, but residential care is still needed for chronically ill and dependent patients. Periodic hospitalizations for chronic mental illness must be viewed in the same way as those for chronic physical illnesses: necessary for control of the illness. The question remains as to whether inpatient care can best be provided by large public institutions or by other kinds of residential facilities. Until adequate alternatives are available, the demise of the state hospital is, indeed, a "premature obituary" (Lamb and Goertzel, 1972). Institutional boundaries must not be sharply drawn, but must instead permit and facilitate movement between institutional and community-based segments of mental health services.

## NOTES

1.  Gardner State Hospital closed in June, 1976, and the regional psychiatric inpatient responsibility for the Gardner catchment areas was transferred to Worcester State Hospital. Westboro State Hospital remains in operation as of September, 1979.
2.  Chronicity was defined as the sum of scores on three hospitalization characteristics: (1) diagnosis (0 = nonpsychotic/1 = psychotic); (2) previous psychiatric hospitalization (0 = no/1 = yes); and (3) length of stay for the index hospitalization (0 = under 1 month/1 = 1–3 months/2 = over 3 months). High scores on the chronicity index reflected psychotic diagnoses with previous psychiatric hospitalizations and longer stays for the index hospitalization.
3.  Posthospital employment status, financial support, and living arrangements were combined into a posthospital lifestyle index ranging from most dependent (not employed, financial support from benefits only, family of origin) to most independent (employed or housewife, financial support from wages only, family of procreation or nonfamily).
4.  Change in lifestyle was determined by differences between the pre- and posthospital versions of the index described in note 3.
5.  The VIRO scale is designed to assess interview behavior. Respondents are rated by interviewers on four dimensions: vigor, intactness, relationship, and orientation. In the present study, selected items from the VIRO were used to measure the respondent's personal presentation. One of the two Vigor items was selected: low energy/high energy. Three of the five Intactness items were used: minimal speech/fluent speech; keen attention/poor attention; fragmented thought/controlled thought. Three of the five Relationship items were included: suspicious/trustful; reluctant participation/eager participation; eager to end session/eager to

continue. One additional item which is not part of the VIRO scale was included: depressed/elated. Each item is scored on a four-point scale. Low scores indicated poor personal presentation. The Orientation items are similar to those concerning time and place from mental status examinations; none were included in the present study.

# PART III

# Persistence and Change

Joseph P. Morrissey
Howard H. Goldman

# 11

# The Paradox of Institutional Reform: Administrative Transition With Functional Stability

This chapter describes and assesses the changes in the structure and functions of Worcester State Hospital (WSH) during the decade of the 1970s.[1] As in past eras, these organizational changes represented adaptive responses to environmental opportunities and constraints and to the strivings of its leaders. However, while the past changes were gradual, the 1970s witnessed the most rapid and paradoxical period of change in the history of the hospital.

Beginning in the late 1960s, Superintendent Myerson made a concerted effort to overcome the ambiguous legacy of WSH by redefining functional boundaries, developing linkages with public and private agencies, and "communitizing" outpatient and aftercare services. These changes were aimed at the transformation of the hospital into a psychiatric treatment institution that could serve as the hub of the public-sector mental health program in central Massachusetts. These goals were consistent with plans of the Massachusetts Department of Mental Health for the future role of its state mental hospitals, and WSH's accomplishments served as a model for the rest of the state.

By the mid-1970s, however, fiscal retrenchment in the state government support for human service programs began to erode the administrative and environmental supports for this pattern of institutional adaptation, and WSH entered a period of rapid decline. State officials saw the dismantling of the Massachusetts state mental hospital system and the reallocation of its resources to area

247

mental health programs as a way of escaping from escalating costs and inflation while promoting the development of a truly community-based mental health service system. As a result, state mental health policy shifted toward the phase-down of state mental hospitals and the transfer of authority from medical superintendents to area program directors. At WSH, Superintendent Myerson's efforts to resist these administrative changes ultimately proved unsuccessful. Following his resignation in late 1977, the medical superintendency of WSH was abolished. Thus ended an uninterrupted tradition dating back to Samuel B. Woodward in the early 1830s. With its passing, two of the basic principles upon which the asylum was originally founded—medical dominance and centralized control—were cast aside. In their place, a new administrative structure—nonmedical and decentralized—was installed.[2] The treatment units based on geographic catchment areas that Myerson had created in 1970 began to operate as "mini-hospitals" under the line authority of area program directors who were not physicians. In addition, many of the hospital's training, research, and regional services were phased out and/or transferred to agencies in the community.

Developments in the "interorganizational field" (Warren, 1967) surrounding WSH also contributed to its decline as the dominant mental health agency in the Worcester area. Under the auspices of the local mental health advisory board, a coalition of agencies that were formerly part of WSH's services network secured a federal Community Mental Health Center grant. This award resulted in the recombination of these agencies under the administrative umbrella of the new center. It also led to the opening of an inpatient psychiatric unit at the state medical school in Worcester. As WSH was administratively disaggregated, a number of its senior medical and other professional staff resigned to accept positions in these new agencies or to enter private practice. In addition, many of the less disturbed and less disadvantaged patients who would have been admitted to WSH were referred to these programs.

Nevertheless, through the close of the 1970s WSH continued to serve as the institution of last resort in the Worcester area. None of its historic functions—treatment, custody, or social control—was completely eliminated. Although many of its former staff, resources, and patients were relocated, WSH still provided care to the most disadvantaged and most disruptive patients. Thus, in spite of extensive changes in the organizational ecology of mental health services, many of the problems of the old institutional order remained unresolved.

## TOWARD INSTITUTIONAL
## TRANSFORMATION

At the time that Massachusetts embarked on its community mental health program in 1966, there were few mental health services outside of its state mental hospitals. This situation was the direct result of the State Care Act of 1904 which gave the Commonwealth exclusive jurisdiction over public provisions for the mentally ill and prohibited localities from operating independent mental health services (Marden, 1968). The Massachusetts Mental Health Planning Project (1965:1) proposed two basic principles for a statewide program of community mental health services: (1) "no distant hospitals" and (2) "a decentralization or dispersion of resources." The plan called for a gradual transfer of resources away from state hospitals into local community services and the phase-down of those state hospitals that were located in remote areas of the Commonwealth. A major reorganization of the Department of Mental Health was undertaken and all cities and towns were grouped into seven mental health regions. Each regional office had a director and staff and performed both management and planning functions. Within each region there were from 5 persons to the "areas" or subregional districts of approximately 200–250,000 population. Ultimately, it was envisioned that each of these areas, in turn, would have their own area offices.

Given the imbalance of resources between institutions and local communities and the lead time needed to create mental health administrative units in each area, a dual role was proposed for the 11 state mental hospitals. Each would serve as a "community mental health center" by providing the essential services mandated by the federal guidelines for such centers (e.g., inpatient, outpatient, emergency, and partial hospitalization) to the area in which it was located while serving as a regional back-up facility for the other areas in its region. WSH was cited as a model of the new state mental hospital envisioned in this plan. While Region II in which it was located encompassed a large part of central Massachusetts, WSH's primary catchment area consisted of the City of Worcester and contiguous towns with a population base in 1965 of about 260,000 persons.

When David Myerson assumed the superintendency of WSH in 1969, however, he inherited an institution that was a mixture of the new and the old (see Chapter 4). Under his predecessor, the hospital had shed many of the custodial practices it had acquired between 1850 and 1950: the resident census had been reduced from 2,850 to 1,050 patients, active treatment programs had substantially shortened the average length of hospitalization, and several hospital-based outpatient and aftercare services had been developed to serve the large number of former patients who resided in the local communities. At a more fundamental level, however, the hospital's ambiguous legacy of serving multiple and contradictory functions remained essentially unaltered. It was still expected to care for many of society's "rejects"—the homeless, the alcoholic, the aged and the senile—as well as indigent persons suffering from acute and chronic psychiatric conditions.

Myerson was one of a new generation of superintendents appointed by Milton Greenblatt, Commissioner of the Department of Mental Health, under whom he had worked during the latter's years as superintendent of Boston State Hospital. Myerson's mandate was to implement the Department's new community mental health policy by reorganizing WSH and moving its services into the community. His charge, in many respects, was to replicate the institutional changes that Greenblatt had introduced at Boston State Hospital (Greenblatt et al., 1971; Schulberg and Baker, 1975).

During his first few years as superintendent, Myerson established a reputation for aggressive and innovative leadership both within the hospital and in the community. He reorganized the inpatient services at WSH into geographic treatment units and broke down the insular structure and functional autonomy of its professional departments. In phasing out the alcoholism treatment program developed by his predecessor, Myerson made it clear to the community that WSH would no longer serve as dumping ground and custodian for the "residual social deviants" (Scheff, 1966) of Worcester and its surrounding towns. The enactment of revised statutes governing involuntary commitments (Bayle, 1971) provided a legal basis for his insistence that WSH was a psychiatric institution and that its distinctive competence resided in the treatment of persons with manifest psychopathological conditions. For the first time since the founding of WSH, the superintendent had legal authority to limit the flow of inappropriate admissions into the institution.

In addition to specifying restrictive admission criteria, the new law invested state hospital superintendents with authority to designate "qualified physicians" who could sign involuntary commitment papers. Myerson quickly seized the opportunity to reinforce the admission standards he was advocating. Unilaterally, he re-

voked the commitment powers of Worcester area physicians knowing that it would create an uproar in the local medical community.
Subsequently, at a special meeting of the Worcester Medical Society, Myerson reassured the physicians that as long as they avoided
indiscriminant dumping of patients, their admission privileges
would be restored.

With no formulated master plan he was able to delimit the role
of WSH while collaborating with other health and welfare agencies
in the development of alternative treatment and rehabilitative services in the community. His dual position as Superintendent and
Director of the Greater Worcester Mental Health Area—though the
roles would ultimately become irreconcilable—provided crucial le-
verage during the early 1970s both in redeploying institutional resources to community programs and in realigning the functional
boundaries of WSH.

Between 1969 and 1973, these efforts led to a marked change in
the utilization of WSH. The resident patient census was reduced
from 972 to 547 (-56 percent) and the annual admissions—which
had steadily risen since 1950—fell from 1465 to 776 (− 53 percent).
Underlying these changes was a dramatic growth in the number
and variety of community-based services in the Worcester area
staffed by WSH personnel (MDMH, 1971). The day hospital, aftercare, and outpatient programs were moved off the grounds of WSH
and relocated in five Neighborhood Opportunity Centers and the
Model Cities Multi-Service Center in the City of Worcester; outpatient clinics were set up at the Worcester City and The Memorial
Hospitals; and a variety of other jointly staffed services were created in collaboration with community health and social welfare
agencies. The latter included consultation to alcoholism and drug
rehabilitation agencies, nursing homes, and community programs
for the elderly. In addition, as services formerly provided exclusively by WSH were "communitized" and moved off the hospital
grounds, new institution-based services were created to serve populations with special needs. These included a 30-bed unit for drug
abusers, the Woodward Day School for emotionally disturbed adolescents (see Chapter 7), the Adolescent Treatment Program (see
Chapter 8), and the Quimby School for retarded and autistic children.

Throughout this period Myerson had the strong support of the
Commissioner, the Region II Director, and the Greater Worcester
Area Mental Health Board. While dedicated to the transformation
of WSH into a high-quality treatment institution, he realized that

this goal was contingent upon the availability of community-based outpatient, aftercare, and rehabilitation programs. Since most of the state appropriations for mental health services were allocated to the state hospitals, Myerson recognized that these resources had to be shared with community agencies if viable programs were to be developed. Through informal understanding and *quid pro quo* arrangements, he was able to "bootleg" staff and funds into community programs. While relinquishing day-to-day supervision to community agency directors, he retained budgetary control over the staff positions that were redeployed to community clinics and other programs. Although at times these arrangements created confused lines of authority and accountability, they sustained a network of community-based services. Between 1973 and 1977, however, his freedom in manipulating the WSH budget in support of institutional as well as community services was gradually curtailed.

### THE END OF MEDICAL SUPERINTENDENCY

The economic downturn of the mid-1970s led to increasing pressures to decentralize state government and to introduce stricter fiscal planning and management accountability into its operations (Goldman, 1976). The placement of the Department of Mental Health (along with other human service departments) under the administrative umbrella of an Executive Office of Human Services led to greater control of mental health planning activities by the executive branch and a reform of the fiscal and organizational structures that were supposed to implement the community mental health legislation of 1966. A new Commissioner of the Department of Mental Health took office in 1973 with the mandate to accelerate the reallocation of resources from institutional to community accounts. Increasingly, state officials in Massachusetts and in the rest of the country adopted a posture of fiscal retrenchment and a policy of removing the state from the business of delivering direct services (c.f., Scull, 1977; Cameron, 1978). With a leveling off of state appropriations, the dismantling of institutional budgets was seen as the only way community services could be financed. In addition, the increase in litigation delineating the rights of mental patients and in judicial intervention in the mental health system made it clear that enormous sums of money would have to be invested in state institutions if they were to meet court-ordered standards of care (Robitscher, 1976). The coalescing of interests among fiscal conservatives, civil libertarians, and community mental health advocates accelerated the national movement toward "deinstitutionalization" and closure of state mental hospitals (Greenblatt and Glazier, 1975; Becker and Schulberg, 1976).

In Massachusetts, these social forces led to the closing of Grafton State Hospital in 1973 (Kahn and Kaplan, 1974) and to the closing of Foxboro State Hospital in 1974. Since Grafton was in the Worcester region, funds from the hospital's budget along with many of its staff were transferred to mental health programs in two areas within Region II: Blackstone Valley and South Central. WSH was assigned regional back-up responsibilities for these two areas and for the Grafton patients who were unable to be placed in community residences. Both of these areas contained several small mill towns and their surrounding rural populations (Fig. 1). In contrast to the Greater Worcester Area, where Myerson had developed a network of outpatient and aftercare services, these towns had few mental health services prior to the closure of Grafton State Hospital. Consistent with his "communitization" policies, Myerson assigned WSH staff to work in these areas on a part-time basis. Over the next few years, however, as community-based services were developed the Blackstone Valley and South Central Area Directors (both nonphysicians) began to accuse Myerson of favoritism in allocating hospital staff to the Greater Worcester Area and to its WSH inpatient unit, rather than to their programs.

In 1975, as the Commonwealth's fiscal crisis deepened, a new governor was elected and he began to call for sweeping reductions in state human services expenditures. The Commissioner and several of the senior staff in the Department of Mental Health were replaced. The new Departmental leadership proceeded to strengthen the administrative capacity of the regional offices. These offices were delegated greater authority for overseeing institutional appropriations and expenditures, and new formats for fiscal planning, management information, and program evaluation were introduced. In central Massachusetts, the psychiatrist who had served as Regional Administrator for nine years resigned. He was replaced by a psychologist whose background was in public education. The regional office staff was also expanded and changed by the recruitment of "systems-oriented" managers without clinical training or prior experience in the state hospital system. Increasingly, as the mandate and administration of the Department changed, Myerson and his fellow superintendents came to be defined as the principal

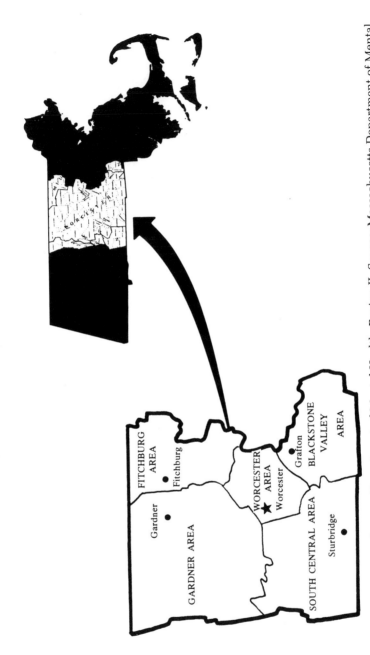

Fig. 11. Massachusetts Department of Mental Health, Region II. Source: Massachusetts Department of Mental Health, Challenge and Response: A Five-Year Progress Report on the Comprehensive Mental Health and Retardation Services Act of the Commonwealth of Massachusetts. Boston, MA: MDMH, 1972, p. 38.

obstacles to the implementation of community mental health services.

In 1976 a major inroad into Myerson's power base was achieved with the closing of Gardner State Hospital; which was also located in Region II (Sills, 1975). The staff and patients on the Fitchburg-Leominister Unit at Gardner were transferred to WSH but they were not placed under the superintendent's control. Clinical and fiscal authority for the unit were assigned to the Fitchburg-Leominister Area Director. WSH was responsible only for providing space and support services (e.g., medical, dietary, and maintenance). Thus, for the first time in its history, the WSH superintendent was no longer exclusively responsible for clinical functions performed at the hospital. The new Region II Administrator and other Area Directors increased their pressure on Myerson to extend this administrative model (which was a prototype of the Department's plan to decentralize the state hospitals) to the Blackstone Valley and South Central area units at WSH as well.

Moreover, the economic recession and level funding of WSH, despite rapid inflation, led to innumerable problems of staff morale, strained resources, and hospital-community conflict (see Chapter 5). Not only were state employees refused a cost of living increase, but welfare support for discharged patients was reduced. WSH admissions began to increase, and the volume of work for the inpatient staff—already spread thin by time commitments to community clinics—became unmanageable. The employee strike in June 1976 was soon followed by allegations of patient abuse in November 1976, which led to several well-publicized inquiries by the District Attorney, state police, and the Worcester Area Mental Health Association. As a result, Myerson became increasingly preoccupied with the hospital's internal management and in defending himself against the encroachment of the Regional Office staff.

Despite these problems, Myerson remained committed to his "communitization" program. As WSH's discretionary funds dwindled, he expanded the hospital's links with community agencies and other sources of funds. The enactment of special education statutes in Massachusetts created new funding opportunities and community supports for the Woodward Day School and the Adolescent Treatment Complex (see Chapter 7 and 8). In addition, the opening of a psychiatric inpatient unit at the Memorial Hospital enabled him to stengthen the network of mental health services in the Worcester area, to enhance the WSH residency training program, and to broach the chasm between the public and private sector (see Chapter 9).

Although selected programs at WSH were able to flourish during the mid-1970s, the hospital as a unitary institution began to decline, and the executive functions of the superintendency were stripped away by administrative fiat. In 1976, the Commissioner ordered the phase-out of all state hospital personnel not assigned to direct patient care and the transfer of their positions or salary equivalents into community program accounts. The implementation of this policy led to a reduction in the central administrative and training staff at WSH, and Myerson lost budgetary control over many of the positions he had informally reassigned to community services. Furthermore, programs and services had to be disaggregated into area-specific modules, and all nongeographic or "regional" treatment services had to be justified repeatedly to the Regional Administrator and Area Directors. While Myerson was being attacked for deteriorating services and patient abuse, his control over the hospital was lessened and he was prevented from developing multi-unit treatment programs for the care of special groups of patients. In January 1977 the Department of Mental Health reiterated its commitment to phasing out the superintendency in its new Five-Year Plan: " . . . it is a major objective of this administration to effect full transfer of authority at the new unit level to the area director in all catchment areas within the next year and a half" (MDMH, 1977:113). In short, by mid-1977, the position of superintendent at WSH had become little more than a legal point of accountability with little authority or opportunity for initiative. In October of that year, Myerson resigned and accepted a position at the University of Massachusetts Medical Center.

During his tenure as superintendent, Myerson tried to adapt the structure and functions of WSH and its network of community services to changing social conditions in a way that would place renewed emphasis on therapeutic as opposed to custodial and social control functions. In this sense, though the specifics of their proposals were quite different, Myerson's efforts were analogous to those of Merrick Bemis who served as WSH Superintendent a century earlier (see Chapter 3). Both men were innovators who tried to resolve the ambiguous legacy of WSH by developing a hybrid structure of centralized administration and decentralized services: Bemis in the form of the "cottage hospital" and Myerson in the form of the "communitized hospital." Both met early success in implementing their plans, but then encountered insurmountable economic and professional–administrative obstacles. In the 1870s, Bemis' plans were defeated because decentralized hospitals were seen as too expensive and as *undermining* the power of the medical super-intendency; in the 1970s, Myerson's plans were defeated because centralized hospitals were seen as too expensive and as *sustaining* the power of the medical superintendency. In each instance, state policies did not allow for diversity in the state hospital system and external definitions of WSH's role and mission prevailed.

Myerson's efforts to promote and sustain WSH as the hub of a network of community-based satellite clinics and rehabilitation programs also approached the futuristic visions of Adolf Meyer and of William Bryan, two other innovative leaders who had guided the hospital in earlier eras (see Chapter 3). Although Meyer promul-gated his views on community psychiatry only after leaving Worcester, Bryan mounted pioneering community programs as an extension of WSH during the 1920s and 1930s at a time when most state mental hospitals were still preoccupied with custodial prac-tices inherited from the late 19th century. These early programs, however, were constrained by the sunk costs of caring for a large institutionalized population and a social climate that emphasized the segregative functions of the hospital. In the early 1950s, the changing climate of opinion and the resurgence of treatment-orient-ed programs allowed for a sharp reduction in the hospital census. Under the direction of Bardwell Flower, WSH once again began to be recognized as a center of innovative patient care and a model community-oriented institution. The slack resources obtained from a declining census and increased budgetary support during the 1960s provided the resource base for Myerson's "communitization" efforts in the 1970s. Just as it appeared that WSH was on the verge of resolving its ambiguous legacy, however, external policies changed and the vision sustained by several generations of WSH leaders was administratively dismantled.

## ADMINISTRATIVE DISAGGREGATION AND DEMEDICALIZATION

Following Myerson's resignation, the responsibilities of the WSH superintendency were divided between two positions—an Assistant Superintendent (Clinical) and an Assistant Superinten-dent (Administrative)—which were filled by the incumbent Assis-tant Superintendent and Steward, respectively. However, these nominal changes exacerbated the internal management problems of the hospital. Traditionally, members of the medical staff discharged

their functions in the name of the superintendent who assumed ultimate responsibility for hospital operations.[3] In Myerson's absence, considerable confusion and conflict arose over whether the
Area Directors (nonphysicians) or the Unit Directors (psychiatrists)
had final responsibility for deciding who would be admitted, who
would be discharged, and who would sign pretrial commitments
from the courts. These ambiguities precipitated a number of conflicts between psychiatrists and area directors and, in one instance,
when an area director insisted that a patient be admitted over the
objections of one of the WSH staff psychiatrists, the psychiatrist resigned.

    In an effort to resolve these disputes and to clarify the long-
range plans of the Department, the Commissioner issued a memorandum in February 1978 stating that the integration of state
hospitals into the community mental health system required " . . .
the dismantling of an institutional structure and the rebuilding of a
structure of community-based care" (Okin, 1978:22). This memorandum provided the first detailed description of the clinical, legal,
budgetary, and management responsibilities that would be assigned
to the Area Directors and the steps that would be taken to supplant
the institutional chain of command over the area-related inpatient
units at each state hospital. The Commissioner indicated that he
would designate these units as "facilities" of the Department and
place them under the charge of their respective Area Directors who
would then have the statutory authority of a superintendent over
the personnel and patients on the unit. "This means that the Area
Director will have hire-and-fire and disciplinary authority over . . .
personnel as well as the legal authority to admit, commit, and discharge patients to and from the catchment area unit" (Okin,
1978:15–16).

    This memorandum stated that the transfer of authority to area
directors would not occur until the state hospitals were decentralized and their inpatient units fully integrated with their respective
area programs. Under the plans outlined, the role of the hospital
administration would shift from its traditional focus on direct patient care to furnishing core support services (e.g., maintenance,
housekeeping, dietary, pharmacy, medical care). In addition, all
professional departments (e.g., nursing, social work, psychology,
occupational therapy) would be disbanded and their supervisory
responsibilities transferred to area program personnel. Treatment
units serving "low-incidence, region-wide populations" (e.g., geriatrics, children, mentally retarded) that could not be absorbed by

area units would be clustered into Regional Services Units under the direction of the Regional Administrators or their designees. The Regional Administrators were given the option of operating the regional and administrative support services with hospital personnel or of developing purchase-of-service contracts with community vendors. Finally, by August 1978, each Regional Administrator was instructed to submit a detailed plan for implementing this changeover.

As part of the planning process for decentralizing WSH, the Regional Administrator began to lobby for the conversion of all psychiatry positions from civil service blocks on the hospital's payroll to a purchase-of-service contract with the University of Massachusetts Medical Center (UMMC). By this time, the psychiatric staff at WSH had been significantly reduced by natural turnover and resignations and the Regional Administrator saw a purchase-of-service contract as a way of demedicalizing the authority structure of the hospital while insuring adequate psychiatric coverage.

In 1976, for example, there were 24 psychiatrists on the staff: 12 residents, 4 junior, and 8 senior psychiatrists. In practice, due to their training and administrative responsibilities, these 24 persons represented only 14 full-time equivalent (FTE) staff: the residents spent half of their time in training and clinical supervision[4] and thus constituted about 6 FTEs; the junior staff spent all of their time in patient care and represented 4 FTEs; and the senior staff (superintendent, assistant superintendent, three unit directors, two residency training directors, and the director of the outpatient psychotherapy clinic) provided 4 FTEs for direct patient care. In July 1977, the psychiatric staff was reduced to 17 persons (8 residents, 4 junior, and 5 senior) for a FTE staff of approximately 10 positions. Three of the senior and two of the junior staff psychiatrists had resigned to accept other positions or to enter private practice. Six residents completed their training, two succeeded to the junior staff, four left the Worcester area, and two new residents were hired.

In the spring of 1977, Myerson affiliated the WSH residency training program with the Department of Psychiatry at UMMC which did not have its own residency program. Similiar to the arrangement he had developed with The Memorial Hospital (see Chapter 9), the UMMC affiliation was designed to meet the new psychiatric accreditation requirements for a first-year medical internship, and to enhance the residency program's training and recruitment capability. After Myerson resigned as WSH superintendent, he joined the Department of Psychiatry at UMMC as Director of Continuing Education. When the Region II Administrator proposed developing a purchase-of-service contract with UMMC, Myerson was receptive to the offer and arrangements were made for transferring administrative and financial responsibility for the residency program from the Department of Mental Health to the Department of Education, which was responsible for the new medical school.

As part of this contract, the staff psychiatrists at WSH were offered a substantial salary increase to transfer their positions to UMMC. However, each psychiatrist would be committed to spend a full 40-hour week in direct patient care at the hospital. Since this arrangement, in effect, would prohibit staff from seeing private patients on "state time" (at WSH, in their private offices, or at The Memorial Hospital inpatient unit) none of the senior staff agreed to the transfer.[5] Three of the junior psychiatrists who did not have a private practice (and for whom the contract represented a salary increase from $20,000 to $40,000) accepted this arrangement. In July 1978, the training program and the three junior psychiatrist positions were transferred to UMMC. Over the next several months, the four remaining senior psychiatrists resigned from the WSH staff.

In January 1979, when the plans for the decentralization of WSH were implemented, five full-time psychiatrists were working at the hospital. None of them had any responsibilities for the administration of the hospital or its area inpatient units; they devoted all of their time to direct patient care. Each was accountable to a nonmedical unit Director who, in turn, reported to one of the four Area Directors. Thus, within 15 months of the demise of medical superintendency, the authority structure of WSH was completely demedicalized.

Consistent with the new policy of the Department of Mental Health, the responsibility of the central administration was limited to providing "housekeeping" and administrative support services, professional departments were abolished, and a Regional Service Unit was established under the direction of the former Chief of Psychology. These services included six geriatric wards, two mentally retarded wards, two educational programs (the Woodward Day School and the Adolescent Treatment Complex), and several clinically related services (dental, laboratory, pharmacy, medical, admissions, vocational rehabilitation, and psychology). Plans were also made effective July 1, 1979 to contract with a private vendor for the operation of the drug treatment unit, to phaseout the psychoendocrine research unit operated by the Psychology Department, and to close the outpatient psychotherapy clinic.

The formal governance structure of WSH was also brought directly under the control of the Regional Administrator. A Regional Executive Committee [composed of the Regional Administrator, two Associate Administrators, four Area Directors, the Assistant Superintendent (Administrative), and the Regional Services Unit Director] was organized to oversee all policy and budgetary matters at WSH and three other state institutions in central Massachusetts. Responsibility for the day-to-day operation of WSH was assigned to a Steering Committee composed of key hospital-based staff [the Assistant Superintendent (Administrative), the Regional Services Unit Director, and the four area Unit Directors.] With these changes, the trend started over a hundred years ago in the 1860s toward evolution of control away from the hospital had reached its ultimate stage, and WSH ceased operating as a self-directed organization with a unitary administrative structure.

## INSTITUTIONAL SUCCESSION

In late 1976, while Myerson and other WSH administrators were attempting to cope with the internal management problems of the hospital, forces were set in motion that would soon radically alter the ecology of mental health services in the Worcester area. Members of the Greater Worcester Area (GWA) Board had become increasingly frustrated with Myerson's execution of his dual responsibilities as Area Director and Superintendent. As Myerson began to spend more of his time on the internal problems of the hospital, the complex of community services that he had helped to create was left in a holding pattern. Some board members also were concerned that the area program in Worcester was lagging behind other areas of the state and that Myerson was not interested in undertaking the systems development work that was needed to fill in the housing, rehabilitative, and other nonmedical service gaps in the local community.

Faced with declining resources, the Department of Mental Health had encouraged its Regional and Area office staff to explore alternatives to state funding in support of community mental health services. The passage of Public Law 94–63 in 1975 extended the national Community Mental Health Centers (CMHC) program, and the Department believed this legislation presented a major opportunity

for shifting some of the burden of community program support
from state to federal budgets (MDMH, 1977:124). In December 1976,
the Regional Administrator invited a representative from the U.S.
Department of Health, Education and Welfare (DHEW) Regional Office in Boston to meet with the GWA Board and representatives
from other local health and welfare agencies to discuss the prospects of CMHC funding. The DHEW representative encouraged the
Board to develop a proposal for a CMHC in the City of Worcester.

In April 1977 the Board selected the Worcester Area Drug Coalition, Inc. as the lead agency to prepare an application for CMHC
funding.[6] The selection was based on the Coalition's demonstrated
expertise in securing federal, state, and local funding; its planning
and management experience in organizing and operating a multi-
agency collaborative; and its program evaluation and monitoring
capabilities. The one potential drawback was its identity as a sin-
gle-purpose agency (i.e., drug abuse) without experience in providing major mental health services. Accordingly, it was reconstituted
as the Worcester Area Community Mental Health Center
(WACMHC), Inc.

As the grant application developed, two opposing viewpoints
on the organizational structure of the WACMHC emerged. Some
members of the planning group favored a highly centralized organization which would provide all of the mandated services, while
others advocated a decentralized model with most of the services
provided under contract with existing agencies. Advocates of the
centralized model argued that it would be easier to administer and
that it would be more responsive to the federal CMHC guidelines
which place a heavy emphasis on a "single portal of entry" and
continuity of care between service elements. Proponents of the decentralized model, on the other hand, felt that it was more consistent with the strong tradition of autonomy and separation that had
dominated inteagency relations in Worcester for many years. Moreover, they argued that the Worcester Area Drug Coalition and the
Worcester Model Cities Program had demonstrated the viability of
multi-agency service delivery networks.

A compromise was negotiated that combined elements of both
models: direct services would be provided on a decentralized basis
by existing human service providers under affiliation contracts
with the WACMHC which would retain centralized administrative,
case management, and client intake functions. It was agreed that
each affiliate agency under the authority of the Center Director
would be directly responsible for the management of its own pro-

gram, including an integrated client data system, development of treatment plans, billing, and financial management. However, a central intake unit staffed by case managers would serve as a "single portal of entry" into the WACMHC. Case managers would screen, evaluate, and assess each client; refer the client to an affiliate agency; cooperate with the affiliate's Clinical Director in developing a plan of treatment; and provide aftercare and client advocacy services. Thus, the "Worcester Model" attempted to coordinate decentralized delivery of services with centralized administration by relying upon case managers to broker client access and movement through the affiliate agencies.

Once the proposed model was accepted the WACMHC requested local human service providers to develop proposals for each of the 12 mandated services except inpatient care. For the latter service, the WACMHC planning group tried to negotiate priority bed agreements with St. Vincent's Hospital (for 14 beds) and The Memorial Hospital (for 6 beds), the two private nonprofit general hospitals with separate psychiatric inpatient units in the Worcester area. Initially, the Chiefs of Psychiatry at each hospital were receptive to this proposal. After reviewing the formal affiliation agreement, however, they declined the offer because of the control that the WACMHC would have over the operation of their inpatient units.

The planning group then sought help from the Chairman of the Psychiatry Department at the UMMC. He indicated that, rather than opening a psychiatric inpatient unit, the medical center had planned to develop a collaborative service wth the general hospitals in Worcester following the model Myerson had developed with The Memorial Hospital. By this time, the WSH Psychiatric Residency Training Program had affiliated with UMMC and plans were already in progress for linking the residency with other hospitals. This collaborative model, however, had not been adopted by choice. The original design for the medical center included plans for an inpatient psychiatric unit but the lack of resources at UMMC and the surplus of psychiatric beds at WSH prevented their implementation. With the prospect of external funding and the political support that would result from affiliation with the WACMHC, the Chairman was able to persuade UMMC officials to reconsider the original plan for operating a separate inpatient unit. He also recognized that an inpatient unit would enhance the status of psychiatry within the medical school. As a result, UMMC applied to the local Health Systems Agency for a Determination of Need to open a 20-

bed unit. This proposal was disapproved because its implementation would increase the number of acute psychiatric beds in Worcester hospitals beyond accepted levels. Subsequently, with the support of the Regional Services Administrator, a plan for phasing out acute beds at WSH was developed that would allow UMMC to open an inpatent unit: for every two beds phased out on the acute wards of the GWA unit at WSH, one bed could be made available at UMMC. In effect, the proposal, subsequently approved by the Health Systems Agency, required the phase out of 40 beds at WSH over a two-year period and the creation of a 20-bed unit at UMMC.

When the final WACMHC proposal was submitted to the National Institute of Mental Health (NIMH) in November 1977, eight affiliates were identified:

1.  Worcester City Hospital (outpatient and emergency services for adults and children)
2.  Crisis Center, Inc. (crisis intervention services)
3.  Chandler Street Center, Inc. (day care services)
4.  Family Health and Social Services, Inc. (outpatient, day care, and alcoholism services)
5.  Worcester Youth Guidance Center, Inc. (outpatient and day care for children)
6.  Jewish Home for the Aged, Inc. (services for the elderly)
7.  Youth Opportunities Upheld, Inc. (temporary shelter for adolescents)
8.  University of Massachusetts Medical Center (inpatient services)

The first three agencies originally formed the core of the Worcester Area Drug Coalition (in which WSH was a key service provider), while the Family Health and Social Services, Inc. operated one of the community clinics and day centers that Myerson had helped to develop with WSH staff. Furthermore, the inpatient service at UMMC was staffed principally by the former psychiatric staff at WSH. Thus, many of the core components of the WACMHC grew out of the infrastructure of services that had been spawned in the early 1970s with resources from WSH.

The proposal was reviewed by NIMH in December 1977 and conditionally approved in January 1978. The conditions reflected the concerns that had been identified in the Health Systems Agency review: (1) the estimated per diem costs for inpatient care at UMMC appeared to be excessive and it was recommended that a request for proposal be circulated to all eligible hospitals to establish competitive costs; (2) inadequate arrangements had been made for transitional residences; and (3) the separate adult outpatient programs at Worcester City Hospital and Family Health and Social Services seemingly would promote a two-tiered system of acute (City Hospital) and chronic (Family Health) care. Subsequently, these conditions were removed on the basis of an amended proposal that justified the UMMC affiliation, identified the New England Fellowship Rehabilitation Alternative, Inc. as an affiliate for a transitional residence, and clarified the anticipated patient mix at the two adult outpatient clinics. With these assurances, the proposal was approved for funding effective November 1, 1978.

The application budgeted the WACMHC's total first-year program at $1,555,000; $800,000 from the federal government, $620,000 from local and state agencies, and $125,000 from third-party revenue. The application was funded at a reduced level of $664,576 using carry-over monies from NIMH's fiscal year 1978 appropriation.

Over the next several months, the development of the WACMHC and the implementation of the Department of Mental Health's plans for the complete decentralization of WSH led to major realignments in the local mental health services network. New organizations were created and old ones coalesced under the administrative umbrella of the WACMHC. The leadership role and centrality of WSH in the local mental health services network declined but it continued to serve its historic functions (especially as a service of last resort) on a reduced scale. Although the "negotiated order" (Day and Day, 1977) in the interorganizational field had not been fully worked out by September 1979, clear signs were present that many of the problems of the old institutional order had yet to be fully addressed.

## Inpatient Services at UMMC

When WACMHC received its notice of grant award, planning for the opening of the 20-bed inpatient unit at UMMC was quickly initiated. A number of logistical problems had to be overcome in equiping a ward for psychiatric patients—cooking facilities, occupational therapy areas, seclusion rooms, etc. In addition, a major staff recruitment effort was undertaken. This effort coincided with DMH's plans for placing the psychiatric staff at WSH on personal services contracts. The Assistant Superintendent (Clinical) and the Director of Residency Training were offered positions on the new unit. The former agreed to become Unit Chief but the latter chose to enter private practice in the Worcester area. Other WSH staff were also recruited for senior clinical and administrative positions on the UMMC inpatient unit, including six psychiatric nurses, a clinical psychologist, and a Unit Director. Thus, when the unit opened in March 1979, 8 of the 28 staff members were former WSH employees.

The new unit was one of the first WACMHC affiliates to become fully operational. During its first five months of operation, 75 patients were admitted to the unit. The average length of stay for these patients was 17.5 days with a range of 1–60 days. Initially, in keeping with the conditions of its Determination of Need, the UMMC unit drew virtually all of its admissions from WSH. Priority was placed on patients being admitted for the first or second time; but in order to cement good relationships with the community, a number of patients with multiple admissions also were accepted. When the Central Intake Unit of the WACMHC opened in May 1979, patients began to be referred to UMMC directly from the community. By September 1979, the UMMC inpatient unit had developed into a high-volume, full-occupancy treatment program and its administrator was already developing plans to increase the unit from 20 to 27 beds.

Although the opening of the UMMC inpatient unit was originally justified in terms of supplanting the acute treatment functions of the GWA Unit at WSH, this aspiration was moderated by the realities of its organizational auspices and by its economic dependence on third-party reimbursements. As part of a medical school and teaching hospital, the new unit had to adapt its program to satisfy a broader set of interests and to the stringent requirements of a Utilization Review Committee whose members were not sympathetic to prolonged patient stays. Moreover, many staff members had been recruited with the inducement of working in a short-stay dynamic treatment unit. These external and internal pressures resulted in the selection of patients with good prognoses, usually first admissions with depressions or other acute psychiatric conditions who could benefit from short-term treatment. In addition, economic realities dictated that only a few patients without private resources or third-party coverage could be admitted. The unit maintained its commitment to the public sector by using psychiatric residents to care for these patients, leaving private patients to the staff psychiatrists.

Thus, within a few months of its opening, the UMMC inpatient unit began to replicate the experiences of The Memorial Hospital

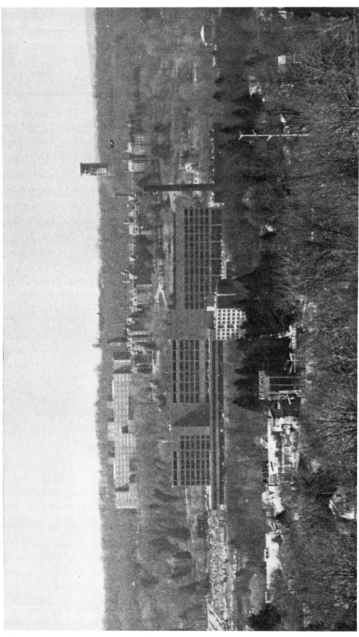

Fig. 12. University of Massachusetts Medical Center, 1980. Following the demedicalization and administrative disaggression of Worcester State Hospital in the late 1970s, the inpatient psychiatric unit at the new University of Massachusetts Medical Center (foreground) emerged as one of its institutional "succesors." The Main Hospital (right rear) and the Bryan Center (left rear) can be seen in the background. Source: Original photograph by Ann Youngstrom.

psychiatric unit both with regard to patient "creaming" practices and the use of residents to care for economically disadvantaged patients (see Chapter 9). Both units also attracted the "cream" of WSH's psychiatric and other clinical staff. As a private-sector institution, The Memorial Hospital justified its selective orientation in terms of the private practice of psychiatry and the needs of the middle-class community for short-term intensive care. As a public sector institution, however, the UMMC unit began to encounter community pressures to function as the "new WSH." In its early months, it was able to justify its selective orientation in terms of its medical school auspices and the availability of the "old WSH" as a back-up institution for unmanageable and indigent patients. In this sense, the division of labor that was emerging between UMMC and WSH was an extension of the "front-ward–back-ward" system of patient and staff assignment in the traditional state mental hospital (Bucher and Schatzman, 1962). The *intra*organizational mechanism for coping with resource scarcity and overwhelming numbers of patients in state institutions was becoming an *inter*organizational adaptation to the same fundamental problems in a diversified and segmented network of public and private institutions.

Thus, the demedicalization and phase-down of WSH promoted the growth of new psychiatric institutions and the relocation of its psychiatric staff in general hospitals. However, the movement of psychiatrists from WSH to the community and the realignment of organizational boundaries in the Worcester area led to the displacement rather than the resolution of the problems and the conflicts of the old institutional order.

### Operational Status of the WACMHC

Although funded at a reduced level, the WACMHC award from NIMH was a combined planning and operations grant.[7] The challenge was to formalize the interagency working relationships implied by the "Worcester Model" while simultaneously developing a service delivery capacity. By September 1979, progress had been made on both fronts, but the organizational viability of the WACMHC was beginning to be tested.

During its first three months, much of the WACHMC's effort was devoted to staff recruitment and completion of affiliation agreements. A gradual phase-in of services was necessitated by the reduction in the size of its federal grant and a delay in receiving its final Determination of Need (DON) from the Massachusetts Public

Health Council, the state-wide advisory board responsible for approving local Health Systems Agency determinations. (The absence of the DON prevented the licensing of affiliates for collection of third-party reimbursements). Certification was received in June 1979, and by September, most of the federally mandated services were operational. The adult transitional residence and children's outpatient services were scheduled for implementation out of second year funding in January 1980.

The WACMHC's core administrative staff and Central Intake Unit were established in the outpatient building at Worcester City Hospital in the offices formerly occupied by its predecessor organization, the Worcester Area Drug Coalition. The emergency, outpatient, crisis intervention, and alcohol detoxification services sponsored by the Hospital and two other affiliates were located in adjacent buildings. In many ways, WACHMC's close physical and organizational ties to Worcester City Hospital were designed to bolster and expand the hospital's ambulatory care functions in the local community. In the 1970s Worcester was one of the most overbedded metropolitan areas in the United States in terms of acute care general hospital beds.[8] When UMMC opened its teaching hospital (99 beds) in 1975 the local Health Systems Agency urged the phase-out of the municipally operated Worcester City Hospital (325 beds), but community interest groups managed to keep it open. The Worcester Area Drug Coalition had contributed to the hospital's survival by expanding its services into drug abuse, a major community concern in the early 1970s. The architects of the WACMHC hoped that, by making the hospital a key element in Worcester's community mental health service network, its chance of survival could be increased.

At the same time, the new center was designed to enrich and expand the capacity and variety of Worcester's community-based mental health services. Under its administrative umbrella a number of new services were established in 1979 and others were in the process of being developed. These included the UMMC inpatient unit, the adolescent shelter operated by Youth Opportunities Upheld, and the adult respite home sponsored by the New England Fellowship for Rehabilitation Alternatives. In addition preexisting agencies such as the Worcester Youth Guidance Center, Family Health and Social Services, and the Jewish Home for the Aged were able to sustain and expand their mental health-related service programs with WACMHC funding.

However, the reality problems of coordinating a large network of autonomous agencies began to surface as the WACMHC neared the end of its first full year of operation.[9] Three areas of conflict— all related to the basic principles of the "Worcester Model"—tested the organizational viability of the WACMHC: (1) the "single portal of entry" or central intake function, (2) the roles and responsibilities of case managers, and (3) the sharing of third party revenue.

In May 1979, as the individual service components became operational, the WACMHC Central Intake Unit began to screen admissions for its affiliates. The initial efforts to extend this function to UMMC led to a number of conflicts. The affiliation agreement between WACMHC and UMMC called for a priorty bed system for WACMHC referrals. However, UMMC staff sought to retain control over its own admissions. An "on-call" system was developed whereby UMMC psychiatrists participated in admission screenings at City Hospital, but in several instances, WACMHC referrals were refused admission to UMMC. Similar boundary control issues emerged in negotiations with the Worcester Youth Guidance Center, the other major psychiatric affiliate of the WACMHC. As part of a children's outpatient contract, WACMHC insisted on admission control through its Central Intake Unit but the Guidance Center objected to the arrangement as a threat to its clinical autonomy. Nevertheless, consistent with its federal mandate, the WACMHC planned to centralize the screening of all admissions to the remaining affiliates, including WSH, by November 1979.

The second incipient problem closely related to centralized intake concerned the roles and responsibilities of WACMHC case managers. Ideally, the "Worcester Model" envisioned case managers as the "glue" that would bond WACMHC affiliates into a comprehensive and continuous network of services. They would participate in the screening, evaluation, and assessment of each client at the Central Intake Unit; refer the client to an affiliate agency; assist the affiliate staff in developing a treatment plan; and provide aftercare and client advocacy services. In practice, WACMHC's early experience with case managers ran into conflict with affiliate autonomy and the reluctance of clinicians to share responsibility with "outsiders." As low-status and relatively untrained workers, case managers found it difficult to "coordinate" higher-status professionals (especially psychiatrists) who were sceptical about their ability to participate in the treatment process.

The third problem involved the financing of case management and central intake functions. During its first year of operation, these services were supported out of the NIMH grant. However, as the federal share of operating expenses declines over the eight-year life of the WACMHC grant, these services will have to be supported by local funds and third-party reimbursements. WACMHC administrators attempted to persuade affiliate agencies to include case management charges in their third-party billings, since these services were not separately reimbursable. However, affiliates were also dependent on third-party reimbursement as a source of their own budgetary needs. In the 1980s, the "acid test" of the "Worcester Model" will turn on the willingness of affiliate agencies to support such core services out of their third party revenue.

Moreover, to insure the economic viability of the new center, WACMHC officials were committed to making services available to clients with private resources or third-party insurance. In their view, the primary burden of caring for chronic patients and persons without resources had to remain with the Department of Mental Health and its local area program. Thus, the division of labor that was beginning to emerge among community and state agencies in Worcester was tending toward an acute resource-rich versus a chronic resource-poor differentiation that tended to perpetuate the historic two-class system of mental health care. The WACMHC was not unique in this regard. For their role in reinforcing this dual system, CMHCs throughout the country have been resoundly criticized (Chu and Trotter, 1974; Bassuk and Gerson, 1977).

In a number of respects, therefore, the tensions and conflicts over resource scarcity, preferential treatment, and centralization versus decentralization of responsibility for mental health services were not resolved by the demedicalization and disaggregation of WSH. Rather, these conflicts were displaced into the community where they became core issues in the effort to create a community-based mental health system out of a loosely connected network of public and private agencies.

## INSTITUTIONAL ADAPTATION AT
## WORCESTER STATE HOSPITAL

In March 1978, the former Executive Director of the Worcester Model Cities Program succeeded Myerson as Director of the Greater Worcester Area (GWA) mental health program. He had extensive experience in community organization and city management as well as the broad human services management orientation that the Department of Mental Health was trying to instill in its regional and area program staff. In his Model Cities position, he had worked closely with Myerson in the development of WSH's neighborhood mental health clinics and had served as a member of the GWA Board. He also had been actively involved in the planning for the WACMHC and was a strong supporter of the hybrid "Worcester Model" eventually adopted as the organizational structure for the new mental health center.

His appointment completed the staffing of the four area mental health programs in the region served by WSH with full-time, non-medical Area Directors. It also coincided with the Department of Mental Health's policy decision to decentralize WSH and transfer line authority over its inpatient units to area directors. Over the next several months, the four Area Directors and the Regional Administrator developed the operating and governance procedures that the Commissioner had stipulated in his memorandum calling for the integration of state hospital units with area mental health programs (Okin, 1978:23–24). In contrast to the three other areas, the GWA did not have the administrative capacity needed for the change-over. Due to budgetary constraints, Myerson had operated the GWA program out of the superintendent's office at WSH, and with the exception of a full-time administrative assistant, he relied upon WSH staff to manage the area program. Accordingly, during this period the new Area Director devoted much of his time to staff recruitment and the development of a separate administrative structure for fiscal control, program monitoring, and resource development. The informal agreements for use of space, staffing, and other resource exchanges that Myerson had developed with community agencies also were converted to formal contracts.

When the WACMHC received approval of its NIMH application, the new Area Director quickly implemented the UMMC Determination of Need formula for bed reduction at WSH. Over the period November 1978–May 1979 two wards (60 beds) on the GWA unit at WSH were closed. Funds from the GWA budget were given to the WACMHC on a contract basis to support its Central Intake Unit and plans were made for this Unit to screen all admissions to WSH beginning in November 1979. Plans were also developed to utilize the WACMHC case management model as a mechanism for followup and aftercare of persons committed to WSH by local courts.

In December 1978, the pace of the Department of Mental Health's planning for state hospital phase-down was accelerated by the Northampton State Hospital consent decree issued by the United States District Court *(Brewster v. Dukakis)* on the basis of a class action suit brought by the Massachusetts Association for Mental Health and the Massachusetts Association for Retarded Citizens against the Commonwealth. The suit cited violations of patients' constitutional and statutory rights to be treated in the less restrictive alternative suitable to their needs. In deciding in favor of the plaintiffs, the judicial decree mandated the establishment of a comprehensive system of community residences, as well as less restrictive treatment, training, and support services for patients at the Northampton hospital. Although the decree was limited to this one institution, the Department began to use this mandate to justify its overall program of state hospital phase-down.

At WSH, as region-wide treatment units and support services were phased out, funds were transferred from hospital to community accounts for purchase-of-service contracts with local vendors. In the GWA, a contract was developed with a nursing home to provide 18 beds for chronic patients and the services of a part-time psychologist to serve as on-site clinical director. A survey of the caseload on the GWA inpatient unit at WSH conducted by the Massachusetts Department of Public Welfare in May 1978 (as part of its Medicare–Medicaid certification review) indicated that approximately one-third of the 140 resident patients were suitable for the type of residences created in Western Massachusetts under the Northampton consent decree. Consistent with the Department of Mental Health's goals for continued census reduction at WSH, the Regional Administrator earmarked an additional $700,000 for transfer from regional to community accounts in fiscal year 1980.

During this period, however, a gap began to emerge between the Department's census projections and the actual caseload at WSH. With the demise of the medical superintendency and the resultant ambiguities surrounding the authority structure of WSH, the stringent monitoring of the admissions service was relaxed and admissions began to rise. In May 1978, the average resident census was 433; by July it had increased to 453, and over the next five months it averaged 447. The hospital had been budgeted for a census of 350 patients in fiscal 1979, and by the early spring the food budget was exhausted. Food was trucked in from a nearby state facility, and eventually funds were borrowed on credit to sustain the dietary department through the end of the fiscal year. An inquiry by the Assistant Superintendent (Administrative) and the Greater Worcester Area Director revealed that for some time the quality of food had been substandard, that poor administration had led to inadequate food service planning, and that WSH had been without a qualified dietitian for nearly two years.[10] In addition, with cutbacks in the central administrative staff, the maintenance of the buildings and wards also had deteriorated.

This situation attracted wide publicity from the local press and news media which resurrected the stories of patient abuse at WSH during 1976 (see Chapter 5). This publicity occurred shortly before the legislative hearings on the Department of Mental Health's fiscal year 1980 budget which proposed major reductions in WSH's regional service account. The state senate appropriations committee voted to restore these cuts, and challenged the Department's overall deinstitutionalization plans as overambitious and detrimental to the quality of care in state institutions.

Other problems also were reaching crisis proportions. Seven residents (all foreign medical school graduates) had been assigned to WSH on a part-time basis as part of the UMMC service contract. In addition to working on the wards and community clinics, the contract called for the residents to cover the admission service on a 24-hour basis and to serve as physician-on-call for emergency services during the evenings. Three of the residents were in their first year of training. While their work was supervised during the day by a senior resident and by Dr. Myerson (who was then serving as liaison between UMMC and WSH), they were on their own during the evenings. After 5 P.M. the resident "on call" at WSH was the backup for all of the public and private mental health services in central Massachusetts. The "buck stopped" in the admitting room at WSH; covering the emergency service was the most difficult and onerous task of the resident.

The inexperience of the first-year residents led to a number of "inappropriate" admissions and unit staff began to complain about the quality of their work-ups and misuse of medication. The residents, in turn, began to complain about their night call schedules and the amount of service work they were expected to perform. The situation became critical in the late spring, when a resident on call failed to respond to an emergency, and a patient died without medical attention. Residents came under fire from the Regional Administrator and from other WSH personnel for gross neglect. As tensions mounted, two of the first-year residents resigned. Faced with a manpower shortage and no prospects for immediate relief (UMMC had not recruited any new residents for the next year), the UMMC-WSH contract for admissions and night coverage was terminated in June 1979.[11]

Under the leadership of the Regional Services Unit Director (the former head of the WSH Psychology Department) a new system of clinical coverage was initiated. The funds that had been allocated to the UMMC residency contract were used to hire additional psychologists and to pay for the services of medical consultants. A clinical psychologist was assigned responsibility for the WSH admission service and medical evaluations were performed under contract by six "on-call" physicians (nonpsychiatrists) from the Worcester area. In the vacuum created by the demedicalization of WSH, psychologists also assumed increased responsibilities for staff supervision, in-service training, and the development of treatment programs on each of the area and regional inpatient units. The Psychology Internship Program, one of the few remaining state hospital-based psychology training programs in the country,[12] was refunded by NIMH in July 1979. These funds allowed for the recruitment of six predoctoral interns, who spent part of their time in clinical work under the supervision of staff psychologists. By September 1979 psychologists (7 staff and 6 trainees) constituted the largest professional group at WSH other than nurses, and they were responsible for many of the clinical functions formerly reserved for the psychiatric staff.

The political "backlash" to the Department of Mental Health's deinstitutionalization program led to a postponement in the designation of Area Directors as "facility heads" which had been scheduled to occur on July 1, 1979. In the wake of the deepening controversey over the deteriorating conditions at WSH and other state institutions, the Regional Administrator asked the Director of the Regional Services Unit at WSH to assume hospital-wide responsibilities as "clinical director." This offer met with strenuous opposition from the four Area Directors, who saw it as the first step toward recentralization of authority at WSH and as contrary to Departmental policy. Their opposition blocked the appointment and reinforced the strong thrust to keep each unit functionally autonomous. These centrifugal forces at the unit level also undermined efforts to maintain the hospital-wide committees and standards required by the Joint Commission for Accreditation of Hospitals. As a consequence, WSH faced the prospects of losing its accreditation and Medicaid–Medicare elegibility.

The longer-term implications of the professional succession from psychiatrists to psychologists at WSH were difficult to discern in September 1979. Informally, the psychologist Director of the Regional Service Unit served as the "superintendent" of the phased-down WSH, but largely in terms of clinical as opposed to administrative matters. His formal authority was limited to the clinical support services that fell under the umbrella of the Regional Service Unit, including the care of about 250 residual patients (geriatrics and the mentally retarded) not assigned to specific area-based inpatient units. Moreover, unlike the medical superintendent, his powers were not defined by statute and he served at the pleasure of the Regional Administrator. He also presided over a precarious resource base. In order to finance community treatment programs, the Department of Mental Health looked to the continued phase-out of regional services at WSH including the Woodward Day School and the Adolescent Treatment Complex (see Chapters 7 and 8). These administrative and fiscal constraints imposed formidable barriers to the rejuvenation of WSH under the control of psychologists.

Yet, as other staff members left WSH for better-paying jobs and more congenial working conditions, the psychologists remained. For them, WSH represented stable employment and the opportunity to assume increased responsibilities in a hospital previously dominated by psychiatrists. Once the loyal advisors of the superintendent (Shakow, 1972), the psychologists now could shape directly the clinical orientation of the hospital. Furthermore, their opportunities for moving into full-time private practice outside of WSH were diminished by the movement of former WSH psychiatrists into the community. In addition, WSH offered an advantageous research and training setting for the psychologists whose work in psychoendrocrinology and related fields was a direct extension of the tradition established by the Schizophrenia Research Program which had brought international renown to WSH during the 1930s and 1940s (see Chapter 3). Thus, they had a vested interest in the continued existence of WSH just as the medical superintendents and their medical staff had before them.

In addition to these personal and professional commitments, the psychologists worked hard to sustain the quality of care at WSH and to rekindle a sense of purpose among an otherwise demoralized patient-care staff. To many observers both within and without the hospital, they were engaged in a losing battle. WSH in 1979 still had responsibility for over 400 patients who needed humane care and the psychologists were convinced that the Department of Mental Health's underfinanced and piecemeal approach to deinstitutionalization would fail to supplant state institutions. They were aware that despite the opening of inpatient units at The Memorial

Hospital (see Chapter 9) and at UMMC, WSH still provided acute care for the indigent and most disturbed patients. Many patients, despite an array of community clinics, could not be maintained indefinitely in the community (see Chapter 10). The development of consultation services in the local courts and revised commitment statutes had not stopped the flow of involuntary commitments to WSH (see Chapter 6). The expansion of nursing home beds in Worcester had not allowed WSH to eliminate completely its geriatric or "back" wards. The Woodward Day School and Adolescent Treatment Complex did not remove the need for high-security beds for adolescents (see Chapters 7 and 8). In addition, the formation of a central intake unit under the auspices of the WACMHC did not supplant the emergency services at WSH. And finally, the shift in responsibility and fiscal control from institutions to the community had not resulted in added resources or adequate support services for the chronically mentally ill.

## THE RESIDUE OF INSTITUTIONAL REFORM

During the decade of the 1970s, the structure and functions of WSH and the organizational ecology of mental health services in the Worcester area underwent a series of dramatic changes. The underlying dynamic revolved around competing definitions of the preferred role and mission of the hospital. In the early 1970s, under the direction of a new superintendent, a number of innovative programs were developed that began to move WSH from a "total" delivery system for the indigent mentally ill and socially incapacitated to the hub of a functionally decentralized network of institutional and community-based mental health services. By attempting to impose treatment-oriented boundaries around its organizational domain and by "communitizing" responsibility for the mentally ill in partnership with other public and private agencies, WSH seemed to be on the verge of resolving its ambiguous legacy. The emergent mental health system in the Worcester area was a hybrid structure of institutional *and* community-based, public *and* private, custodial *and* treatment-oriented services of first *and* last resort.

In the mid-1970s, the environmental supports for this pattern of institutional adaptation were eroded by fiscal retrenchment and changing policies concerning the preferred locus of care for the mentally ill. These forces led to the demedicalization and disaggregation of WSH and the growth of new organizations in the interorganizational field surrounding WSH. In the process, WSH lost many of its staff, patients, and resources. Although the resultant diversification and expansion of the local mental health system enhanced the overall quality and variety of services, the new system led to the displacement rather than the resolution of the conflicts and problems of the old institutional order. WSH continued to serve as the institution of last resort for the most disadvantaged, the most disturbed, and the most disruptive patients in the Worcester region. From an administrative perspective, WSH had been transformed, yet it retained its basic functions (treatment, custody, and social control) and continued to face persistent problems (resource scarcity, limited autonomy, and ultimate responsibility for the most difficult patients). Therein lies the paradox of organizational change and institutional endurance.

### NOTES

1. The observations in this chapter are based on the authors close involvement with events at Worcester State Hospital from 1974 through 1978. Throughout this period Howard Goldman served as a psychiatric resident at the hospital under the auspices of the Brandeis-Worcester Training Program in Social Research and Psychiatry (see Klerman et al., 1979) and, from 1975 through 1978, Joseph Morrissey served as Research Director of the Training Program. Supplemental information on developments in the Worcester area through September 1979 was obtained by the senior author from in-depth interviews with several key informants at WSH and at other community agencies.

2. Our usage of the terms "nonmedical" and "demedicalization" throughout this chapter deserves special comment. We emloy these terms to designate the end of medical superintendency at WSH and the transfer of legal authority for its operation from physicians to nonphysicians.

   There is another way in which these terms are used in the social science literature, however. Some authors speak of "medicalization" with reference to the process of defining deviant behavior as illness and mandating or licensing physicians to treat it (c.f., Conrad, 1975; Conrad, 1979; Melick et al., 1979). In this tradition, "demedicalization" would imply the process of removing certain behaviors from legitimate medical definition and intervention.

   As noted later in this chapter, although a process of professional succession from psychiatrists to psychologists did occur in the aftermath of WSH's deinstitutionalization, physicians and psychiatrists were still involved in hospital treatment programs. While psychologists were committed to the expansion of treatment into psychosocial dimensions, it was not clear that they had supplanted the traditional "medical model" at WSH. Moreover, with regard to the mental health service system as a whole, the relocation of psychiatrists from WSH to general hospitals in the community led to the solidification of acute care under medical auspices. This is only one example of the administrative transition with functional stability aluded to in this chapter.

3. Even during the medical superintendency of WSH, the hospital was governed by an informal "dual authority" structure composed of the medical–psychiatric and business–maintenance staff. For a discussion of the antecedents and consequences of dual lines of authority in state mental hospitals and general hospitals, see Belknap (1956) and Smith (1958).

4. The psychiatric residents, together with the junior staff (typically psychiatrists who had recently completed their training), performed most of the service duties at WSH. Theoretically, 50 percent of a resident's time was devoted to "training" but the purely clinical demands were too great to make this allotment of time practical. Residents had clinical responsibilities on the acute and chronic wards and in the community clinics operated by WSH. They were also expected to provide 24-hour psychiatric coverage of the hospital and the admitting unit, processing emergency and routine admissions. When psychiatric residents finished their formal training and became members of the junior staff, they could expect a reduction in the burden of emergency coverage. Furthermore, succession to the senior staff freed the psychiatrist from all but supervisory admissions duty and occasional direct clinical services on a ward or in an outpatient clinic. This succession and the concomitant reduction in service responsibility was essential to maintaining a viable medical staff at WSH.

5. Salaries for public-sector psychiatrists were relatively low in Massachusetts and public service was difficult and often professionally unrewarding. In exchange for administrative, training, supervisory, and limited clinical responsibility, senior staff spent part of their 40-hour week in private practice. This was not officially sanctioned but had been common, and had received the tacit consent of the Department of Mental Health. These arrangements could continue only as long as the Department supplied WSH with psychiatric positions and as the psychiatric residents accepted the imbalance of the service load and the rules of staff succession.

6. The Drug Coalition had been organized in 1971 in response to a sudden increase in drug-related crimes in Worcester, and the paucity of specialized services for the treatment of drug abusers. Originally funded by the Worcester City Council, the Coalition subsequently received a National Institute of Drug Abuse grant to serve as an umbrella structure for a local drug abuse program. Worcester City Hospital contributed its former outpatient clinic for a drug rehabilitation program, a methadone withdrawal center, and a drug crisis center that was operated jointly by the Coalition and the Worcester Model Cities Program. In collaboration with the Coalition, Myerson opened a 30-bed drug detoxification and treatment unit at WSH and provided staff assistance and training services to the City Hospital program.

   In July 1979, however, responsibility for drug treatment programs was to be assumed by the Department of Mental Health and the Worcester Drug Coalition would be disbanded. Accordingly, the opportunity to apply for the CMHC grantee agency came when the Coalition was faced with administrative extinction. For a classic study of such "organizational goal succession," see Sills (1957).

7. Some federally funded CMHCs receive initial grants for program planning before the receipt of staffing monies to operate services. The WACMHC, however, received a joint operations–planning grant.

8. In 1979, according to statistics compiled by the Central Massachusetts Health Systems Agency, Worcester's eight general hospitals (including the teaching hospital at the University of Massachusetts Medical Center) had 9.0 beds per

thousand population, whereas the national norm advocated by federal regulatory agencies was 4.0 beds per thousand population (Personal communication from R. Higgins, Executive Director, Central Massachusetts Health Systems Agency, Shrewsbury, MA).

9. There is an extensive literature on the problems and pitfalls associated with voluntary coordination strategies in interorganizational planning and service delivery. For a review and discussion of these issues see Warren (1973), Warren et al. (1974); Rein (1970), Morris and Hirsch-Lescohier (1978), and Aldrich (1978).

10. This situation reflects the "zero-sum mentality" discussed in Chapter 5 by which staff salaries are often met at the expense of patient welfare.

11. The contract between WSH-UMMC for the services of staff psychiatrists remained in effect when the resident contract was terminated. In September 1979, UMMC officials were negotiating an arrangement whereby psychiatric residents would spend a six-month rotation at WSH as part of their training.

12. The psychology training program at WSH was also one of the first of its kind in the country and it served as a model for many other state hospitals. For a discussion of its origins and development, see Shakow (1970).

Joseph P. Morrissey
Howard H. Goldman
Lorraine V. Klerman

# 12
# The Enduring Asylum

Time is sort of river of passing events, and strong is its current; no sooner
is a thing brought to sight than it is swept by and another takes its place,
and this too will be swept away.

*Marcus Aurelius* (c. 170 AD)

The more things change, the more they remain the same.

*Alphonse Karr* (1849)

From its founding in 1830, Worcester State Hospital (WSH) has
mirrored the cyclical pattern of reform and retrenchment, of hope
and despair, which has characterized institutional care of the mentally ill in America. Just as its institutional history provides unique
insights into the environmental and organizational forces that have
led to the endurance of public asylums for the past 150 years, its recent deinstitutionalization experiences reveal, in microcosm, the
social forces that will insure their continued existence in some
form. In this concluding chapter, the meaning and significance of
the Worcester story for the larger mental health field will be reviewed and evaluated.

Current evidence indicates that like earlier attempts at institutional reform, deinstitutionalization as practiced in the 1970s failed

to develop a system of humane care for the chronically mentally ill. This assessment will be supported by a review of the parallels in the cycles of institutional reform, in the context of the fundamental social forces that have conditioned American social policy toward the care of the mentally ill. This review, in turn, will highlight the enduring functions of state mental hospitals and the fundamental changes required for the dissolution of the two-class system of care in this country. Short of a major technological breakthrough in understanding the causes and cures of mental disorders, progress toward the development of a truly humane system of mental health care requires a commitment of societal resources commensurate with the personal and social costs of these intractable problems. Moreover, such a system will remain elusive until mechanisms are developed to overcome the fragmentation of the current service network and the penchant to polarize the organizational and ideological approaches to the problem of mental illness.

### CYCLES OF REFORM: PERSISTENCE AND CHANGE

Since the reform movements of Horace Mann and Dorothea Dix at WSH that led, in turn, to the rise and proliferation of state mental hospitals in the early and middle decades of the 19th century, American social policy toward the care of the mentally ill has been a reflection of social values and ideologies. The belief that man could be perfected by manipulating his social and physical environment, the reformist zeal of Evangelical Protestantism, and the spirit of *noblesse oblige* were prominent features of the social climate at the time of the founding of WSH. As a seed bed of moral treatment during its first decades of operation, it provided the model that was followed by the rest of the nation and established the precedent for the state to assume exclusive responsibility for the indigent mentally ill. As the intellectual, social, and technological base of society changed, however, so too did the structure and functions of the institutions devoted to the care and treatment of the mentally ill.

The lack of an effective technology for treating large numbers of chronically ill patients drawn from lower class and immigrant groups, and the consequent decline in the rates of therapeutic success associated with hospitalization, gradually transformed WSH and other public mental hospitals from small, therapeutic asylums into large, human warehouses that provided cheap custodial care and segregation for the mentally ill, the medically infirm, the aged, and a miscellany of other social rejects. The cause of the "therapeutic asylum" became an ambiguous legacy of the past and a rhetoric for periodic institutional reform. Institutional change, however, was administrative and contextual, emphasizing the locus more than the modes of care and treatment. Some reformers favored large, centralized institutions; others advocated small, decentralized facilities such as general hospitals and other community-based settings. Over the past 150 years, while the pendulum of social and institutional reform oscillated between these extremes, a sharply divided two-class system for mental health care emerged and became firmly entrenched.

A careful analysis of these institutional reforms indicates that the social forces that shaped American social policies toward the mentally ill have remained largely unaltered. Social policies are principles or courses of action designed to influence the overall quality of life in a society; the circumstances of living of individuals and groups in that society; and the nature of intrasocietal relationships among individual groups, and society as a whole (Gil, 1973). Such policies operate through three interrelated, universal processes or societal mechanisms:

1. *Resource development:* the generation of life-sustaining and life-enhancing material and symbolic resources, goods, and services;
2. *Division of labor:* the allocation of individuals and groups to specific statuses (social positions) within the total array of societal tasks and functions, involving corresponding roles, and prerogatives intrinsic to these roles; and
3. *Distribution of rights:* the assignment to individuals and groups of specific rights to resources, goods, and services through general and specific entitlements, rewards, and constraints.

The mental health referents of these key processes are readily identifiable in relation to the characteristics of the organizations and clientele which constitute the mental health service system in its historical and contemporary context. In the late 18th and early 19th centuries, the general hospital became the first medical institution to care for the mentally ill in America, supplementing other social institutions, such as the family and the almshouse. The early general hospitals developed "insane departments" and later built separate asylums, many of which have become today's private mental hospitals. The general hospital did not become the dominant model because it was unable to provide care for the indigent insane who had become a great burden to their community. The public mental hospital was created to meet this need.

Accordingly, since the mid-19th century, mental health care has been divided into a public and a private sector (*resource development*). Public resources were allocated for the establishment of separate asylums for the indigent mentally ill; private resources were used almost exclusively to build facilities for paying patients. Following this initial schism, organizations within each sector developed specialized functions (*division of labor*) to serve different populations. Some facilities primarily treated acutely ill patients, while others provided predominantly long-term custodial care to the chronically disturbed. Some hospitals accepted only voluntary patients, while others were licensed to detain patients involuntarily. The differentiation of voluntary and involuntary care reflected not only a *division of labor*, but also a difference in the *distribution of rights*, in this case, the right to liberty and to refuse treatment. Further, because of the unequal distribution of rights to resources, the separation into public and private sectors also meant that each sector served a different population. State hospitals cared for the disadvantaged patients, while private hospitals treated the advantaged patients. This distribution of rights to resources, in turn, weighed the right to treatment in favor of the advantaged. As the care system evolved, private sector facilities tended to specialize in providing treatment to wealthier, acute, quiet, primarily voluntary patients. The state hospitals were left to provide long-term custodial care to poor, chronic, disturbed, involuntary patients. The differentiation of the mental health care delivery system during the past century has resulted in a pluralism of institutions, patient populations, methods of treatment, and professional ideologies.

The failure of institutional reforms throughout this period at WSH and elsewhere resides in their ad hoc or "cosmetic" nature (Talbott, 1978): changes *in* rather than changes *of* this dual system of care. An early effort to alter the institutionalization of the mentally ill occurred in the 1860s and early 1870s in the form of the cottage hospital movement. Merrick Bemis, the medical superintendent at Worcester, was one of the principal spokesmen and innovators in the effort to decentalize state hospitals in a way that would sustain their role in caring for all social classes and ethnic groups while providing humane custody of the chronically ill in family-like residences (see Chapter 3). Professional and economic considerations led to the defeat of Bemis' proposals (and of similar proposals in other locales) and the institutionalization of the mentally ill continued unabated. As a consequence, well-to-do families resorted to private facilities for the care of the mentally ill members and state hospitals became filled with lower class and ethnic minorities.

Subsequent reforms followed a similar course. The mental hygiene movement of the early 20th century was originally dedicated to improving the care and treatment of mental hospital patients (Deutsch, 1944). Much of its impetus came from Adolf Meyer, who formulated many of his ideas while working at WSH. As it matured, however, the movement began to concentrate on prevention in the form of early detection and treatment of mental disorders. The movement spawned the development of psychopathic hospitals within the state system for the reception and evaluation of acute cases, but most admissions were still funneled into large custodial institutions. The lasting contribution of the movement, however, were the child guidance clinics and parental education programs which were championed as interventions that would reduce the need for mental hospitalization. As Gruenberg and Archer (1979:488) note, however,

> (I)n hindsight . . . it is clear that the child guidance clinics were treating, as best they could, a new set of problems that had not before received psychiatric attention—disorders of childhood. They enlarged the spectrum of cases receiving attention; but they were not arresting later psychoses through early effective treatment on a significant scale.

The middle-class biases of the mental hygiene movement and the rejection of the poor by private social welfare and psychiatric agencies has been apparent for decades (Davis, 1939; Hollingshed and Redlich, 1958; Hunt et al., 1958; Cloward and Epstein, 1965; Fisher, 1969). Likewise, the Community Mental Health Center movement initiated in the early 1960s quickly became oriented to meeting the needs of a new or "underserved" clientele in local communities that rarely consisted of people with severe mental disorders who often needed inpatient care (Chu and Trotter, 1974; Cameron, 1978; Bassuk and Gerson, 1978; Scherl and Macht, 1979). And the more recent state hospital "deinstitutionalization" movement of the early 1970s, justified as a broad-based plan to provide humane care for the chronically mentally ill, has led to their abandonment in the eyes of many critics (Reich and Segal, 1973; Kirk and Therrien, 1975; Rose, 1979; Gruenberg and Archer, 1979).

These reform movements shifted attention from one administrative solution to another, from institution to community and from centralized to decentralized services. Each expanded and diversified the mental health system but none fundamentally changed the two-class system of care.

The evidence of cyclical patterns in the social and institutional reforms at WSH as well as in the mental hospital arena as a whole, however, goes much deeper. There are a number of striking parallels in the processes as well as the outcomes associated with the two principal "reforms" of the past 150 years: the rise of state mental hospitals, or "institutionalization," and their apparent demise, or "deinstitutionalization." These parallels can be found in the exaggerated success claims of the early advocates of both reform movements and in the two distinct phases within which the reforms were carried out.[1]

With regard to exaggerated success claims, each movement was launched with little or no appreciation of the practical limits to which the core ideas could be pushed. In the case of the mental hospital movement of the 19th century, institutionalization proved beneficial only for milder and acute cases of mental illness; moral treatment had little success with chronic, long-term cases. The early successes of moral treatment at WSH, however, spawned the diffusion of asylums throughout America even as the original hospitals were floundering under the pressure of an ever-expanding chronic caseload. Proponents of institutionalization, such as Dorothea Dix and Samuel Woodward, were so wedded to the idea that environmental change and removal to state hospitals was instrinsically beneficial (Rothman, 1971), that institutions continued to be built regardless of their deteriorating quality of care and inadequate resources.

In the case of the community mental health movement of the mid-20th century, the development of new psychosocial techniques (e.g., milieu therapy, therapeutic communities, "open hospitals") and later the discovery and widespread use of psychoactive drugs made deinstitutionalization or community-based treatment possible for relatively acute cases of mental disorder. Research documented the value of short-term hospitalization and alternatives to hospitalization for acute episodes, but there was little research evidence that the new technologies could reverse the course of chronic deterioration in long-stay patients (Klerman, 1977; Gruenberg and Archer, 1979). Community mental health ideologues, nonetheless, saw the state hospital census decline following 1955 as evidence that the majority of patients could benefit by transfer to the community, with little appreciation for the absence of life-support systems needed to maintain chronic patients outside of these hospitals. Social science research on conditions in many state hospitals (e.g., Goffman, 1961), also contributed to "... the romantic notion that all chronic deterioration was the product of institutional life" (Klerman, 1977:624). Shifting the locus of care by removing chronic patients to community settings rested on naive environmentalist assumptions similar to those advanced in favor of mental hospitalization in the 19th century (Caplan, 1969).

With regard to phases of reform, both the mental hospitalization and the community mental health movements were initially stimulated by therapeutic innovations but were ultimately accelerated by political-economic considerations. In the 19th century, the mental hospital movement got underway during the era of moral treatment (roughly between 1830 and 1855) when humane psychosocial treatment in small, intimate asylums led to high rates of recovery for persons who were ill less than a year. In the 20th century, the community care movement (roughly between 1950 and 1965) was occasioned by the resurgence of psychosocial treatment approaches and early release policies (Gruenberg and Archer, 1979), and then by the use of psychotropic medications (Klerman, 1977). Active treatment programs and renewed optimism about the treatability of mental disorders led to dramatic census declines in state hospitals throughout the country.

Although political-economic factors played a crucial role in the subsequent development of each movement, it was the growing belief in the incurability of mental disorders and the pervasive therapeutic nihilism of the late 19th century that led to expansion of large custodial mental hospitals, while it was the near-opposite belief—that the technological advances of chemotherapy provided an effective basis for treating all state hospital patients in the community—that transformed the community care movement into a program of "deinstitutionalization" in the past decade. History has shown that both beliefs were misleading. With the apparent failure of moral treatment, concern shifted to providing custodial care for the largest number of patients at the lowest possible cost in large centralized institutions removed from the mainstream of community life. Contrary evidence, such as the Park-Eastman studies at Worcester State Hospital which clearly showed that with proper care a significant number of patients recovered without relapse (see Chapter 3), was ignored and the burden for caring for the mentally ill and other social problem cases was shifted from local communities to the state.

In the late 1960s, under the banner of "deinstitutionalization," state hospital phase-down became "a slogan and a de facto policy decision" (Klerman 1977:624). The coalescing of interests among community mental health advocates, civil libertarians, and fiscal conservatives led to a sharp break with the state hospital reform movement of the 1950s and early 1960s. As Gruenberg and Archer (1979:500) note, the

> *.* . . recognition that [state hospitals] can sometimes do more harm than good . . . developed into a belief that they can never do any good . . . (T)he court decision that mental patients must be treated in the "least restrictive care" setting has been interpreted to mean that any care is less restrictive than state mental hospital care, even though these hospitals can often provide care with less restriction on the patient's life than can nursing homes, adult residence hotels, and general-hospital, locked psychiatric wards.[2]

Moreover, as Klerman (1977:624) relates:

> . . . right-wing fiscal conservatives were interested in reducing the budgets of state governments. If they could shift the fiscal burden of responsibility to the Federal level, they did so. Transferring a patient into a nursing home meant that the cost was borne by Medicare, and discharging patients into the community, even if the were sent to state-subsidized boarding homes, was still less expensive per diem. If the patients could be certified as disabled, they were eligible for Social Security, with costs being borne in large part by Federal rather than state or local funds."

The result was a rapid depopulation of state mental hospitals despite little documentation of the relative cost-benefit ratio of deinstitutionalization. Thus, in a number of respects, recent reforms in mental health care have committed the counterpoint error of the late 19th century: assuming that all patients would benefit by release to the community, while ignoring evidence that many chronic patients require some kind of institutional care for the rest of their natural lives (see Chapter 10; Klerman 1977; Gruenberg and Archer, 1979). Moreover, the claims that community care would be more cost-efficient than state hospitals—so appealing to the fiscal conservatives who endorsed rapid deinstitutionalization policies—have proved to be exaggerated (Arnhoff, 1975). "Although the release of patients to the community," as Mechanic (1978b:6) points out, "is always less expensive in direct care costs than other alternatives if this is all that is done, required welfare expenditures and indirect social costs to the patients, their families and the community measured by patient deterioration, disruption of family life, and social control problems may be large. Effective community care requires not only adequate medical services and the provision of supportive services but also efforts in teaching patients coping skills that enhance their social capacities and life satisfactions."

The Group for the Advancement of Psychiatry (GAP, 1978:339–340) has also noted the marked parallels in the ideological, social, and economic climate of society a hundred years ago and the current post-deinstitutionalization era:

(The) ideological emphasis *then* on the interpersonal and humanistic understanding of the mentally ill was replaced by an emphasis on cellular and brain pathology and on classification of mental illness. *Now*, the humanistic concern for mental patients, which reappeared in the middle years of this century, is endangered by preoccupation with advances in psychobiology and psychopharmacology.

Educationally, the inspired leaders of moral treatment failed *then* to train successors to counteract the pessimistic view of mental illness that evolved with the development of scientific medicine. *Now*, the pioneers in community care have failed to train new leaders and new clinician-administrators prepared to accept the responsibility for the formulation of new policies and for the development and operation of community programs for psychiatric rehabilitation.

Culturally, the advocates of moral treatment, dependent on familiar interpersonal relationships, were not prepared *then* to adapt their treatment approach to the mentally ill members of a mass of immigrants who differed in language, socioeconomic status, and education. *Now*, the advocates of community care, also dependent on familiar types of interpersonal relationships, have not sufficiently adapted their treatment approach to the growing demands of new consumer groups, recent migrants from a broad range of ethnic and cultural backgrounds, and people such as drug abusers who have been diverted from the correctional system.

*Then*, the locus of segregation of the mentally ill was shifting from jails and almshouses to state hospitals away from our communities. *Now*, the locus of segregation is again shifting, this time from state hospitals to ghettoes and residential care facilities still isolated from our communities.

*Then*, rising costs and financial distress caused cutbacks in hospital services and virtually made moral treatment impossible to carry out. *Now*, recession and inflation have led to cutbacks in community care that have made its ambitious goals virtually impossible to attain.

These parallels are disturbing and suggest that history may be repeating itself, that the hope that the chronic mentally ill in this country will be rehabilitated or at least given humane and dignified care is being abandoned, and that they are doomed either to return to custodial institutional care or to drift, rejected and unattended, in the back-waters of our cities.

In a number of respects, therefore, the ambiguous legacy of institutional care is now being supplanted by the ambiguous legacy of community care. In the past decade, the gap between the ideal of a community-based mental health system and its reality has widened considerably. Similar to the early private asylums, CHMCs and general hospitals have not provided the comprehensive care required for chronic as well as acute patients; social and rehabilitative services have not been put into place; and the state hospital system has been dismantled prematurely. Rather than "deinstitutionalization" a process of "transitutionalization" has occurred in many instances, with "back wards" moved to nursing homes (Schmidt et al., 1977) and other residential care facilities (Reich and Segal, 1973) and "front wards" moved to general hospitals and CMHCS (Windle and Scully, 1976). Thus segregation of the mentally ill persists in a new ecological arrangement.

These observations are not meant to imply that nothing has changed in the American mental health system, nor that the changes have not been beneficial to many patients. Indeed, the past two decades have witnessed dramatic increases in outpatient services, private-sector care, and community-based services (c.f., Kramer, 1977; Redlich and Kellert, 1978; Regier et al., 1978; Klerman, 1979). Nevertheless, as long as social forces shape policies toward the mentally ill, the basic functions of the state mental hospital will continue to be needed even if the institutions are phased down, consolidated, or closed. The following section will examine briefly the enduring functions of the state mental hospital in the present and future mental health care system.

## THE MULTIPLE FUNCTIONS OF STATE
## MENTAL HOSPITALS

It is overly simplistic to view the history of the public mental hospital as a fall from the "grace" of moral treatment into the "snakepit" of custodialism. It is certainly true that Worcester State Hospital and the institutions modeled after it never lived up to the exaggerated expectations of their founders. However, neither is it accurate to regard the public asylum as "dead" (Talbott, 1978) or even as an institutional failure—its "premature obituary" has been noted elsewhere (Lamb and Goertzel, 1972). The endurance of public asylums beyond the era of moral treatment attests to the multiple "usages" (Perrow, 1978) or functions they came to serve for the larger society, for their staff, and for other community organizations. Although officially a medical institution in which treatment was presumed to be the legitimate, announced purpose, in practice, the actual functions served by state mental hospitals were (1) to provide inexpensive custody, control, and segregation of persons who were disruptive of social order or burdensome to their families; (2) to provide stable employment and health-welfare benefits for their staff (and, historically, they did serve as the arena for the professionalization of psychiatry); (3) to provide a cottage industry in towns with few or no other economic resources; and (4) to operate as a backup or "dumping ground" for cases deemed inappropriate or unacceptable by other health and welfare organizations and community practitioners (Belknap, 1956; Fowlkes, 1975; Bachrach, 1976; Goldman, 1978). In each of these respects, state mental hospitals for the past century or more have been remarkably successful as "tools" (Perrow, 1972) or resources for realizing the purposes of a variety of internal and external interest groups.[3]

Within the last two decades, however, many of the political-economic supports for the social functions of state hospitals have been altered by the opportunities to transfer patients to community settings and the financial burden of their care from state to Federal and local government budgets, by the growth of the nursing home and other rehabilitation service industries, and by the proliferation of general hospital psychiatric units and community mental health centers as alternative practice settings for the professional staff of these institutions. However, despite the rapid depopulation of state hospitals, most continue to exist (albeit "creamed," "dumped upon," and "exposéd"). Their residual social functions are still needed and they have not been supplanted by other institutions.

## TB Sanitoriums: A Case of Successful Deinstitutionalization

It is instructive in this regard to contrast the deinstitutionalization of tuberculosis (TB) sanitoriums with the depopulation of state mental hospitals. Historically, both institutions performed similar functions: treatment, social control, and custody of patients suffering from chronic conditions for which there were no effective cures. Therapy consisted of removal to a healthful environment which promoted recovery. Enforced segregation of the patient from the family and the community was justified on the basis of societal protection from contagion (TB) or imminent danger (mental disorder).

Both institutions provided "homes" for the indigent victims of chronic disease, often on a life-long basis. The proliferation of both institutions was a product of the Industrial Revolution, with its concomitant urbanization and changes in population density. There is also evidence that aspects of what Goffman (1961) characterized as "total institutions" could be found in TB sanitoriums as well as mental hospitals (Wittkower, 1955; Roth 1965).

However, there were marked differences in the etiology, morbidity, and mortality associated with TB and the mental disorders. By the 1880s, it had been established that TB was a unitary disease and its specific cause (the tubercle bacillus) had been isolated, although no effective therapy was available (Des Prez, 1975). In the early years of the 20th century, TB was the leading cause of death with rates on the order of 200 per 100,000 and morbidity was widespread, though reliable data were unavailable (Dublin, 1958). In contrast, mental patients rarely died of their illness and they accumulated much more rapidly in public institutions. With the exception of disorders such as pellagra and syphilis, the causes of mental illness have been elusive and, with advances in scientific understanding, substantial evidence for their multiple as opposed to unitary origins has mounted (Sobel, 1979). In the late 1940s and early 1950s, there were 400 TB sanitoriums operating under public and private auspices with an average daily resident population of over 60,000 patients and annual admissions in excess of 80,000 (American Hospital Association, 1977:4). During the same time period, state and county mental hospitals numbered 322 with a resident population of over 500,000 patients and annual admissions of over 150,000 persons (NIMH, 1979).

The phase-out of TB sanitoriums was occasioned by the development of a cure for the disease which reduced the risk of contagion and decreased its chronic morbidity. The technological breakthrough occurred in 1947 when streptomycin was established as a truly effective antituberculous drug. In 1953, isoniazid was demonstrated to be even more effective, and TB became a medically curable illness in most cases. As Des Prez (1975:392) points out: "(S)ince patients on treatment became rapidly noninfectuous and required little bed rest or specialized therapeutic methods ... the need for sanatoriums disappeared, and tuberculosis became, perhaps for the first time, the legitimate province of the general physician and general hospitals." Since the tuberculin skin test and chest x-ray already provided reliable case-finding methods, the new chemotherapy made TB susceptible to public health control measures. Responsibility for treatment was gradually transferred to community general hospitals and outpatient clinics and the TB sanitoriums were closed or converted to other uses. Between 1950 and 1960, the number of TB sanitoria declined by 40 percent (from over 400 to 238) and, by 1976, their decline had reached nearly 95 percent, with only 21 still in operation as respiratory disease hospitals (American Hospital Association, 1977:4).

Although occurring roughly over the same time period, the "deinstitutionalization" of state mental hosital stands in marked contrast to the disappearance of the TB sanitoriums. The impact of technological breakthroughs in the treatment of mental disorders, such as electroconvulsive therapy in the late 1930s and 1940s and psychoactive drugs in the mid-1950s, differed from the effect of the new treatments for TB. The neuroleptics (antipsychotic and antidepressive medications) improved patient management and helped reduce the length of hospitalization by controlling the symptoms of acute conditions, but they did not cure mental disorders, nor did they substantially prevent chronicity. The causes of mental disorders remain elusive and psychiatric epidemiology still lacks effective case-finding techniques (Cassel, 1966). In the past few decades, however, significant progress has been made in understanding schizophrenia—the condition that alone accounted for most of the long-term state hospital population—and it now appears to be several different diseases, brought on by multiple causes, involving heredity, brain structure, brain chemistry, and physical and social environmental factors (Sobel, 1979). "There is no 'schizococcus'— no single agent that causes schizophrenia," as Nathan Kline (Sobel, 1979:1) notes, "and so there will be no 'magic bullet' found as cure." Nonetheless, armed with the new psychiatric technology and the political-economic supports described above, the community mental health and deinstitutionalization movements led to the decrease of state hospital resident populations by 365,000 patients (or 65 percent) between 1955 and 1975. Released patients on drug maintenance have been described as "better but not well" (Klerman, 1977) but new forms of chronicity have been created in the community, which raise a number of disturbing social and ethical issues about the policy of deinstitutionalization (c.f., Chapter 10; Crane, 1974; Arnhoff, 1975; Scheff, 1976; Klerman, 1977; Koenig, 1978). Moreover, as of 1975, despite the rapid depopulation of state hospitals during the late 1960s and early 1970s, only a handful of these institutions (primarily in California and Massachusetts) had been closed (Greenblatt and Glazier, 1975).

## Enduring Functions of State Mental
## Hospitals

Today, state mental hospitals continue to serve their historic patient care and social control functions, albeit at a reduced level. Data available from the National Institute of Mental Health (Goldman and Rosenstcin, 1979) indicate that:

1. These hospital still serve a substantial acute care function. In 1975 approximately 400,000 admissions (duplicated count), consisting largely of persons from socially and economically disadvantaged backgrounds, were recorded by the 313 state and county mental hospitals in the United States;
2. These hospitals still serve a major social control function through civil, criminal, and emergency commitment. In 1972, some 200,000 persons were admitted to these hospitals on involuntary status; and
3. These hospitals still serve a sizeable custodial care function. In 1975 there were some 100,000 to 125,000 resident patients in state hospitals who could not be moved permanently into community facilities, either because they were "inappropriate" (too disturbed or too disturbing) for current types of residential alternatives or because the alternatives are not available.

Thus, despite the rhetoric of deinstitutionalization, public resources are still required to maintain state mental hospitals. Many disadvantaged patients are still barred from admission to nonpublic facilities because of a lack of resources to pay for care and treatment. Courts, police, private physicians and other agencies continue to commit mental patients involuntarily to public hospitals because most nonpublic facilities do not have (or seek) licenses to treat involuntary cases. In addition, a substantial residue of the most difficult and undesirable patients remain to be cared for in the state mental hospitals because nonpublic facilities refuse to accept (or keep) them even if they are able to pay and are admitted voluntarily. From their inception, state hospitals have served as a buffer or (less euphemistically) "dumping ground" for the mental health and social welfare system, and this role continues to be performed today. As Shore (1979:770) notes, the relationship between state hospitals—the "institutions of last resort"—and the rest of the mental health system involves a "tacit social contract":

> Maintenance of the system of private entitlement depends upon the co-existence of a public system in which the quality of care is infinitely di-

lutable by the addition of new patients to a fixed resource pool. Thus the private sector of psychiatry needs the public institutions as they are currently set up and is subtly but strongly motivated not to look too deeply into their functioning.

The state mental hospital is not unique in this regard. Similar organizations or parts of organizations can be found in the medical care system (c.f., Roth and Eddy, 1967 on chronic disease hospitals), the public school system (c.f., Carlson, 1965 on "special" classrooms for the educationally handicapped), higher education (c.f., Clark, 1960 on community colleges), and in many other direct service arenas. By managing the "failures" and tough problem cases in each institutional sphere, these organizations allow other more powerful or prestigious agencies to provide high-quality services to carefully selected client groups.

The expansion of a pluralistic (public–private, acute–chronic, inpatient–outpatient) mental health services system has occurred at the expense of the state mental hospitals. While the phase-out of many of these institutions—especially those established during the era of institutionalization as overflow chronic care facilities in remote rural areas—can be justified on clinical, administrative, and fiscal grounds, it is clear that the closure of *all* state hospitals is premature. To date, the private sector has accepted the more acute, less disturbed, voluntary patients with financial resources, leaving the public sector with the residue of the patient population. The growth of the nursing home industry and the development of alternative community residences has reduced the number of long-term chronic patients who once languished on back wards in state mental hospitals. However, many authorities question the categorical claims that their relocation has led to demonstratable benefits. Indeed, rather than "deinstitutionalization," the process has often resulted in their "transinstitutionalization" or movement from one debilitating environment to another (Talbott, 1979b).

The existence of a "pluralism" of services—so enticing in the context of the American political creed—has had unanticipated or counter-intuitive consequences for the state mental hospital. The Joint Commission on Mental Illness and Health (1961) had encouraged the expansion of the mental health system, including the proliferation of community mental health centers and psychiatric units in general hospitals. The Community Mental Health Centers Act of 1963 largely ignored the state mental hospital but it created the expectation that the new centers would prevent hospitalization and would provide aftercare for patients released from these hospitals.

Likewise, there was a hope that psychiatric units in nonpublic general hospitals would assume the acute inpatient function of state mental hospitals. Neither expectation has been realized fully. Further, the expansion of mental health services siphoned away professional staff and the most treatable patients from the public hospitals. This "creaming" left them to perform an increasingly more difficult set of tasks with diminished resources. Rather than replacing the state mental hospital, however, the proliferation of community-based facilities reinforced the role of the public asylum as a 24-hour backup and institution of last resort and ultimate responsibility. The continued existence of the state hospitals permits other facilities and practitioners to maintain the privilege of treating a selected target population, referring the most difficult problems and abdicating responsibility for the least desirable and most costly patient care (Chapter 9; Shore, 1979; Shore and Shapiro, 1979). The endurance of the two-class system of care throughout these administrative change processes can be attributed to the persistence of the fundamental social forces that have shaped policies toward the care of the mentally ill for the past century.

## PREREQUISITES FOR FUNDAMENTAL
## REFORM

"Images of the future," as Paul Starr (1978:175) reminds us, "are usually caricatures of the present. They inflate some recognizable features of contemporary life to extravagant proportions, and out of fear or hope respond to every vagary of historical experience, as if it were a sign of destiny." So it is with images of the mental health service system. After a brief period of quiesence in the late 1970s, calls for the closure of state mental hospitals are again being heard.[4] To avoid the shortcomings of the past, however, it is imperative for policy makers and planners to consider the prerequisites for fundamental reform in the American mental health care system. Until effective cures are developed for the major mental disorders—thereby allowing state hospitals to take their place alongside TB sanitoriums in museums for archaic social institutions—the residual functions of state hospitals, and the two-class system which they anchor, can only be supplanted by fundamental changes in the resource base, division of labor, and distribution of rights (Gil, 1973) underlying current policy toward mental health care.

Consistent with this view, Goldman et al. (1979) have pointed out that a viable plan for the elimination of state mental hospitals will require three broad-based reforms:

1. A comprehensive *national health insurance* program for inpatient as well as ambulatory care, and the expansion of services in general and private mental hospitals to accomodate 400,000 additional admissions of severely disturbed patients;
2. A shift in the locus of *involuntary care* into the private sector or into specialized correctional facilities, or more radically, its outright abolition at all mental health facilities; and
3. A comprehensive *national social insurance* program for essential psycho-social rehabilitation services, and the expansion of intermediate care facilities or psychiatric nursing homes for more than 100,000 very disturbed chronic patients.

The first and third proposals would go a long way toward eroding the economic underpinnings of the present two-class system of care. Comprehensive health and social insurance programs would enrich the resource base of the mental health system and alter the distribution of rights to resources. Insurance benefits would enfranchise the disadvantaged and thereby universalize the purchase of services in the private sector. This would presumably shift the burden of acute care farther away from the public sector and the state mental hospitals toward general hospitals and Community Mental Health Centers. In addition, broad insurance benefits for long-term as well as short-term care would be required to encourage community residential and aftercare facilities to increasingly become involved in chronic care functions once left by default almost exclusively to state institutions. Moreover, these health benefits would have to be complemented by a comprehensive social insurance program or some other mechanism for insuring that the chronically mentally ill have access to the psychosocial, recreational, and vocational supports needed for optimal functioning (c.f., Group for the Advancement of Psychiatry, 1978; Sharfstein, 1978; Turner and TenHoor, 1978, President's Commission, 1979; Schulberg, 1979; Talbott, 1979a).

Alterations in the resource base and distribution of resources alone, however, would not be sufficient to shift the division of labor completely away from state mental hospitals. Before public asylums could be closed, their role in civil and criminal commitment would have to be supplanted. The elimination of all forms of involuntary care would obviate the problem by fundamentally altering the division of labor as well as the distribution of rights, both to seek as well as to refuse treatment. Although the abolition of involuntary care is strongly advocated by some critics of current psychiatric practice (e.g., Szasz, 1968) its near-term occurrence would seem unlikely. Short of this dramatic change, the closure of state mental hospitals could be facilitated by the transfer of responsibility for civil and criminal commitment to private facilities or specialized correctional units. However, such transfers would have to avoid the simple "dumping" of difficult cases from one institutional sphere to another and the associated risks of "criminalizing" the mentally disordered (c.f., Abrahamson, 1972; Rachlin et al., 1975; Stelovich, 1979). Otherwise, policymakers may inadvertently recreate the very conditions in local jails and prisons that led Dorothea Dix and other 19th-century reformers to crusade for the decarceration of the insane and their relocation in separate asylums.

The implementation of these reforms, by opening equitable access to the private sector and by sharing the burdens of involuntary treatment among a pluralism of providers, would allow for the closing of state mental hospitals. Unlike the case of the TB sanitoriums, however, the patient care functions now served by state mental hospitals would not cease to exist. Short of a major therapeutic breakthrough, provisions in some type of organized inpatient setting will still have to be made for the violent, the seriously disordered, and the chronically disabled. *Thus, under present circumstances, even if state hospitals were closed, the residual functions of public asylums—relabeled and relocated within the boundaries of different organizations—would endure in the resultant system of care.*

Clearly, it is one thing to recognize the scope of the fundamental changes that are required for the closure of state mental hospitals and the dissolution of the two-class system of care; it is quite another to design and implement the organizing and financing mechanisms that will lead to their accomplishment. Without a firm grasp of the ultimate goals toward which public policy should be directed, however, technical planning often deteriorates into the search for administrative "fixes" for pressing problems. Moreover, as is made abundantly clear from the history of Worcester State Hospital, the failures of institutional reform in American mental health care have often resided in their unidimensional or segmental approach to a multidimensional and recalcitrant set of problems. In the absence of a critical assessment of the "goodness of fit" between proffered solutions and the magnitude of the problems of

mental health care, each generation endorsed proximate solutions
that soon became the basis for another cycle of institutional reform.
To avoid the failures and partial successes of the past, policymakers and planners must be sensitive to the potential for unanticipated consequences in the implementation of fundamental reforms.
These reforms transcend the capacities of any individual community or state, acting alone—they necessitate a comprehensive national
policy based on public–private sector collaboration. Even then, a
number of organizational, professional, and civic problems will
have to be addressed and resolved, especially if a truly humane system of care for the chronically mentally ill is to emerge in the aftermath of deinstitutionalization.

## CHRONIC MENTAL PATIENTS: THE NEXT
## CYCLE OF REFORM?

It is fashionable to offer proposals for reform on the assumption that current modes of service delivery constitute a "nonsys-
tem" that requires "rational" realignment (e.g., Talbott, 1979b).
While it is true that pluralism in the mental health service arena
has promoted the growth of a fragmented or loosely connected network of agencies, it is naive to assume that interorganizational relationships in this network are either nonrational or easily
realigned. There is a deeply rooted, "natural system" underlying
this network (see Chapter 5). It is organized according to the special
interests of individual agencies and professional groups if not the
recognizable needs of the populations in need of mental health
care.[5] Moreover, many of the specific proposals under active consideration for transforming this network into a more comprehensive
and continuous delivery system to meet the needs of the chronically mentally ill may well have opposite effects. The impact of national health insurance is one case in point.

Many mental health administrators and policy-makers look forward to a national health insurance program to solve the financing
problems for all forms of mental health care. While an insurance
program with liberal psychiatric benefits (most proposals now are
exceedingly conservative with regard to psychiatric care) would
help to subsidize short-term acute psychiatric care in general hospitals, it would have little impact on the care of the chronically
mentally ill (Astrachan et al., 1976; Sharfstein, 1978). Moreover, it
would promote the "medicalization" of mental health care and its

transfer to the general hospital. While many observers see these trends as the ultimate solution to present problems in the delivery of acute care, they may exacerbate rather than mitigate the problems of chronic care. The medical profession has a long-standing bias toward acute ("curing") versus chronic ("caring") services and a narrow concern for the medical rather than the health status of its clients. Accordingly, fueled by insurance reimbursements, a general hospital model of psychiatric practice might solidify the retreat from chronic mental patients whose problems involve a myriad of social as well as medical deficits. "Housing, opportunity for some significant activity, and protected arrangements for interpersonal relationships," as Morris (1978:17) notes, "constitute essential, tangible [social] support elements that, for this population, must be provided . . . if the mentally disabled are to cope with the uncertainties and hostilities of 'making it' among their largely able-bodied fellow human beings."

Consistent with the earlier recommendations of the Joint Commission on Mental Illness and Health (1961), some observers advocate the change-over of state mental hospitals into chronic care institutions to serve the chronically mentally ill and other long-term care populations with physical and social disabilities. Such a policy might help to destigmatize the mentally ill. It would also provide a broader base for developing the nonmedical, social support programs needed in common by all chronically disabled populations. And it would provide a socially constructive use for the capital plant of many state hospitals. However, the costs as well as the benefits of this policy must be carefully assessed. Chronic-care institutions, for example, may blur the distinctive needs of the mentally ill and blunt the formation of the political constituencies that other observers see as essential for effective relief in a pluralist political system (Talbott, 1978; Scherl and Macht, 1979). In addition, the growing recognition that chronic patients are susceptible to episodic relapses suggests that a rigid separation of the acute and chronic care systems may exacerbate problems in continuity of care for the chronically mentally ill. Should this occur, it may well substitute a "two-caste" system (acute versus chronic) for the present two-class system of care.

In the view of some professionals, just as effective treatment today requires a combination of psychopharmacological and psychosocial interventions (Klerman, 1977), an effective organization of the mental health system requires the integration of hospital and community care (e.g., Morris, 1978). According to Gruenberg and Archer (1979:500):

> Even the best community mental health service cannot provide the type of long-term psychiatric attention that is most beneficial to chronic seriously mentally ill patients, even if it has a close cooperative relation with an inpatient service . . . What is needed is a unified clinical team, to take responsibility for conducting aftercare and follow-up after its own decision to release. If, when these team members readmit, they themselves continue the treatment of the same patient within the inpatient service, they will not have any grounds for feeling that someone else had failed the patient, and will learn to respond realistically to what they can do for that particular patient.

The integrated team was a core feature of the state hospital-based community mental health services developed in New York by Hunt and Gruenberg (c.f., Gruenberg, 1974) and of the services developed at Worcester State Hospital by Flower and Myerson in the 1960s and early 1970s (see Chapters 3, 4, 10, and 11). These programs were casualties of the deinstitutionalization movement, but they represent prototypic models that will have to be reevaluated in the emergent mental health system.

The recent diversification of the mental health system has fragmented rather than integrated the care of chronic patients. There are many proposals that seek to overcome these problems, ranging from centrally funded but decentralized services to administratively unitized, comprehensive service agencies (c.f. Talbott, 1978). However, the relative merits and benefits of these administrative structures remain to be carefully evaluated:

> . . . a multiple provider, pluralist system with many relatively small units may meet the innumerable wants and needs of a large and diverse population much more satisfactorily than a large hegemony of integrated or tightly controlled subunits. Good data is simply lacking to decide when small units may be more flexible, effective, and responsive, and for what conditions of distress, and when large units can overcome the cumbersomeness of size through mobilization of resources. Efforts have been made to isolate and define conditions suitable for large-scale human service organization and conditions favorable for small-scale organization, but convincing evidence for or against any one paradigm is lacking (Morris and Hirsch-Lescohier, 1978:28).

Nor are financing mechanisms the only barrier to developing a responsive delivery system for the chronically mentally ill. It has been noted, for example, that the fragmentation of acute, hospital-based care and chronic, community-based care has occurred in the mental health services of the National Health Service in Britain where economic barriers have been removed (Jones, 1979). "We have learned," as Mechanic (1975:314) also reports, "that health delivery systems, even when they involve no financial barriers to care erect a variety of other social and psychological barriers that keep certain patients out of their systems or induce a lack of continued participation and cooperation. There is a wide variety of ways in which services come to be rationed: by the resources provided to deal with a given patient load, and the limitation of these resources; by the location of sites of care, and the difficulties involved for patients and their families in reaching such locations; by creating social distance between providers and patients; by over-professionalization and other barriers to communication; by wasting time to obtain services and other noneconomic costs that divert those who particularly have ambivalence about using services to begin with; and by the stigmatization of patients and their families."

Traditionally, little prestige or professional fulfillment has been associated with the care of the chronically ill. Organizations as well as their professional staff have tended to disassociate themselves from such clients.[6] The prospects for a more responsive delivery system in the future will turn on the extent to which humane custodial and supportive care is legitimized as socially and professionally important and, equally challenging, the extent to which functions and caring services are subsidized rather than particular organizations or professional groups. That is, the elusive goal of a client-centered versus an organizational–professional centered delivery model may be the *sine qua non* of humane care for the chronically mentally disabled. The task in this case resides in the design of treatment organizations that can respond to the needs of chronic mental patients while avoiding pressures toward the extremes of "elitism" (i.e., creaming, and the selective acquisition of "nice" clients) or "dumping ground" (i.e., serving as repositories for patients unwanted by other agencies).

As part of the growing trend for government at both the federal and state levels to disengage from the provision of direct patient services, it appears that many programs will be financed by "purchase-of-service-contracts" between state mental health authorities and human service vendors (both public and private) at the local community level. The underlying rationale is that a system of incentives can thereby be created that will induce local agencies to take responsibility for the needs of chronically disabled patients in a manner that is presumed to be more cost-effective than institutionally based programs. In the longer run, it is hoped that these programs will evolve into a totally community-based mental health service delivery system.

Whether the reliance on marketplace mechanisms in the mental health arena will actually lead to a more responsive and comprehensive service delivery system remains to be carefully evaluated. An opposite effect is equally plausible. Namely, confronted with year-to-year performance contracts, vendor agencies may resort to "creaming" practices whereby the tough problem cases are rejected in favor of those clients who will show up as "successes" in end-of-year performance reviews (see Chapter 8). In other words, without explicit provisions to the contrary, purchase-of-service arrangements may operate as *disincentives* for taking on chronic cases that require disproportionate amounts of staff time and effort relative to the probability of ever demonstrating effective outcomes. Moreover, these initiatives are being launched at a time when the resource base for mental health service programs is shrinking. Given the press of other social problems that have received even fewer societal resources to date and the ominous citizens tax revolt now sweeping the country (Talbott, 1979c), the goal of community-based mental health services seems even more remote than it did in the recent past. Ironically, the transfer of responsibility to the community without secure, long-term funding may make the mentally disabled more vulnerable to the capriciousness of public opinion on the question of who and what deserves to be funded from the public treasury. Will community groups today accept responsibilities that their counterparts rejected 150 years ago? The chronically mentally ill are even more resource-poor, more heterogeneous, and more anomic now than they were then. And, in no small measure, the current climate of public opinion mirrors the socioeconomic forces and social prejudices that eroded the support base of the early public asylums.

Will history repeat itself again? The administrative changes of recent years have improved the care of many patients and current proposals offer hope to many more. However, unless this generation of policymakers address the problems of mental health care as reflected in the institutional history of Worcester State Hospital, the public asylum will endure as a repository for the unwanted. Short of fundamental change, today's "solutions" will surely become the target of another cycle in institutional reform.

## NOTES

1. Many radical critics of the efforts at intitutional reform in the mental health field (e.g., Scull, 1977) fail to recognize the discontinuities between origins (starting mechanisms) and outcomes (maintenance mechanisms). By noting the repressive features that often characterize the outcomes or end states of reform, they erroneously infer that these consequences were part of the original motives and intentions of early reformers. To argue from outcomes to motives is not only a logical fallacy but it also distorts the historical record of mental hospitals in America (c.f., Grob, 1977; Grob, 1978). For a similar assessment of Piven and Cloward's (1971) critique of the functions of public welfare, see Higgins (1978).

2. As Mechanic (1978b:6) points out, the institutionalism syndrome can be found in varying degrees in a variety of settings: "(M)ost discussions of deinstitutionalization are misleading in their failure to differentiate the impact of varying community settings on the quality of life of patients and the course of their illnesses and handicaps." Moreover, social science research in the past decade suggests that Goffman's (1961) depiction of state hospitals as "total institutions" may be accurate only for large hospitals—that are extremely bureaucratic, understaffed, and underfinanced—rather than an inevitable feature of institutional care (see Goldstein, 1979:399–401).

3. Perrow (1978) suggests that the conventional view of human service agencies in mainstream organizational theory—that they are rational instruments in pursuit of announced goals—is a "mystification" of reality. Rather, he argues that all organizations are resources for a variety of group interests within and without the organization, and the announced purposes (e.g., therapy, treatment), while they must be met to some limited degree, largely serve as legitimating devices for these interests.

   This view is compatible with Carlson's depiction of state mental hospitals, prisons, and public schools as *domesticated organizations*. "By this is simply meant," Carlson (1965:266) notes, "that they are not compelled to attend to all of the ordinary and usual needs of an organization . . . they do not compete with other organizations for clients; in fact a steady flow of clients is assured. There is no struggle for survival for this type of organization. Like the domesticated animal, these organizations are fed and cared for. Existence is guaranteed. Though this type of organization does compete in a restricted area for funds, funds are not closely tied to quality of performance. These organizations are domesticated in the sense that they are protected by the society they serve. Society feels some apprehension about domesticated organizations. It sees the support of these organizations as necessary to the maintenance of the social system and creates laws over and above those applying to organized action in general to care for domesticated organizations."

   And, in another context, Perrow (1972:184) comments on the consequence of their protected status: "(P)risons, mental hospitals, and many small welfare agencies exist to show that *something* is being done about some problems, but few care just what it is or how effective it is; those who control the organization's resources (legislators, religious boards, etc.) care only that the 'something' should not involve scandals and should not cost too much."

4. In November 1979, following growing criticisms of the Commonwealth's deinstitutionalization plans and the deaths of several patients in state hospitals, the Commissioner of the Massachusetts Department of Mental Health established a Blue Ribbon Commission to make recommendations on the future of the eight remaining state mental institutions (Dietz, 1979a). A few weeks later, he proposed the abolition of the state mental hospital system and the creation of inpatient units in existing general hospitals and private psychiatric hospitals (Dietz, 1979c), and announced plans for a pilot program at a general hospital in the Boston area (Dietz, 1979e). His proposals met with divided reactions (Dietz, 1979d) and the prospects for their full implementation were uncertain at the close of 1979. In a separate action, the Commissioner of the Department of Mental Hygiene in New York requested legislative authorization to close 2 of that state's 24 mental hospitals (Goldman, 1979).

5. The work of Warren et al. (1974) on the model cities program (including mental health agencies) provides a comprehensive understanding of the social order underlying community health and welfare networks. The authors indicate the ways in which an "institutionalized thought structure"—shared interagency paradigms on the nature of clients, the ameliorative steps that should be taken, and the basic soundness of the existing system—serves to stablize the status quo and protect agency domains and prerogatives.

6. The critique of professions has been a prominent theme in recent literature. The most trenchant critic of medicine has been Ivan Illich (c.f., Illich, 1976; Illich et al., 1977) but his assessment extends to professions in general, namely, modern professional activity has a debilitating rather than enhancing effect because it is designed to "manufacture" needs in accord with professional satisfactions rather than client interests. Other insightful evaluations of professions can be found in Freidson (1970), Yarmolinsky (1979), and Starr (1979).

Wilfrid L. Pilette

# Epilogue

Monday is always the hardest. At least it seems so. While driving to work, I plan on there having been two admissions, one runaway, and several other problems during the weekend. Maybe a patient refused to return from a weekend pass. Maybe a patient required seclusion because of assaultive or suicidal behavior. Or maybe a patient got stoned on alcohol or street drugs. There are other more unpleasant possibilities, which I try not to think about.

Problems pile up on weekends because there is no clinical staff on duty then and only custodial care is available to a large number of patients who always need much more than that. Although several patients have been on weekend passes or shorter passes off the hospital grounds, most have had to cope with the boredom and frustration of spending a weekend in an unpleasant place—Worcester State Hospital.

On entering the hospital the first person I meet is a severely retarded young man who shouts gibberish at me. The next person I run into is an older patient who asks me for a cigarette. A moment later I skip over a puddle of urine as I hurry up the stairs to my unit. The hospital's unpleasant air—dank and stinking of urine, body odor, and harsh cleaning agents—is only noticeable to me on Monday mornings.

This statement originally appeared in The Boston Globe, January 27, 1980, under the caption "One Psychiatrist's Monday at a State Mental Hospital." Reprinted with permission of the editor.

307

While walking down the corridor to my office I exchange a few pleasant hellos with patients and staff and I receive a few unfriendly stares and two loud calls from patients who demand to be spoken to immediately.

By the time I get to my office, I have a few minutes to file some articles I've brought in with me and to do some paper work. As clinical director of our unit, I could use a full-time secretary, but I only have access to our one overworked ward clerk, who must act as receptionist, secretary and clerk for the whole unit. So I dictate very few letters, writing most of them in longhand. I've noted that my office is cold today. Last week it was too warm.

It is now 9:30 A.M. and time for our clinical staff to gather for rounds. We have one hour to discuss changes in the legal status of some patients, requests for privileges and passes, and problems over the weekend.

We are told that a patient was brought back to the unit by the police after he threatened suicide while on a pass. Two hours after his return he demanded to leave the unit again, was refused, and then broke our only guitar. Another patient, a transfer from Bridgewater State Hospital who has been grossly psychotic for two weeks, was put in seclusion for seven hours after he assaulted another patient. An older female manic patient presented problems all weekend as she repeatedly attempted to make sexual contact with the former Bridgewater patient. An acutely psychotic young male required treatment for side effects (severe rigidity and restlessness) from his antipsychotic medication. A chronic patient was caught "cheeking" her medication and a young male is suspected of having stolen another patient's jacket.

All these problems must be reviewed and reassessed, and decisions must be made as to how to deal with them presently. We also must review and interview the two patients who were admitted during the weekend.

The first patient is 6 ft. 5 in., weighs over 200 pounds, and required four policemen to bring him into the hospital last night in an acute psychotic state. He is presently in restraints in a seclusion room, and because he was given antipsychotic medication at 5 A.M. he is sleeping for the first time in three days. We will not wake him.

The second patient is a middle-aged woman who was found wandering the streets and could only tell the police that her apartment was unsafe to live in because her upstairs neighbor was the devil. When we interview her, she tells us a little more. She says the neighbor-devil is a young man and he has been pumping an odorless, invisible gas into her apartment. She tells us we should lock him up and she demands to be discharged. She will stay with us for further evaluation.

After rounds, I have a half-hour for ward work and then I meet with our four medical students for group supervision. We discuss their problems in caring for their assigned patients. Each student has been assigned four patients and has been given much latitude in carrying out their evaluations, treatments, and dispositions.

We give the students the opportunity to manage interesting and difficult patients. The range of psychopathology on our unit is awesome. We have adolescent patients as young as 15. We have adult patients as old as 73. We have antisocial personalities sent (sometimes "dumped") by the courts. We have epileptics, phobics, hysterics, hypochrondriacs, anorexics, diabetics, alcoholics, drug abusers, and the mentally retarded. We have demented patients, delirious patients, incontinent patients, and a pedophile. We also have borderline personalities (the most difficult), manics, depressives, and schizophrenics. Our schizophrenics cover all the major categories of the syndrome.

Some of the above are also moochers, hoarders, con-artists, kleptomaniacs, hypersomniacs, insomniacs, sleep walkers, bed wetters, fire setters, exhibitionists, foul mouths, screamers, biters, pinchers, punchers, and kickers.

We are indeed running "a one-room schoolhouse" of psychiatry. So we offer our students a unique opportunity to learn about mental illness.

The students are usually awkward, anxious, and just plain scared stiff during their first week on our unit. They then quickly learn to use psychiatric jargon to control their fears. But during the last few weeks of their six-week rotation, they have become comfortable with their patients. They are now clearly committed to treating them as people and have learned to relish their small improvements.

My meeting with the students is the "fun part" of my day. I am stimulated by their enthusiasm and curiosity. I could not tolerate my job without the opportunity to teach them what I have learned. My 90 minutes with them pass by very quickly.

It is now 12:30 and time for me to go to lunch with our unit director. He is the administrative head of our unit. He deals with the area director, the hospital's executive committee, the unions, outside agencies, and the 44 employees on our unit.

He is supposed to leave me free to deal with the clinical management of the unit and he does so. He is also leaving. I am becoming quite used to seeing unit directors leave. He has been with us for a little over two years. Unit directors often don't last that long. They tend to burn out quickly or they are forced out. They are told to develop new programs both inside and outside the hospital, but they are given little power and less pay. They are blamed for increases in the patient census, even though staffing blocks have been taken from them. They are blamed for lots of things, including the incompetence of some of their staff, whom they can't fire. Unit directors take a lot of heat off psychiatrists—but they leave. So at lunch, today we will continue to discuss the uncertain future of our unit.

On returning to the hospital at 1:30, I am told that a patient has stopped taking his medication and has handed in a "three-day letter," that is, he has written a request to leave the hospital and we now have up to three days to decide whether to petition the court for his commitment.

Even though he is still clearly psychotic, we will probably let him go. Because his wife is willing to let him return home, she will be able to provide for his basic needs for food and shelter. And because he is not suicidal or homicidal, he is clearly not commitable. We expect he will become more psychotic at home and will be returned to us soon for his sixth hospitalization.

Because I have no hospital committee meeting this afternoon, I have a couple of hours to see patients and to prepare a report for a pharmacy committee meeting on Wednesday.

Our head nurse informs me that our newest patient is now awake and has been let out of restraints and seclusion. I talk to him briefly and note that he is not hostile or threatening and is mostly coherent. He is showing a nice, quick response to his medication.

Later, while talking to a patient in the corridor, another patient, a 52-year-old woman, pats my bottom as she walks by mumbling to herself. When I glance at her, I think I see her wink.

At 4 P.M. it is time for our Community Meeting. We bring everybody together—patients and staff—for up to one half-hour. We hold this meeting every two weeks. It can be dull, depressing, wild, exciting, frightening, uplifting, or frustrating. Sometimes it is all of these things.

We're providing a forum in which anyone can speak out about any issue concerning our getting along together. It is difficult to get the patients to attend to this task. Since they are more likely to fo-

cus on purely personal problems, they must be reminded frequently to discuss personal issues with their primary therapists.

The meeting may include as many as 50 people. Patients often
become more bizarre or disorganized when provided with such a
large audience. But sometimes they amaze us all with their sensitivity, articulation, and wisdom.

Today's meeting is uneventful. We stop it after 20 minutes. The
patients then go to supper and the staff meets for a brief after-group
"rehash" discussion.

At 4:45 P.M. I meet with a nurse and an occupational therapist
who are co-leaders of a weekly group therapy session. They also
carry one or two patients apiece as primary therapists. We discuss
their individual patients and their groups.

They sometimes have difficulty finding four or more patients
who are comfortable enough and coherent enough to tolerate and to
benefit from their group sessions. They would like to have eight
such patients available regularly. Sometimes they do. Both of them
are dedicated, bright, enthusiastic, and stimulating. It is a pleasure
to work with them. We have perhaps 15 such people among our
staff and I derive much personal satisfaction and support associat-
ing with them.

I work only four days a week here and I am paid adequately.
Most of our staff work more than I do and for much less money.
Their workload is enormous.

These are the facts: Our small unit will have about 275 admissions this year. This is an increase of almost 50 over last year.
Despite the recent media propaganda declaring the deinstitutionalization of our state hospitals to be a great success, our
admission rate has risen; 275 admissions is an enormous workload
for our staff. Our patient census is 38 today. We have been over 40
much of the time in the past few months. The "acceptable" bed capacity for our unit is 27. One year ago we had 11 R.N.s and 13
L.P.N.s. Today we have 7 R.N.s and 5 L.P.N.s

Our smaller staff must not only treat a larger number of patients than previously, the patients have become more difficult to
manage.

Improved community-based facilities have been able to treat
more patients with moderately severe illnesses. As a result, it is
widely held that those patients who are currently hospitalized in
state hospitals are generally more chronically and severely ill, more
violent, and more complicated. At a time when our commissioner
has called for the closing of our state hospitals, we have an increas-

ing admission rate, more difficult patients, and less staff. To us, his plan seems doomed to fail, and when it does we expect to be the scapegoats. In the past those of us who work in state hospitals have too often been scapegoated to explain away the Commonwealth's unwillingness to provide adequately for the needs of its mentally ill.

The needs of our patients are enormous and our work is very difficult. We do not need to be condemned in the press, to be abandoned by our department and legislators, and to have hiring freezes imposed on us. What we need is public understanding, political support, and financial help.

It is now close to 6 P.M., and I go to the nursing station to review the chart of a newly admitted patient and to check the afternoon lab reports. I see the new patient briefly. She is quiet and stable. We will observe her further before determining her diagnosis and treatment.

On returning to my office, I have one last phone call to make. I must inform a father about his son's current status. We are attempting once again to place his son in a halfway house. His last stay there several weeks ago lasted one day. He was returned to us so quickly because he refused to follow the house rules and because he threatened to kill a staff person.

His father cannot understand why the halfway house staff insisted that he follow the rules like everyone else.

I call the father every week because he is politically influential and must be given special attention. He has recently been quoted in the press as saying that his son was abandoned by us several times in the past, that he was thrown out of the hospital without any follow-up care. His remarks as well as many other similar ones carried in the press recently have diminished the already sagging morale of all state hospital workers.

Massachusetts state hospitals have been called "oppressive." Our own commissioner has compared the present situation of our patients to the "boat people" of Southeast Asia.

A state senate leader has compared the conditions in our state hospitals to Walpole State Prison. The senator then announced that his special committee had uncovered 18 unexplained deaths in state facilities and he declared he was "greatly disturbed by the casual way the Department of Mental Health has treated the deaths." A lawyer appearing before his committee testified that seclusion and physical and chemical restraint are used "mostly for institutional convenience." Understandably, such statements leave all us state hospital workers feeling condemned and abandoned.

The patient's father is now telling me that he hopes his testimony will have helped to secure added funds for our hospital. I tell him that his son has just signed a new contract and we hope he will be ready to return to the halfway house in two weeks. I do not tell him that he continues to avoid soap and water as much as he can and that his body odor can be smelled 20 feet away.

While putting on my coat to go home, I quickly calculate that I answered three pages and six phone calls today and I was cursed at four times. And since I didn't discharge anyone, our census is climbing again. But no one threatened to kill me or to sue me today and I didn't have to order the seclusion or physical or chemical restraint of any patient.

All in all, it's been a pretty good Monday.

# BIBLIOGRAPHY

Abrahamson, M.
1972    "The criminalization of mentally disordered behavior: A possible side effect of a new mental health law." Hospital and Community Psychiatry 23:101–105.

Aldrich, H.
1978    "Centralization versus decentralization in the design of human service delivery systems: A response to Gouldner's lament." Pp. 51–79 in R. Sarri and Y. Hasenfeld (eds.): The Management of Human Services. New York: Columbia University Press.
1979    Organizations and Environments. Englewood Cliffs, NJ: Prentice-Hall.

Aldrich, H. and D. Herker
1977    "Boundary spanning roles and organizational structure." Academy of Management Review (April):217–230

Al-Khazaraji, M., E. Al-Khazraji, and N. Carlson
1970    Social Conditions and Social Needs in a Public Housing Neighborhood: Great Brook Valley, Worcester, Massachusetts. Worcester, MA: Worcester Community Data Center, College of the Holy Cross.

American Federation of State, County, and Municipal Employees
1975    Deinstitutionalization: Out of Their Beds and Into the Streets. Washington, D.C.: The Federation.

American Hospital Association
1977    Guide to Health Care Institutions. Chicago: American Hospital Association.

Anthony, W. and G. Buell
1973    "Psychiatric aftercare clinic effectiveness as a function of patient demographic characteristics." Journal of Consulting and Clinical Psychology 41:116–119.

Anthony, W., G. Buell, S. Sharratt, and M. Althoff
1972 "Efficacy of psychiatric rehabilitation." Psychological Bulletin 78(6):447–456.

Arnhoff, F.
1975 "Social consequences of policy towards mental illness." Science 188:1277–1281.

Astrachan, B., D. Levinson, and D. Adler
1976 "The impact of national health insurance on the tasks and practice of psychiatry." Archives of General Psychiatry 33 (July):785–793.

Bachrach, L.
1976a Deinstitutionalization: An Analytical Review and Sociological Perspective. Rockville, MD: National Institute of Mental Health.
1976b "A note on some recent studies of released mental hospital patients in the community." American Journal of Psychiatry 133 (January):73–75.
1978 "A conceptual approach to deinstitutionalization." Hospital and Community Psychiatry 29 (September):573–578.

Barton, R.
1966 Institutional Neurosis, 2nd. Ed. Baltimore: Williams and Wilkins.

Barton, W.
1962 Administration in Psychiatry. Springfield, IL: Thomas.

Bassuk, E. L. and J. Gerson
1978 "Deinstitutionalization and mental health services." Scientific American 238:46–53.

Bayle, S.
1971 "Chapter 888," Massachusetts Journal of Mental Health 1 (Winter):1–4.

Beck, B.
1979 "The limits of deinstitutionalization." In M. Lewis (ed.): Social Problems and Public Policy: A Research Annual, Vol. 1 Greenwich, CT: JAI Press.

Becker, H. S., B. Geer, D. Riesman, and R. Weiss (eds.)
1968 Institutions and the Person: Papers Presented to Everett C. Hughes. Chicago: Aldine.

Becker, A. and H. Schulberg
   1976   "Phasing out state hospitals—a psychiatric dilemma."
          New England Journal of Medicine 294 (January):255–
          261.

Belknap, I.
   1956   Human Problems of a State Mental Hospital. New York:
          McGraw-Hill.

Bittner, E.
   1967   "The police on skid-row: A study of peace keeping."
          American Sociological Review 32 (October):699–715.

Bockoven, J. S.
   1956   "Moral treatment in American psychiatry." Journal of
          Nervous and Mental Disease 124 (August–Septem-
          ber):193–95.
   1972   Moral Treatment in Community Mental Health. New
          York: Springer.

Boisen, A.
   1960   Out of the Depths: An Autobiographical Study of Men-
          tal Disorders and Religious Experience. New York:
          Harper.

Borus, J.
   1978   "Issues critical to the survival of community mental
          health." American Journal of Psychiatry 135 (Septem-
          ber):1029–1035.

Brill, H. and R. Patton
   1957   "Analysis of 1955–56 population fall in New York State
          mental hospitals during the first year of large-scale use
          of tranquilizing drugs." American Journal of Psychiatry
          114:509–517.
   1959   "Analysis of population reduction in New York State
          mental hospitals during the first four years of large scale
          therapy with psychotropic drugs." American Journal of
          Psychiatry 116:495–508.
   1962   "Clinical statistical analysis of population changes in
          New York State mental hospitals since the introduction
          of psychotropic drugs." American Journal of Psychiatry
          119:20–35.
   1966   "Psychopharmacology and the current revolution in
          mental health services." Pp. 288–295 in Proceedings of
          the Fourth World Congress of Psychiatry, Part I. Amster-
          dam: Exerpta Medica Foundation.

Brill, H. and B. Malzberg
  1962    Statistical Report Based on the Arrest Records of 5, 354
          Male Ex-patients Released From New York State Mental
          Hospitals During the Period 1946–1948. Mental Hospi-
          tal Service Supplement 153. Washington, D.C.: Ameri-
          can Psychiatric Association.

Bryan, W. A.
  1936    Administrative Psychiatry. New York: Norton.

Bucher, R. and L. Schatzman
  1962    "The logic of the state mental hospital." Social Prob-
          lems 9 (Spring):337–349.

Bucher, R. and A. Strauss
  1961    "Professions in process." American Journal of Sociology
          66 (January): 325–334.

Byers, E. S., S. Cohen, and D. D. Harshbarger
  1978    "Impact of aftercare services on recidivism of mental
          hospital patients." Community Mental Health Journal
          14:26–34.

Cameron, J. M.
  1978    "Ideology and policy termination: Restructuring Califor-
          nia's mental health system." Pp. 301–328 in J. V. May
          and A. B. Wildavsky (eds.) The Policy Cycle. Beverly
          Hills, CA: Sage.

Caplan, R. B.
  1969    Psychiatry and the Community in Nineteenth Century
          America. New York: Basic Books.

Carlson, R.
  1965    "Environmental constraints and organizational conse-
          quences: The public school and its clients." Pp. 262–
          270 in D. E. Griffiths (ed.): Behavioral Science and Edu-
          cational Administration, 63rd Yearbook of the National
          Society for the Study of Education. Chicago: University
          of Chicago Press.

Cassel, J.
1966    "Social class and mental disorders: An analysis of the limitations and potentialities of current epidemiological approaches." Pp. 42–53 in Mental Health and the Lower Social Classes. Tallahassee: Florida State University, Study No. 49.

Central Massachusetts Special Education Collaborative
1979    SHEP Proposal, Project Liaison. Worcester, MA: The Collaborative (duplicated).

Child Guidance Association of Worcester
1979a   Application for Social Worker Case Management Services to Adolescents. Worcester, MA: Child Guidance Association (duplicated).
1979b   Application for Inpatient Adolescent Facility. Worcester, MA: Child Guidance Association (duplicated).

Chu, F. and S. Trotter
1974    The Madness Establishment. New York: Grossman.

Clark, B.
1960    The Open Door College: A Case Study. New York: McGraw-Hill.

Cloward, R. A. and I. Epstein
1965    "Private social welfare's disengagement from the poor: The case of family adjustment agencies." Pp. 623–644 in M. Zald (ed.): Social Welfare Institutions. New York: Wiley.

Conrad, P.
1975    "The discovery of hyperkinesis: Notes on the medicalization of deviant behavior." Social Problems 23 (October):12–21.
1979    "Types of medical social control." Sociology of Health and Illness 1:1–11.

Crane, G.
1974    "Two decades of psychopharmacology and community mental health: Old and new problems of the schizophrenic patient." Transactions of the New York Academy of Sciences 36:644–656.

Davis, A., B. Gardner, and H. Gardner
1941    Deep South: A Study of Caste and Class. Chicago: University of Chicago Press.

Davis, K.
1939    "Mental hygiene and the class structure." Psychiatry 1:55–65.

Day, R. and J. Day
1977    "A review of the current state of negotiated order theory: An appreciation and critique." Sociological Quarterly 18 (Winter):126–42.

Des Prez, R.
1975    "Tuberculosis." Pp. 391–396 in P. Beeson and W. McDermott (eds.): Textbook of Medicine, 14th Edition. Philadelphia: Saunders.

Deutsch, A.
1937    The Mentally Ill in America: A History of Their Care and Treatment from Colonial Times. New York: Columbia University Press.
1944    "The history of mental hygiene." In American Psychiatric Association, One Hundred Years of American Psychiatry. New York: Columbia University Press.
1948    The Shame of the States. New York: Harcourt, Brace.

Devereux, G.
1939a   "Maladjustment and social neurosis." American Sociological Review 4:844–851.
1939b   "A sociological theory of schizophrenia." Psychoanalytic Review 26:315–342.
1942    "The social structure of a schizophrenic ward and its therapeutic fitness." Journal of Clinical Psychopathology 6 (October):231–265.

Dietz, J.
1979a   "Deinstitutionalization debate: Plan for mental patients faces stiff fight." The Boston Globe (November 22):1.
1979b   "Mental health system blasted." The Boston Globe (December 4):17, 23.
1979c   "State urged to shut its mental hospitals." The Boston Globe (December 12):1, 26.
1979d   "Call to abolish mental hospitals brings intensely divided reaction." The Boston Globe (December 16):1.

1979e "Hospital in Somerville to pioneer mental plan." The Boston Globe (December 19):1.

Dix, D. L.
1975 On Behalf of the Insane Poor. New York: Arno Press.

Dublin, L.
1958 "The course of tuberculosis mortality and morbidity in the United States." American Journal of Public Health 48 (November):1439–1448.

Earle, P.
1887 The Curability of Insanity: A Series of Studies. Philadelphia, PA: Lippincott.

Editorial
1852 Boston Medical and Surgical Journal 45:537.

Esquirol, E.
1960 Des Passions. Cited in E. T. Carlson and N. Dain: "The psychotherapy that was moral treatment." American Journal of Psychiatry 117:519–524.

Etzioni, A.
1975 "Deinstitutionalization: The latest public policy fashion." Human Behavior (September):12–13.

Ewald, W. M.
1978 First-Year Evaluation Report, State Hospital Education Project, Central Massachusetts Special Education Collaborative. Worcester, MA: Potter and Ewald Associates (duplicated).

Feldman, P., T. Sadtler, R. Lipman, and L. Schiff
1979 "Phasing down state hospitals: Integrated versus nonintegrated services." Hospital and Community Psychiatry 30(5):334–337.

Fisher, B. M.
1969 "Claims and credibility: A discussion of occupational identity and the agent-client relationship." Social Problems 16:423–433.

Fowlkes, M.
   1975    "Business as usual—at the state mental hospital." Psy-
           chiatry 38:55–64.

Frankfather, D.
   1974    "Background and position paper on mental health care
           for the elderly." Unpublished final report. Rockville,
           MD: National Institute of Mental Health.

Freidson, E.
   1970    The Profession of Medicine. New York: Dodd Mead.

Freud, S.
   1957    "Five lectures on psycho-analysis." Pp. 3–56 in J. Stra-
           chey (ed.): Standard Edition of the Complete Psycholog-
           ical Works of Sigmund Freud, Vol. II (1910). London:
           Hogarth.


Geller, J. and E. Lister
   1978    "The process of pretrial commitment for psychiatric
           evaluation: An analysis." American Journal of Psychia-
           try 135:53–60.

General Accounting Office
   1977    Returning the Mentally Disabled to the Community:
           Government Needs to Do More. Washington, D.C.: Unit-
           ed States General Accounting Office.

Gil, D.
   1973    Unraveling Social Policy. Cambridge: Schenkman.
   1976    "Resolving issues of 'social' provision in our society."
           Paper presented at the Annual Program Meeting of the
           Council on Social Work Education, Philadelphia, PA.

Goffman, E.
   1961    Asylums. New York: Doubleday.

Goldman, A.
   1979    "Closing of two hospitals sought by mental health com-
           missioner." The New York Times (November 20):B5.

Goldman, H. H.
   1977a   "Conflict, competition, and coexistence: The mental
           hospital as parallel health and welfare systems." Ameri-
           can Journal of Orthopsychiatry 47:60–65.

1977b    Psychiatry in the General Hospital. Waltham, MA: Florence Heller School, Brandeis University.
1977c    "Using hospital staff to provide aftercare: Kudos and criticism." Hospital and Community Psychiatry 28 (June):461–2.
1978     Within and Between: The Role of the Psychiatric Resident in the Psychiatric Unit in the General Hospital. Unpublished doctoral dissertation. Heller School, Brandeis University.

Goldman, H. and M. Rosenstein
1979     "Pluralism and hospital psychiatry: The future of the state mental hospital revisited I. The continuing role of the state mental hospital." Rockville, MD: Division of Biometry and Epidemiology, National Institute of Mental Health (unpublished).

Goldman, H., C. Taube, and D. Regier
1979     "The present and future role of the state mental hospital." Rockville, MD: Division of Biometry and Epidemiology, National Institute of Mental Health.

Goldman, W.
1976     "Change in a state department of mental health: A view from within." Administration and Mental Health 4 (Fall):2–9.

Goldstein, M. S.
1979     "The sociology of mental health and illness." Annual Review of Sociology 5:381–409.

Gossett, J., D. Barnhart, M. Lewis, and V. Phillips
1977     "Follow-up of adolescents treated in a psychiatric hospital." Archives of General Psychiatry 34:1037–42.

Gove, W. R. and T. Fain
1973     "The stigma of mental hospitalization." Archives of General Psychiatry 28:494–500.

Greenblatt, M. and E. Glazier
1975     "The phasing out of mental hospitals in the United States." American Journal of Psychiatry 132 (November):1135–1140.

Greenblatt, M., M. Sharaf, and E. Stone
1971     Dynamics of Institutional Change. Pittsburg: University of Pittsburg Press.

Greenley, J. R. and S. A. Kirk
1973    "Organizational characteristics of agencies and the distribution of services to applicants." Journal of Health and Social Behavior 14 (March):70–79.
1976    "Organizational influences on access to health care." Social Science and Medicine 10:317–322.

Grob, G. N.
1966    The State and the Mentally Ill: A History of Worcester State Hospital in Massachusetts, 1830–1920. Chapel Hill: University of North Carolina Press.
1973    Mental Institutions in America: Social Policy to 1875. New York: The Free Press.
1977    "Rediscovering asylums: The unhistorical history of the mental hospital." Hastings Center Report 7 (August):33–41.
1978    "Public policy making and social policy." Paper presented at the Conference on the History of Public Policy in the United States, Harvard University Business School, November 3–4.

Group for the Advancement of Psychiatry
1978    The Chronic Mental Patient in the Community. New York: GAP.

Gruenberg, E.
1966    Evaluating the Effect of Community Mental Health Services. New York: Milbank Memorial Fund.
1974    "The social breakdown syndrome and its prevention." Pp. 697–711 in S. Arieti (ed.): American Handbook of Psychiatry. New York: Basic Books.

Gruenberg, E. and J. Archer
1979    "Abandonment of responsibility for the seriously mentally ill." Milbank Memorial Fund Quarterly/Health and Society 57 (Fall):485–506.

Guze, S., R. Woodruff, and P. Clayton
1974    "Psychiatric disorders and criminality." Journal of the American Medical Association 227 (February):641–642.


Hartmann, E., B. Glasser, M. Greenblatt, M. Solomon, and D. Levinson

1968     Adolescents in a Mental Hospital. New York: Grune and Stratton.

Higgins, J.
1978     "Regulating the poor revisited." Journal of Social Policy 7 (April):189–198.

Hofstadter, R.
1955     The Age of Reform. New York: Vintage Books.

Hollingshead, A. and F. Redlich
1958     Social Class and Mental Illness: New York: Wiley.

Holmes, O. W.
1891     Medical Essays 1842–1882. Boston: Houghton Mifflin.

Hughes. E. C.
1939     "Institutions." Pp. 283–347 in R. E. Park (ed.): An Outline of the Principles of Sociology. New York: Barnes and Noble.

Hunt, R. G., O. Gurrslin, and J. Roach
1958     "Social status and psychiatric service in a child guidance clinic." American Sociological Review (February):81–83.

Hyde, R.
1962     "The Massachusetts branch hospital plan." Pp. 28–35 in Decentralization of Psychiatric Services and Continuity of Care. New York: Milbank Memorial Fund.

Illich, I.
1976     Medical Nemesis: The Expropriation of Health. New York: Pantheon.

Illich, I., I. Zola, J. McKnight, J. Caplan, and H. Shaskin
1977     Disabling Professions. London: Marion Boyars.

Janowitz, M.
1975     "Sociological theory and social control." American Journal of Sociology 81 (July):82–108.

Joint Commission on Mental Illness and Health
1961     Action for Mental Health. New York: Basic Books.

# Bibliography

326           *Bibliography*

Jones, K.
1979    "Deinstitutionalization in context." Milbank Memorial Fund Quarterly/Health and Society 57 (November):552–569.

Kahn, N. and R. Kaplan
1974    Phase-Out of Grafton State Hospital: Interim Report. Boston, MA: Massachusetts Department of Mental Health.

Kastenbaum, R., and S. Sherwood
1972    "ZERO: A scale for assessing the interview behavior of elderly people." Pp. 166–200 in D. P. Kent et al. (eds.), Research Planning and Action for the Elderly. The Power and Potential of Social Science. New York, Behavioral Publications.

Kennedy, J., J. N. Mitchell, L. V. Klerman, and A. Murray
1976    "A day school approach to aggressive adolescents." Child Welfare 55:712–724.

Kinard, E. M. and L. Klerman
1980    "Changes in life style following mental hospitalization." Journal of Nervous and Mental Disease (forthcoming).

Kirk, S. A.
1976    "Effectiveness of community services for discharged mental hospital patients." American Journal of Orthopsychiatry 46:646–659.
1977    "Who gets aftercare? A study of patients discharged from state hospitals in Kentucky." Hospital and Community Psychiatry 28:109–114.

Kirk, S. A. and J. R. Greenley
1974    "Denying or delivery services." Social Work 19 (July):439–447.

Kirk, S. A. and M. E. Therrien
1975    "Community mental health myths and the fate of former hospitalized patients." Psychiatry 38:209–217.

Klerman, G. L.
1977    "Better but not well: Social and ethical issues in the deinstitutionalization of the mentally ill." Schizophrenia Bulletin 3:617–631.

1979    "National trends in hospitalization." Hospital and Community Psychiatry 30 (February):110–113.

Klerman, L., J. Morrissey, and H. Goldman
1978    "Training psychiatrists in social research: Problems and prospects." Archives of General Psychiatry 35 (December):1469–1473.

Koenig, P.
1978    "The problem that can't be tranquilized: 40,000 mental patients dumped in city neighborhoods." The New York Times Magazine (May 21):14–17.

Kramer, M.
1977    Psychiatric Services and the Changing Institutional Scene, 1950–1985. Rockville, MD: National Institute of Mental Health, Series B., No. 12.


Lamb, H. R. and V. Goertzel
1971    "Discharged mental patients—are they really in the community?" Archives of General Psychiatry 24:29–34.
1972    "The demise of the state hospital—a premature obituary." Archives of General Psychiatry 26:489–495.

Leeman, C. P.
1980    "Involuntary admissions to general hospitals: Progress or threat?" Hospital & Community Psychiatry 31 (May):315–318.

Leeman, C. P. and H. S. Berger
1980    "The Massachusetts Psychiatric Society's position paper on involuntary psychiatric admissions to general hospitals." Hospital & Community Psychiatry 31 (May):318–324.

Lipsitt, P. D., D. Lelos, and A. L. McGarry
1971    "Competency for trial: A screening instrument." American Journal of Psychiatry 128 (July):105–109.


Marden, R.
1968    "Boston." Pp. 341–406 in R. H. Connery, The Politics of Mental Health: Organizing Community Mental Health in Metropolitan Areas. New York: Columbia University Press.

Marsh, L. C.
1932    "Practical aspects of psychiatry for the general practi-
        tioner." New England Journal of Medicine 206:1337–
        1342.
1933    "An experiment in the group treatment of patients at the
        Worcester State Hospital." Mental Hygiene 17:396–416.
1935    "Group therapy and the psychiatric clinic." Journal of
        Nervous and Mental Disease 82:381–393.

Massachusetts Department of Mental Health
1972    Challenge and Response: A Five-Year Progress Report
        on the Comprehensive Mental Health and Retardation
        Services Act of the Commonwealth of Masachusetts.
        Boston, MA: Massachusetts Department of Mental
        Health.
1974    Code of Human Services, Chapter 2, Part 200. Boston,
        MA: Massachusetts Department of Mental Health.
1977    The Five-Year State Plan for Mental Health Services.
        Boston, MA: Massachusetts Department of Mental
        Health.

Massachusetts Hospital Association
1976    Report of the Task Force on Psychiatric Services. Bur-
        lington, MA: Massachusetts Hospital Association (mi-
        meo).

Massachusetts Mental Health Planning Project
1965    Mental Health for Massachusetts. Boston, MA: Mental
        Health Planning Project.

Massachusetts Superior Judicial Court
1978    Superintendent of Public Buildings of Worcester, Com-
        monwealth of Massachusetts. Case No. SJC 114. Judg-
        ment affirmed January 17th.

Massachusetts Supreme Court
1977    Holger Schonning, Superintendent of Public Buildings.
        Plaintiff vs. People's Church Home, Inc. Defendant. Civ-
        il Act No. 7188 entered January 28th.

McCranie, E. W. and T. A. Mizell
1978    "Aftercare for psychiatric patients: Does it prevent re-
        hospitalization?" Hospital and Community Psychiatry
        29:584–587.

McGarry A., W. Curran, P. Lipsitt, D. Lelos, R. Schwitzgebel, and A.
Rosenberg

1973 Competency to Stand Trial and Mental Illness. DHEW Publication 74–103. Rockville, MD: National Institute of Mental Health.

McKinlay, J.
1975 "Clients and organizations." Pp. 339–378 in J. McKinlay (ed.): Processing People: Cases in Organizational Behavior. New York: Holt, Rinehart and Winston.

Mechanic, D.
1969 Mental Health and Social Policy. Englewood Cliffs, NJ: Prentice Hall.
1978a Medical Sociology, 2nd Edition. New York: Free Press.
1978b "The community integration of the mentally ill: Problems in deinstitutionalization." Madison, Wisconsin: Center for Medical Sociology and Health Services Research, University of Wisconsin (mimeo).
1978c "Alternatives to mental hospital treatment: A sociological perspective." Pp. 309–320 in L. Stein and M. Test (eds.): Alternatives to Mental Hospital Treatment. New York: Plenum.

Melick, M. H. Steadman, and J. Cocozza
1979 "The medicalization of criminal behavior among mental patients." Journal of Health and Social Behavior 20 (September):228–237.

Meyer, A.
1896 "A short sketch of the problems of psychiatry." American Journal of Insanity 53, in E. Winters (ed.): The Collected Papers of Adolf Meyer, Vol. 2:273–282. Baltimore: Johns Hopkins University Press, 1950–52.
1921 "The integrative function of a hospital laboratory—retrospect and prospect." State Hospital Quarterly VI (1920–21), in E. Winters (ed.): The Collected Papers of Adolf Meyer, Vol. 2:78–89. Baltimore: Johns Hopkins University Press, 1950–52.

Milbank Memorial Fund
1962 Decentralization of Psychiatric Services and Continuity of Care. New York: Milbank Memorial Fund.

Miller, E. J. and A. K. Rice
1970 Systems of Organization: The Control of Task and Sentient Boundaries. London: Tavistock

Miller, J. and L. Ohlin
　1976　　"The new corrections: The case of Massachusetts." Pp. 154–175 in M. K. Rosenheim (ed.): Pursuing Justice for the Child. Chicago: University of Chicago Press.

Miller, K. S.
　1976　　Managing Madness: The Case Against Civil Commitment. New York: Free Press.

Morowitz, H.
　1975　　"Social implications of a biological principal." Hospital Practice 10:155–156.

Morris R.
　1977　　"Integration of therapeutic and community services: Cure plus care for the mentally disabled." International Journal of Mental Health 6 (Winter):9–26.

Morris, R. and I. Hirsch-Lescohier
　1978　　"Service integration: Real versus illusory solution to welfare dilemmas." Pp. 21–50 in R. Sarri and Y. Hasenfeld (eds.): The Management of Human Services. New York: Columbia University Press.

Morrissey, J.
　1976　　"Environmental constraints and organization consequences: Boundary control, case mix, and staff conflict in a state mental hospital." Paper presented at the 71st Annual Meeting of the American Sociological Association, New York City.
　1979　　"Keeping patients out: Organizational and policy implications of emergent state hospital deinstitutionalization practices." Paper presented at the Southern Sociological Association, Atlanta, GA.

Morrissey, J. and R. Tessler
　1980　　"Selection processes in state mental hospitalization: Policy issues and research directions." In M. Lewis (ed.): Social Problems and Public Policy: A Research Annual, Vol. 2. Greenwich, CT: JAI Press.

Morrissey, J., R. Tessler, and L. Farrin
　1979　　"Being 'seen but not admitted': A note on some neglected aspects of state hospital deinstitutionalization." American Journal of Orthopsychiatry 49 (January):153–156.

Morrissey, J. and W. Jones
1977    "Research in social work: Interorganizational analysis."
        Pp. 1194–1199 in J. Turner (ed.): Encyclopedia of Social
        Work, 17th Edition. Washington, D.C.: National Associ-
        ation of Social Workers.

Murray, J. T.
1979    "Ethical issues in a state psychiatric hospital." Psychiat-
        ric Annals 9:83–91.

Myerson, A.
1939    "Theory and principles of the 'total push' method in the
        treatment of chronic schizophrenia." American Journal
        of Psychiatry 95:1197–1204.

Myerson, D.
1953    "An approach to the 'Skid Row' problem in Boston."
        New England Journal of Medicine 249:646–649.
1956    "The 'Skid Row' problem: Further observations on a
        group of alcoholic patients, with emphasis on interper-
        sonal and the therapeutic approach." New England
        Journal of Medicine 254 (June 21):1168–1173.
1966    "Origins, treatment and destiny of skid-row alcoholic
        men." New England Journal of Medicine 275 (August
        25):419–425.
1972    "Can institutionalization be prevented?" Massachusetts
        Journal of Mental Health 2:17–26.
1975    "Does history have to repeat itself? A study of reforms at
        the Worcester State Hospital." Unpublished manuscript.

Myerson, D., C. Nadeau, R. Stratton, and M. Kaplan
1974    "The phasedown of the Worcester State Hospital." Mas-
        sachusetts Journal of Mental Health 5:45–56.

Nagi, S.
1974    "The organizational context of evaluation: When norms
        of validity fail to guide gate-keeping decisions in service
        organizations." Pp. 53–78 in W. C. Sze and J. G. Hopps
        (eds.): Evaluation and Accountability in Human Service
        Programs, Cambridge: Schenkman.

National Association of State Mental Health Program Directors
   1979      "Heavy state budget swing to community $$ away from
             institutions. . . . 1976." State Report (January 17).
National Institute of Mental Health
   1974      Where Is My Home? Proceedings of the Conference on
             the Closing of State Mental Hospitals. Menlo Park, CA:
             Stanford Research Institute.
   1979      Provisional Patient Movement Data for State and County
             Mental Health Hospitals. Rockville, MD: Division of
             Biometry and Epidemiology, National Institute of Men-
             tal Health.


Okin, R.
   1978      "Integration of the state hospital into the community
             mental health system." Executive Memorandum, Febru-
             ary 15. Boston, MA: Massachusetts Department of Men-
             tal Health.


Park, R. E. (ed.)
   1939      An Outline of the Principles of Sociology. New York:
             Barnes & Noble.
Park, R. E. and E. W. Burgess
   1921      Introduction to the Science of Sociology. Chicago: Uni-
             versity of Chicago Press.
Perrow, C.
   1965      "Hospitals: Technology, structure and goals." Pp. 910–
             971 in J. March (ed.): Handbook of Organizations. Chica-
             go: Rand McNally.
   1972      Complex Organizations: A Critical Essay. Glenview, IL:
             Scott Foresman.
   1978      "Demystifying organizations." Pp. 105–122 in R. Sarri
             and Y. Hasenfeld (eds.): The Management of Human
             Services, New York: Columbia University Press.
Phillips, L.
   1968      Human Adaptation and Its Failures. New York: Aca-
             demic Press.

Piven, F. and R. Cloward
 1971    Regulating the Poor: The Functions of Public Welfare.
         New York: Vintage Books.
President's Commission on Mental Health
 1979    Final Report. Washington, D.C.: President's Commission
         on Mental Health.

Rachlin, S., A. Pam, and J. Milton
 1975    "Civil liberties versus involuntary hospitalization."
         American Journal of Psychiatry 132:189–191.
Redlich, F. and S. Kellert
 1978    "Trends in American mental health." American Journal
         of Psychiatry 135 (January):22–28.
Regier, D., I. Goldberg, and C. Taube
 1978    "The defacto mental health services system." Archives
         of General Psychiatry 34 (June):615–693.
Reich, R. and L. Siegel
 1973    "Psychiatry under seige: The chronically mentally ill
         shuffle to oblivion." Psychiatric Annals 3 (Novem-
         ber):35–55.
Rein, M.
 1970    "Coordination of social services" Pp. 103–137 in M.
         Rein: Social Policy. New York: Random House.
Robey, A.
 1965    "Criteria for competency to stand trial: A checklist for
         psychiatrists." American Journal of Psychiatry 122 (De-
         cember):616–612.
Robitscher, J.
 1976    "Moving patients out of hospitals—In whose interest?"
         Pp. 141–176 in P. Ahmed and S. C. Plog (eds.): State
         Mental Hospitals: What Happens When They Close.
         New York: Plenum.
Róheim, G.
 1940a   "Freud and cultural anthropology." Psychoanalytic
         Quarterly 9:246–255.
 1940b   "Society and the individual." Psychoanalytic Quarterly
         9:526–545.

1943    The Origin and Function of Culture. Monograph No. 6. New York: Nervous and Mental Disease Monographs.

Rose, S.
1979    "Deciphering deinstitutionalization: Complexities in policy and program analysis." Milbank Memorial Fund Quarterly/Health and Society 57 (Fall):429–460.

Roth, J.
1965    Timetables: Structuring the Passage of Time in Hospital Treatment and Other Careers. Indianapolis: Bobbs-Merrill.

Roth, J. and E. Eddy
1967    Rehabilitation for the Unwanted. New York: Atherton.

Romano, V.
1974    "Institutions in modern society: Caretakers and subjects." Science 183:722–725.

Rosen, P., L. Peterson, and B. Walsh
1980    "A community residence for severely disturbed adolescents: A cognitive-behavioral approach." Child Welfare 59 (January):15–25.

Rothman, D. J.
1971    The Discovery of the Asylum. Boston: Little-Brown.

Rowland, H.
1938    "Interaction processes in a state mental hospital." Psychiatry 1:323–337.

1939    "Friendship patterns in a state mental hospital." Psychiatry 2:363–373.

Rubin, B.
1972    "Prediction of dangerousness in mentally ill criminals." Archives of General Psychiatry 27 (September):397–407.

Saran, B. M., M. Klien, and E. Benay
1978    "Pretrial commitment." American Journal of Psychiatry 135 (July):872–873.

Schatzman, L. and A. Strauss
1966    "A sociology of psychiatry: A perspective and some organizing foci." Social Problems 14 (Summer):3–16.

Scheff, T.
1966    Being Mentally Ill: A Sociological Theory. Chicago: Aldine.
1976    "Medical dominance: Psychoactive drugs and mental health policy." American Behavioral Scientist 19 (January–February):299–317.

Scherl, D. J. and L. B. Macht
1979    "Deinstitutionalization in the absence of consensus." Hospital and Community Psychiatry 30 (September):599–604.

Schmidt, L., A. Reinhardt, R. Kane, and D. Olsen
1977    "The mentally ill in nursing homes: New backwards in the community." Archives of General Psychiatry 34:687–691.

Schooler, N. R., C. G. Solomon, H. Boothe, and J. O. Cole
1967    "One year after discharge: Community adjustment of schizophrenic patients." American Journal of Psychiatry 123:986–995.

Schulberg, H.
1979    "Community support programs: Program evaluation and public policy." American Journal of Psychiatry 136 (November):1433–1437.

Schulberg, C. and F. Baker
1975    The Mental Hospital and Human Services. New York: Behavioral Publications.

Scull, A.
1977    Decarceration: Community Treatment and the Deviant— A Radical View. Englewood Cliffs, NJ: Prentice Hall.

Selznick, P.
1957    Leadership in Administration. New York: Row Peterson.

Shah, S. A.
1974    "Some interactions of law and mental health in the handling of social deviance." Catholic University Law Review 23 (Summer):674–719.
1975    "Dangerousness and civil commitment of the mentally ill: Some public policy considerations." American Journal of Psychiatry 132 (May):501–505.

Shakow, D.

1929      Attendant Survey. Worcester, MA: Psychology Depart-
          ment, Worcester State Hospital, unpublished memoran-
          dum to William A. Bryan, May 28.

1938a     Project Outline for a Personnel Survey of the Worcester
          State Hospital. Worcester, MA: Psychology Department,
          Worcester State Hospital, unpublished memorandum to
          William A. Bryan.

1938b     The Criteria By Which a Mental Hospital Should be
          Judged. Worcester, MA: Psychology Department,
          Worcester State Hospital, unpublished memorandum to
          William A. Bryan, May 11.

1938c     Personnel Problems at Worcester State Hospital.
          Worcester, MA: Psychology Department, Worcester
          State Hospital, unpublished memorandum to William
          A. Bryan, October 24.

1968      "On the rewards (and, alas, frustrations) of public ser-
          vice." American Psychologist 23 (February):87–96.

n.d.      The Contributions of the Worcester State Hospital and
          Post-Hall Clark to Psycho-analysis. Bethesda, MD: Lab-
          oratory of Psychology, National Institute of Mental
          Health, unpublished manuscript.

1972      "The Worcester State Hospital research on schizophre-
          nia (1927–1946)." Journal of Abnormal Psychology
          Monograph 80 (August):67–110.

1978      "Clinical psychology seen some 50 years later." Ameri-
          can Psychologist 33 (February):148–158.

Sharfstein, S.

1978      "Will community mental health survive in the 1980s?"
          American Journal of Psychiatry 135 (November):1363.

Shore, M.

1979      "Public psychiatry: The public's view." Hospital and
          Community Psychiatry 30 (November):768–771.

Shore, M. and R. Shapiro

1979      "The effect of deinstitutionalization on the state hospi-
          tal." Hospital and Community Psychiatry 30 (Septem-
          ber):605–608.

Sills, D.

1957      The Volunteers. Glencoe, IL: Free Press.

Sills, M.
  1975    "The transfer of state hospital resources to community programs." Hospital and Community Psychiatry 26:577–81.

Smith, H.
  1955    "Psychiatry: A social institution in process." Social Forces 33 (May):468–472.
  1957    "Psychiatry in medicine: Intra or interprofessional relationships." American Journal of Sociology 63 (November):285–289.
  1958a   "Two lines of authority—the hospital's dilemma." Pp. 468–477 in E. G. Jaco (ed.): Patients, Physicians, and Illness. New York: Free Press.
  1958b   "Contingencies of professional differentiation." American Journal of Sociology (January):410–414.
  1968    "Crisis in an institutional network: Community health care." Pp. 157–164 in H. S. Becker et al. (eds.): Institutions and the Person. Chicago: Aldine.

Sobel, D.
  1979    "Schizophrenia: Vast effort focuses on four areas." The New York Times (November 13):C1–2.

Soskis, D. A., T. Harrow, and T. P. Detre
  1969    "Long-term follow-up of schizophrenics admitted to a general hospital psychiatric ward." Psychiatric Quarterly 43:525–534.

Srole, L.
  1977    "Gheel, Belgium: The natural therapeutic community, 1475–1975." Pp. 111–130 in G. Serban and B. Astrachan (eds.): New Trends of Psychiatry in the Community. Cambridge: Ballinger.

Stanton, A. and M. Schwartz
  1954    The Mental Hospital. New York: Basic Books.

Starr, P.
  1978    "Medicine and the waning of professional sovereignty." Dedalus 107 (Winter):175–193.

Steadman, H.
  1972    "The psychiatrist as a conservative agent of social control." Social Problems 20 (Fall):263–271.

Stelovich, S.
1979 "From the hospital to the prison: A step forward in deinstitutionalization?" Hospital and Community Psychiatry 30 (September):618–620.

Stone, A.
1975a Mental Health and the Law: A System in Transition. Rockville, MD: National Institute of Mental Health.
1975b "Overview: The right to treatment—coments on the law and its impact." American Journal of Psychiatry 132 (November):1125–1134.
1978 "Comment on J. L. Geller and E. D. Lister, The process of Criminal Commitment for pretrial psychiatric examination: An evaluation." American Journal of Psychiatry 135 (January):61–63.

Strauss, A., L. Schatzman, R. Bucher, D. Ehrlich, and M. Sabshin
1964 Psychiatric Ideologies and Institutions. New York: Free Press.

Szasz, T.
1968 Law, Liberty, and Psychiatry, New York: Collier Books.

Talbot, J. A.
1978 The Death of the Asylum. New York: Grune and Stratton.
1979a The Chronic Mental Patient. Washington, D.C.: American Psychiatric Association.
1979b "Deinstitutionalization: Avoiding the disasters of the past." Hospital and Community Psychiatry 30 (September):621–624.
1979c "The impact of proposition 13 on mental health services in California." Hospital and Community Psychiatry 30 (October):677–685.

Thompson, J.
1967 Organizations in Action. New York: McGraw-Hill.

Turner, J. and W. TenHoor
1978 "The NIMH community support program: Pilot approach to a needed social reform." Schizophrenia Bulletin 4:319–348.

Walsh, B. and P. Rosen
 1979    "A network of services for severely disturbed adolescents." Child Welfare 58 (February):115–125.

Warren, R.
 1967    "The interorganizational field as a focus for investigation." Administrative Science Quarterly 12 (December):396–419.
 1973    "Comprehensive planning—some functional aspects." Social Problems 20 (Winter):355–364.

Warren, R., S. Rose, and A. Bergunder
 1974    The Structure of Urban Reform. Lexington, MA: D. C. Heath.

Watson, J.
 1939    "Psychotherapy for the poor: A state–city cooperative enterprise in the field of mental hygiene." Mental Hygiene 23:558–566.

Webster's
 1949    New Collegiate Dictionary. Springfield, MA: Merriam.

Wenk, G. A., J. Robinson, and G. Smith
 1972    "Can violence be predicted?" Crime and Delinquency 18 (October):393–402.

White, W. C., W. G. McAdoo, and L. Phillips
 1974    "Social competence and outcome of hospitalization: A preliminary report." Journal of Health and Social Behavior 15:261–266.

Windle, C. and D. Scully
 1976    "Community mental health centers and the decreasing use of state mental hospitals." Community Mental Health Journal 12:239–243.

Wing, J.
 1962    "Institutionalism in mental hospitals." Journal of Social and Clinical Psychology 1 (February):38–51.

Winston, A., H. Pardes, D. Papernik, and L. Breslin
 1977    "Aftercare of psychiatric patients and its relation to rehospitalization." Hospital and Community Psychiatry 28:118–121.

Wittkower, E.
 1955    A Psychiatrist Looks at TB. London: Staples.

Wolkon, G. H.
  1970    "Characteristics of clients and continuity of care into
          the community." Community Mental Health Journal 6
          (Fall):215–221.

Woodward Day School
  n.d.    The Woodward Day School: A Program of Worcester
          Youth Guidance Center, Worcester State Hospital,
          Worcester Public Schools. Worcester, MA: Woodward
          Day School.
  n.d.    Woodward Day School Satellite. Worcester, MA: Wood-
          ward Day School.

Woolley, F. R. and R. L. Kane
  1977    "Community aftercare of patients discharged from Utah
          State Hospital: A follow-up study." Hospital and Com-
          munity Psychiatry 28:114–118.

Worcester State Hospital
  1835    Annual Report, Vol. 3. Worcester, MA: Worcester State
          Lunatic Hospital.
  1847    Annual Report, Vol. 15. Worcester, MA: Worcester State
          Lunatic Hospital.
  1849    Annual Report, Vol. 17. Worcester, MA: Worcester State
          Lunatic Hospital.
  1865    Annual Report, Vol. 33. Worcester, MA: Worcester State
          Lunatic Hospital.
  1879    Annual Report, Vol. 47. Worcester, MA: Worcester State
          Lunatic Hospital.
  1881    Annual Report, Vol. 49. Worcester, MA: Worcester State
          Lunatic Hospital.
  1883    Annual Report, Vol. 51. Worcester, MA: Worcester State
          Lunatic Hospital.
  1921    Annual Report, Vol. 89. Worcester, MA: Worcester State
          Hospital.
  1924    Annual Report, Vol. 92. Worcester, MA: Worcester State
          Hospital.
  1929    Annual Report, Vol. 97. Worcester, MA: Worcester State
          Hospital.
  1930    Annual Report, Vol. 98. Worcester, MA: Worcester State
          Hospital.
  1932    Annual Report, Vol. 100. Worcester, MA: Worcester
          State Hospital.

1937     Annual Report, Vol. 105. Worcester, MA: Worcester State Hospital.

1941     Worcester State Hospital Messinger, January 15. Worcester, MA: Worcester State Hospital.

1977     Report of the Committee to Study Patient Abuse. Worcester, MA: Worcester State Hospital (mimeo).

1978     Task Force Report on Children's Services at Worcester State Hospital. Worcester, MA: Worcester State Hospital (mimeo).


Yarmolinsky, A.
1978     "What future for the professional in American society." Dedalus 107 (Winter):159–174.


Zitrin, A., A. Hardesty, E. Burdock, and A. Drossman
1976     "Crime and violence among mental patients." American Journal of Psychiatry 133 (February):142–149.

# INDEX

Social workers, 73
  in ATC, 181, 183
  in aftercare services, 234
  in community-based programs, 116, 119–120
  and 1870s reform movement, 62
  at Memorial Hospital, 213, 215
  at WDS, 163, 174
  at WSH
    areatization and, 121
    in old institutional system, 103, 105
    recruitment of (1910s), 73
    training of, under Bryan, 76
    unitization and assignment of, 113
Socio-ecological perspective on organizational boundaries, see Organizational boundaries, socio-ecological perspective on
Somaticism, 19, 41–42, 57
  failure of, 64
  Meyer rejects, 65
  Southard and, 71
  Woodward and, 24, 25
Southard, Elmer Ernest, 71, 74
SSI, see Supplemental Security Income
Staff
  ATC, admissions and, 183–185
  CLEAT, 187
  community-based mental health program, 136–137
  Memorial Hospital, 203, 207–208, 212
  UMMC inpatient services, 265–266, 268
  WDS, 163, 173
    and dealing with aggressive behavior, 169, 170
    and discharge policy, 168
    and educational program, 171, 172
  WSH
    under Bryan, 75
    Meyer and, 65, 67–69
    Myerson on, 102–103
    unitization and, 112–114
    1852, 34
    1940s, 86
    1970–1979, 274–276
  and 1976 strike, 132–134, 140, 255
  See also Attendants; Mental health assistants; Nurses; Organizational

boundaries, socio-ecological perspective on; Physicians, Psychiatrists; Psychologists; Social workers
Starr, Paul, 296
State government control
  care of mentally ill falls under exclusive (1900s), 70–71, 74
  over admissions (1840s; 1850s), 4
  Massachusetts State Care Act and, 90
  Perkins and, 83–84
  See also Funding and budget; and specific Massachusetts state government departments and agencies
State Hospital Educational Project (SHEP), 165, 173–175
State mental hospitals, 2–7
  critics of, 62–64
  early, 2
  effects of deinstitutionalization on, 2–3, 5–7
  See also Deinstitutionalization
  enduring functions of, 294–296
  growth of, 45–48, 51
  and hospital-based community care, 300–301
  multiple functions of, 290–296
  need for change in, 10–12
  See also Institutional reform
  as social institutions, 8–10
  See also specific state mental hospitals
Strauss, A. L., 140
Strike, 1976, 132–134, 140, 255
Superintendency
  under attack (1870s), 62–64
  basis for selection of superintendent (19th century), 29
  declining autonomy of (1940s), 84
  effects of Massachusetts General Law on control over admissions and, 108
  end of (1970s), 252–257, 273
  eroding power of (1900s), 70
  in old institutional system, 106–107
  Myerson on, 98–99
  shifting authority of, to area program directors (1970s), 246